Contact Lens
Principles and Practice

Contact Lens
Principles and Practice

Kirti Singh MD, DNB, FRCS (E)

Director Professor
Department of Ophthalmology
Guru Nanak Eye Centre
Maulana Azad Medical College and associated hospitals
New Delhi, India

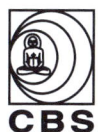

CBS Publishers & Distributors Pvt Ltd

New Delhi • Bengaluru • Chennai • Kochi • Kolkata • Mumbai
Hyderabad • Nagpur • Patna • Pune

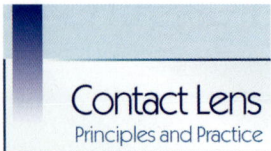

Contact Lens
Principles and Practice

ISBN: 978-93-86478-06-1

Copyright © Author and Publisher

First Edition: 2017

Published by Satish Kumar Jain and produced by Varun Jain for

CBS Publishers & Distributors Pvt Ltd

4819/XI Prahlad Street, 24 Ansari Road, Daryaganj, New Delhi 110 002, India.
Ph: 23289259, 23266861, 23266867   Website: www.cbspd.com
Fax: 011-23243014   e-mail: delhi@cbspd.com; cbspubs@airtelmail.in.

Corporate Office: 204 FIE, Industrial Area, Patparganj, Delhi 110 092
Ph: 4934 4934   Fax: 4934 4935   e-mail: publishing@cbspd.com; publicity@cbspd.com

Branches

- **Bengaluru:** Seema House 2975, 17th Cross, K.R. Road,
  Banasankari 2nd Stage, Bengaluru 560 070, Karnataka
  Ph: +91-80-26771678/79   Fax: +91-80-26771680   e-mail: bangalore@cbspd.com
- **Chennai:** 7, Subbaraya Street, Shenoy Nagar, Chennai 600 030, Tamil Nadu
  Ph: +91-44-26680620, 26681266   Fax: +91-44-42032115   e-mail: chennai@cbspd.com
- **Kochi:** Ashana House, No. 39/1904, AM Thomas Road, Valanjambalam,
  Ernakulam 682 016, Kochi, Kerala
  Ph: +91-484-4059061-62-64-65   Fax: +91-484-4059065   e-mail: kochi@cbspd.com
- **Kolkata:** 6/B, Ground Floor, Rameswar Shaw Road, Kolkata-700 014, West Bengal
  Ph: +91-33-22891126, 22891127, 22891128   e-mail: kolkata@cbspd.com
- **Mumbai:** 83-C, Dr E Moses Road, Worli, Mumbai-400018, Maharashtra
  Ph: +91-22-24902340/41   Fax: +91-22-24902342   e-mail: mumbai@cbspd.com

Representatives

- **Hyderabad** 0-9885175004   - **Nagpur** 0-9021734563
- **Patna** 0-9334159340   - **Pune** 0-9623451994

Printed at: HT Media, Noida, UP, India

to

---

my parents, whose steadfast belief
in me made me realize my potential.
They laid the foundations on which I hold my head high.

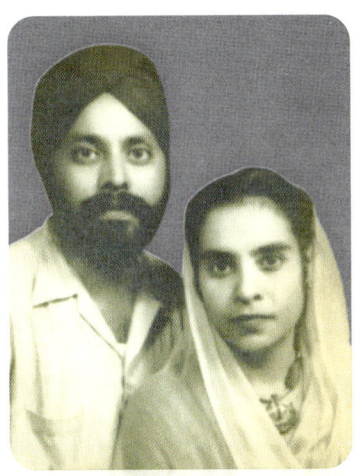

Ms Parkash Kaur
Er. S Kartar Singh

Foreword

I am honored to write the Foreword to this book on principles and practice of contact lens, which has been beautifully written by Dr Kirti Singh. With increasing use of contact lenses in the world, it has become extremely pertinent for every ophthalmologist as well as optometrist to have a proper understanding of this subject. The field of contact lens is constantly changing with newer research broadening its scope.

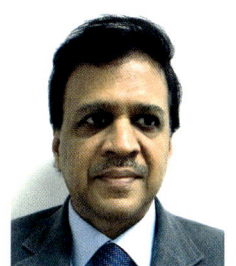

The author has put in tremendous effort in providing comprehensive knowledge of contact lenses starting from basics to fitting in special situations. She heads the contact lens and low vision aid services at a major ophthalmic centre in the country for the last two decades. She has also been trained at Moorfields Eye Hospital, London, in pediatric lens fitting.

The initial section on anatomy and physiology is of paramount importance for better understanding of principles of contact lens wear. Contact lens fitting methodology has been discussed at length with systematic approach to the patient. Specialized section on fitting in difficult situations will help ophthalmologists and optometrists handle challenging case scenarios with ease.

Also, contact lens related complications have been highlighted which is very important for every clinician to be familiar with. Beautiful clinical photographs of contact lens fitting and evaluation are given throughout the book, which would guide the residents to a great extent. Finally contact lens care, which is often neglected by the patients as well as residents, has been concisely put up.

This book is ideally suited for PG students, ophthalmologists as well as optometrists, so I would recommend it for all those who require practical knowledge in the field of contact lenses.

Atul Kumar MD, FAMS
Chief and Professor of Ophthalmology
Dr RP Centre for Ophthalmic Sciences
(WHO Collaborating Centre for Prevention of Blindness)
All India Institute of Medical Sciences
New Delhi, India

Padma Shri and Dr BC Roy Awardee
Hon Advisor Ophthalmology, Government of India
Hon Consultant to Armed Forces Medical Services

Preface

Contact lenses have evolved over decades to the current era of sophistication. This small disc of plastic has succeeded in transforming vision and, therefore, lives of many visually incapacitated patients. It is most often used as a visual correction device for refractive errors where it replaces the less trendy spectacles. Recent advances in corneal mapping and topography have opened new vistas for contact lens use and helped in its metamorphosis from a cosmetic visual aid to a vision restoring intervention. Concomitant to these advances, it has been a phenomenal refinement in lens material and design, that has proved a boon for patients of keratoconus, aphakia, post-keratoplasty and corneal irregularities.

Contact lens fitting is a complex, painstaking but rewarding art, which most ophthalmologists have forgotten and it is majorly left to optometrists to handle this intervention. The increased complexity of diseases and conditions managed by contact lenses has created an increasing need for an integrated inter-sectoral approach. For this to happen, both ophthalmologists and optometrists need to work in tandem by understanding intricacies of the disease process and patient expectations. This book has been conceived with the hope of reviving interest of the fellow ophthalmologists in this lost art and help optometrists upgrade their knowledge and skills about *Contactology*, an art of lens fitting based on scientific knowledge. I am hopeful that it will make the path of adventurous fitters easier, as they move beyond the realm of comfortable fitting for simple myopia and hypermetropia to more complex situations.

Years of work in the contact lens clinic of a major eye hospital in India, gave me enough expertise to learn the finer strokes and nuances of this art. It was not easy to learn and master this subject due to lack of available literature and focus during postgraduate training. Furthermore, in resource-limited conditions like ours, maximum focus of training is doctor-centred with supporting technical groups, like optometrists, lacking a structured or standardized training. So it was not surprising that in this journey, I often felt alone as not many of my peers or students would be interested in this field which has a great potential to help people live their lives fully by optimizing their visual needs. My training at Moorfields Eye Hospital, London, in pediatric lens fitting under tutelage of Prof Roger Buckley helped me rectify this and enabled me to take bolder steps in lens fitting.

Fitting children has been most rewarding and I have watched children whom I fitted as infants grow into strapping adolescents with pride and humility. I feel blessed in touching lives of these young children, for whom this lens transcends from being a mere visual aid to the key unlocking the portals of higher education and ensuring enhanced quality of life.

The book has been divided into three sections: • Principles and Basic Fitting; • Specialized Contact Lens Fitting; and • Complications and Care. There is an attempt to make each chapter easy to comprehend with the aid of pictures and diagrams. The initial part of each chapter deals with relevant applied anatomy, physiology or clinical aspects of the topic followed by technical details, fitting methodology.

Kirti Singh

Acknowledgements

I am grateful to my husband Dr Varinder Singh who has supported all my trials and tribulations and endured the many nights of my burning midnight oil to write this book. I am indebted to my sister Dr Manjeet Kaur who has been a solid cheerleader throughout my career. I acknowledge my mentors and peers who helped me in this journey. Above all, I salute the Almighty, architect of vision, whose blessings enabled me to serve as His instrument to restore the miracle of sight.

I am thankful to my chief, Prof Kamlesh (Director, Guru Nanak Eye Centre), for his vision and encouragement in publishing this book. I am thankful to Dr Paul Rose BOpt, BSc, FNZCLP, the creator of Rose K lens design, for his help in writing the Rose K aspect lens fitting. I am extremely grateful to Ms Jyoti Dave-Singh, Advisor, India MENICON/David Thomas Contact Lenses Ltd, UK, for her meticulous checking and editing of the chapter on keratoconus. I acknowledge the help given to me by Lynn White MSc, FC Optom of Ultravision CLPL, UK, in writing the section on kerasoft lens. I am thankful to Mr Rajesh (optometrist) and Sr Kiran Sharma Dip Nursing of Guru Nanak Eye Centre for their help in the logistics of this book. I acknowledge the contributions of Mr Gagan Sahni, optometrist; Mr Abhilekh Aneja, Senior Faculty Optometrist, Department of Contact Lens, Dr Shroff's Charitable Eye Hospital; and Monica Chowdhary BSc, MSc, Professor and Head, Department of Optometry and Visual Sciences, Amity University, Gurgaon.

Last but not the least, I thank Mr YN Arjuna and the entire team of CBS Publishers & Distributors for guidance and critical appraisal of this book.

This book is a homage to my patients whose life this little magical disc has been able to transform.

Kirti Singh

Contents

Section III: Complications and Care

Principles and Basic Fitting

1. Need for Contact Lenses

2. Voyage of Contact Lenses

3. Contact Lens Basics: Terminology, Optics, Relevant Anatomy and Physiology

4. Instruments used in Contact Lens Fitting

5. Fitting Methodology

6. Fitting a Rigid Contact Lens

7. Fitting a Soft Contact Lens

Reader's Note

CHAPTER 1

Need for Contact Lenses

The last couple of decades have witnessed a phenomenal increase in usage of contact lenses for correction of refractive errors, primarily myopia. There is a worldwide increase in myopia cases, particularly in East and Southeast Asia,[1-3] with almost every fifth case of visual impairment in the Indian subcontinent having refractive error.[4-7] The linkage of myopia to near work, video display terminal and reduced outdoor activities,[1,5] (current lifestyle of our youth), is expected to translate into further increase in the refractive errors. As a result of these refractory errors, an estimated 80–100 million patients worldwide use elective contact lenses currently.[8] Contact lenses remain the preferred option for visual correction for these, particularly among young adults, not only due to their cosmetic acceptance, improved visual field and spatial resolution but also because of their use that facilitates many sporting activities and opens certain professions, closed to the bespectacled impaired vision persons.[8,9]

With the evolution of refractive surgery and improved corneal imaging, there is a higher and early diagnosis of irregular corneas and corneal ectasia, thus adding a host of other conditions for customized contact lens fitting. In response to this increasing requirement for contact lens rehabilitation, customized refinements in both material and design have comeup, like Rose K™, Kerasoft™, minisclerals, and Mc Asfeer lenses to mention a few.

Choosing the right lens material, shape, design aligned to patient requirement, requires a knowledge of the current resources and fitting techniques by ophthalmic fraternity and allied fields.[10] Chapters are arranged sequentially to help the reader learn the language of *Contactology,* from basic to specialized fittings, so as to enable him to do optimal, targeted fitting.

With increasing lens usage one may expect increased complications, and a recent analysis of 1255 contact lens users documented a 20% prevalence rate of complications, particularly among students, soft lens wearers and those with excess wear.[11] The multiplicity of complications listed should not discourage the new fitter as they in no way detract the therapeutic efficacy of lenses, but should make him aware that adopting safe care practices and stringent follow up protocols would prevent and/or control almost all complications. The section dealing with complications and care seeks to provide the relevant information to the readers on this aspect.

REFERENCES

1. He M, Xiang F, Zeng Y, Mai J, Chen Q, Zhang J, Smith W, Rose K, Morgan IG. Effect of Time Spent Outdoors at School on the Development of Myopia Among Children in China: A Randomized Clinical Trial. JAMA. 2015 Sep 15; 314(11):1142–8.

2. Matamoros E, Ingrand P, Pelen F, Bentaleb Y, Weber M, Korobelnik JF, Souied E, Leveziel N. Prevalence of Myopia in France: A Cross-Sectional Analysis. Medicine (Baltimore). 2015 Nov;94(45):e1976.

3. Chin MP, Siong KH, Chan KH, Do CW, Chan HH, Cheong AM. Prevalence of visual impairment and refractive errors among different ethnic groups in schoolchildren in Turpan, China. Ophthalmic Physiol Opt. 2015 May;35(3):263–70.

4. Haq I, Khan Z, Khalique N, Amir A, Jilani FA, Zaidi M. Prevalence of common ocular morbidities in adult population of Aligarh. Indian J Community Med. 2009 Jul;34(3): 195–201.

5. Saxena R, Vashist P, Tandon R, Pandey RM, Bhardawaj A, Menon V, Mani K. Prevalence of myopia and its risk factors in urban school children in Delhi: the North India Myopia Study (NIM Study). PLoS One. 2015 Feb 26;10(2):e0117349.

6. Dandona R, Dandona L, Srinivas M, Giridhar P, McCarty CA, Rao GN. Population-based assessment of refractive error in India: the Andhra Pradesh eye disease study. Clin Experiment Ophthalmol. 2002 Apr;30(2):84–93.

7. Krishnaiah S, Srinivas M, Khanna RC, Rao GN. Prevalence and risk factors for refractive errors in the South Indian adult population: The Andhra Pradesh eye disease study. Clin Ophthalmol. 2009;3:17–27.

8. Roth HW. Contact Lens complication. Etiology, Pathogenesis, Prevention, Therapy. Thieme, New York, 2003.

9. Contact lenses. In:Cantor LB, Rapuano CJ, Cioffi GA. Clinical Optics. Basic and clinical Science Course. American Academy of Ophthalmology 2015–16, 151.

10. Lee YC, Lim CW, Saw SM, Koh D. The prevalence and pattern of contact lens use in a Singapore community. CLAOJ. 2000 Jan;26 (1):21–5.

11. Nagachandrika T, Kumar U, Dumpati S, Chary S, Mandathara PS, Rathi VM. Prevalence of contact lens related complications in a tertiary eye centre in India. Cont Lens Anterior Eye. 2011 Dec;34(6):266–8.

Reader's Note

Reader's Note

CHAPTER 2

Voyage of Contact Lenses

HISTORY OF CONTACT LENSES

The genesis of contact lenses started with the idea of neutralizing corneal refractive error with water. This was the brainchild of the versatile genius Leonardo da Vinci, whose 1508 pencil drawings depict glass shells full of water resting on the eye.[1] However, it took almost four centuries for his ideas to be implemented and it was in 1801 that Thomas Young employed the same idea to correct his own myopia using a homemade device of a glass tube filled with water, attached with wax to a lens taken from his old botanical microscope. He used this tube on his eye, in an attempt to replace his myopic cornea with a regularly ground lens. This idea was refined by Sir John Herschel in 1830, who gave the concept of placing spherical lenses over cornea for correcting refractive errors and suggested making such lenses using impressions of corneal surface. To him is thus accorded the status of being the *father of contact lenses*.[2]

The first actual lens was, however, made in 1888 by Adolf Fick using blown glass shells and was called the *Kontaktbrille*. After using this lens, he made the important observations of corneal clouding, conjunctival/limbal injection and recommended inserting an air bubble behind the lens to reduce this clouding. The concept of lens disinfection and adaptation was also given by him. In the same year, Eugene Kalt used such a lens for the first time to improve the vision of a keratoconus case,

after cauterizing the cone with silver nitrate. This prompted Thomas Lohnstein, himself a keratoconus patient, to develop lens cups filled with saline (*water spectacles or hydrodiascope*) which could be worn successfully for a few hours.[3] A high myope of 14 D, August Müller in 1889 suggested confirming posterior lens surface to corneal surface by utilizing capillary attraction of tears to ensure lens adherence. He recommended incorporation of an edge lift to lens, to enhance tear circulation under the lens and used the newly introduced cocaine as a local anaesthetic during the fitting procedure.

It was in early twentieth century that Carl Zeiss manufactured the first trial set of lenses to correct keratoconus from lathe-cut moulds. The commonest problem faced by these early pioneers was corneal oedema after lens wear, which was named *Sattler's veil* after the gentleman who studied this phenomenon extensively.[4] It took many years before the physiological reasons for this was found to be hypoxia and negative hydrostatic pressure which led to modifications in lens material.[5–7]

Material and Type of Lenses

In 1930, Röhm and Haas Company (USA) isolated a novel plastic from an acrylic resin base called *Plexiglass*. This forerunner of polymethyl methacrylate (PMMA) was sold to US aviation industry and used to manufacture cockpit roofs of fighter plans during Second World War. This fact led to the amazing serendipity of inertness of this material in a fighter pilot, Gordon Cleaver's eye after his plane was bombed. Mr Cleaver was operated upon by Sir Harold Ridely of Moorfields Eye Hospital, London, who during subsequent 18 operations in the same patient noted that the embedded perspex material itself caused no inflammation in the blinded right eye. Dr Ridley then used this material to create the first intraocular lens in 1949, thereby converting a blinding adversity into a stupendous medical discovery. The same material in the form of an IOL was later on used to treat traumatic cataract in Mr Cleaver's only seeing left eye.

This material was taken up by John Crawford and Rowland Hill of Imperial Chemical Industries (ICI) in 1934 and modified to polymethyl methacrylate (PMMA), which rapidly replaced glass as the material of choice for making a contact lens. The reasons for this were: Low specific gravity of this material which made it lighter, less prone to low riding coupled with ease of manufacture, allowing thinner designs to be produced. The material was also malleable to alterations and modifications.

In 1936, William Feinbloom created a hybrid contact lens with corneal portion made of glass and scleral skirt of translucent plastic.[8] This was followed by impression moulded scleral lenses by Ernest Mullen and Theodore Obrig. Obrig was also responsible for using fluorescein dye to stain post lens tear film and evaluating lens fit using cobalt blue filter.

Corneal lenses were first made by Kevin M Tuohy in 1946 using PMMA with dimensions of 10–11 mm diameter and 0.4 mm thickness. Since fit was found to be flatter than optic cap of cornea, a peripheral curve was incorporated to keep upper edge of lens from impinging on sclera which was called the "scleral flange".

In 1954, Otto Wichterle and Drashoslav Lim of Prague experimented with plastics simulating living tissue which could be made into orbital implants. During the process, they discovered a stable transparent gel, polyhydroxyethyl-methacrylate (PHEMA). This water-absorbing polymer which was permeable to nutrients and metabolites, turned out to be unstable. Addition of a xerogel altered this polymer to hydroxyethyl methacrylate (HEMA), which could be hydrated without affecting its physical properties. This started the era of hydrogels/HEMA lenses manufacturing using centrifugal moulding or spin-casting technology.

The first rigid gas permeable (RGP) lenses was made of cellulose acetate butylrate, by J Teissler of Czechoslovakia in 1937. However, Norman Gaylord, a polymer chemist and Leonard Seidner, an optometrist are credited to be the fathers of RGP lens as they were the ones to experiment with silicone and fluorocarbon materials which gave the property of oxygen permeability to the RGP lens. It was in 1972 that they submitted a patent for a copolymer of polysiloxanyalkyl acrylic ester with an alkyl acrylic ester.[9] Within a few years, Walter E Becker developed his silicone elastomer contact lens and in 1970s, Ron Seger and Wayne Trombley of Dow Corning (USA) designed silicone elastomer Silsoft™ lens, to be used as daily wear in refractive errors and as extended wear for aphakia.

The concept of a disposable lens was mooted by Orlando A Battista (USA) in 1978. He used a collagen material which later proved to be unstable and dissolved in human tear enzymes. Later Michael Bay successfully used high water content hydrogel materials as an alternative. In 1987, Etafilcon A material (58% water content) was approved as disposable lens material and packaged in disposable 'blister' packs which evolved into Acuvue™ Lenses.

This brief history detailing evolution of contact lenses over centuries, reflects intense work, firm resolve and *never say die* attitude of men driven to survive all odds.

REFERENCES

1. CodexD of Leonardo 's notebooks ; Ravaisson Mollien. Les manuscripts de Leonardo de Vinci, 1881–91.
2. Sir Stewart Duke Elder. Contact Lenses. In System of Ophthalmology Vol 5, Ophthalmic optics and refraction. London. Henry Kimpton, CV Mosby, 1970: 713–92.
3. Heitz R. *Leonardo da Vinci did not invent contact lenses*. CLAO J. 1983; 9(4): 313–6.
4. Sattler. Dtsch. Med. Wschr. 1931, 57: 312.
5. Anderson. Technique of fitting Contact Lenses. Minneap 1944.
6. Dallos. Br J Ophthalmol 1946, 30: 607.
7. Ruben. Trans Ophthalmic Soc UK 1967, 87(27): 643, 661, 1967.
8. Knoll HA. *William Feinbloom: Pioneer in plastic contacts*. CL Forum. 1977; 1(8): 29–32.
9. Sposato P. *Father of the RGP lens*. CL Spectrum. 1986;1(3): 50–2.

Reader's Note

CHAPTER 3

Contact Lens Basics: Terminology, Optics, Relevant Anatomy and Physiology

This chapter deals with the common terms and nomenclature employed in contact lens practice. A section of relevant anatomical and physiological aspects of lens wear on ocular surface is added along with an overview of indications of contact lens (CL) wear.

Contact lens blank: A lens blank is a solid block of polymer formed from a mixture of crosslinked monomers. It is the raw material from which a contact lens is fashioned.

Single cut lens: The front surface of a single cut lens comprises a single continuous curve with back surface having one or more curves. The number of curves on the back surface name the lens as being monocurve, bicurve or multicurve.

Base curve: Radius of curvature of optic zone of the posterior surface of contact lens.

Overall diameter: These are lens dimensions from one edge to the other.

Optic zone: This area carries the optical power and is the entire front surface in a single cut lens and minus the carrier zone for a lenticular lens. On back surface, it is the diameter minus width of peripheral and intermediate posterior curves.

Peripheral and intermediate posterior curves: These are present on posterior surface of lens and provide gradual flattening of lens from base curve to lens edge so as to conform to the aspheric cornea.

Sagittal depth: Perpendicular distance from central posterior portion of lens to lens diameter. Figure 3.1 depicts the various part of a contact lens.

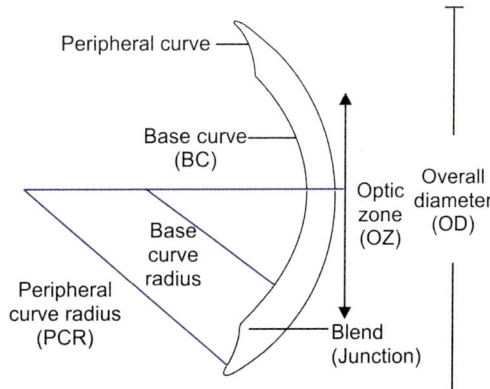

Fig. 3.1: Diagram depicting parts of a monocurve contact lens

Power: It is the focal length of contact lens in air and is determined by difference in power of central anterior curve to central posterior curve.

Oxygen permeability (Dk): Expressed as coefficient of variation, it is the property of the lens polymer to transmit gaseous substances especially oxygen. It is written as Dk value, where D = diffusion coefficient and k = solubility coefficient or solubility of gas in the material. Oxygen permeability is a property inherent and specific to the lens material.

Oxygen transmissibility (Dk/L): Expressed as Dk/L, it refers to the oxygen permeability/exchange of a lens of given thickness where Dk = oxygen permeability and L = lens thickness. Oxygen exchange across a lens is proportionate to oxygen permeability of polymer (Dk value) and inversely related to lens thickness. The central thickness of a – 3.0 D contact lens is taken as standard by most lens manufacturers. Oxygen requirement of cornea under a CL has been calculated to be Dk/t = 24 for daily wear and Dk/t = 87 for extended wear.[1] Poor oxygen transmission during lens wear causes hypoxic corneal changes like epithelial microcyst, endothelial blebs and poly-megathism. Carbon dioxide retention under a CL results in an acidic pH which reduces efficiency of endothelial pump leading to corneal oedema.

- Oxygen permeability = Dk value

$$Dk = \frac{Amount\ of\ oxygen \times thickness}{Lens\ area \times time \times pressure\ difference}$$

- Oxygen transmissibility Dk/t = Dk/central lens thickness

Water content: Crosslinked monomers used in a CL result in a porous structure which is able to retain water. Water-holding capacity of a lens in turn is directly proportional to its oxygen permeability, with a 20% increase in water content serving to double the oxygen permeability. Water content alters durability, thickness, with wearers of higher water content lenses being more vulnerable to changes in atmospheric humidity. Anatomical and optical parameters of high water content lens alter significantly in dry dusty environments and/or dry eye conditions.

Wettability: Soft lenses are hydrophilic in nature and absorb water depending on their hydration level. Rigid gas permeable lenses, on the other hand, are either hydrophobic, proportionate to silicone content or partly hydrophilic. Despite the umbrella of a wetting agent incorporated in the silicone impregnated rigid lens, such lenses dry more

rapidly and bind more lipid containing tear debris. In situations of diminished tear flow, these debris adhere to back surface of lens, generate friction during blink-induced lens movements and a gritty feel.

Sessile drop/water-in-air test: This test is used to measure contact lens wettability. It measures angle θ (theta) between a tangent drawn to surface of drop at its point of contact with the horizontal test surface. A zero angle implies completely wettable surface and a large angle >90° implies a poorly wettable surface (Fig. 3.2). Poor water adherence lenses with large θ values have poor vision quality, are prone to deposits and uncomfortable to wear.[2]

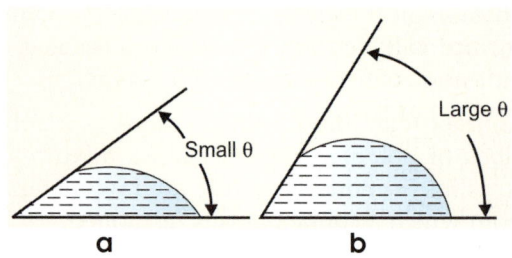

Fig. 3.2: (a) Small wetting angle θ (theta): Greater wettability, enhanced comfort; (b) Large wetting angle: Lesser wettability, poorer comfort

Light transmission and refractive index are optical property measures and *heat resistance and lens flexure* are measures of mechanical property of lens material.

RELEVANT APPLIED ANATOMY AND PHYSIOLOGY

Corneal Refraction and Haemostasis

Cornea is the principal optical surface accounting for two-thirds refractive power of the eye. It is a meniscus lens with a mean front apical radius of 7.8 mm, back apical radius of 6.5 mm, a refractive index of 1.376 and power of 43.27 D (Fig. 3.3). The *visual axis* is line joining fixation point to fovea and passes through the nodal point of eye. **Fixation axis** is line joining fixation point to center of rotation of eye. **Optic axis** is the line through nodal point in which optical center lies (Fig. 3.4).

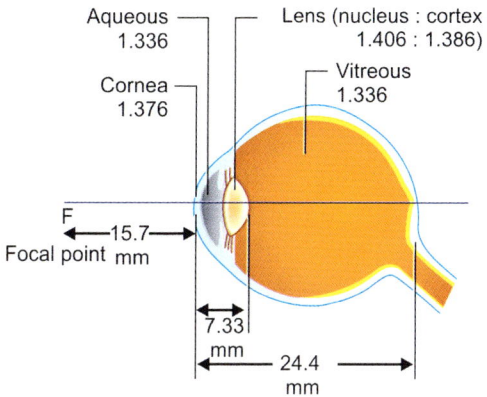
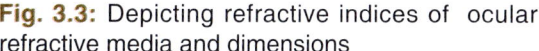

Fig. 3.3: Depicting refractive indices of ocular refractive media and dimensions

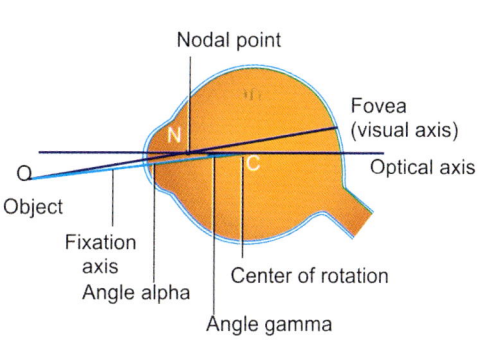

Fig. 3.4: Depicting various axis of eye and nodal point

The optically non-homogeneous cornea is composed of 78% water, 15% collagen, 5% other proteins, 1% glycosaminoglycans (GAGs) and 1% salts. Basement membrane and Descemet's membrane both consist of type IV collagen and stroma of type III collagen.

The corneal epithelium tear film interface with atmospheric air is the most important optical surface due to maximum difference in refractive index (air versus corneal epithelium). To serve this important refractive function, this layer needs to be renewed regularly so as to remain vital. This is made possible by continual migration and transformation of limbal stem cell along with surface desquamation. Thus two movement streams occur constantly at corneal surface, a horizontal one from limbus to center and a vertical one from basal cells lying on basement membrane to its surface during the process of desquamation. The vertical movement is called "corneal epithelial cellular turnover" and usually takes seven days to complete. Contact lens wear disturbs this homeostatic control, impedes cell migration, reduces surface epithelial cell shedding, prolongs basal cell retention and decreases epithelial proliferation. This in turn causes a stagnant and thinner central corneal epithelium.[3]

Sensory Supply of Cornea

Cornea is a highly sensitive organ and is supplied by ophthalmic division of trigeminal nerve. The corneal nerves enter from limbal area in anterior and middle stromal layers, run forwards radially and become more superficial in central area.

Corneal Topography

Normal cornea has a prolate surface, which means paracentral flattening starting from a steeper center, which is more on nasal side. Asphericity is the degree of peripheral flattening or steepening from apical radius of curvature and is expressed as eccentricity (e) or the shape factor (p). This asphericity is partly responsible for reduction of spherical aberration and for a circle, the asphericity value is 0. The ellipsoid cornea has e values between 0.41 and 0.58, average being 0.47. Based on asphericity, cornea can be divided into three regions:

a. Central corneal cap of 4 mm diameter which is decentered nasally by 0.2–0.6 mm and superiorly by 0.2 mm.

b. Mid-peripheral region of greater flattening.

c. Peripheral region with a positive asphericity.

To match this prolate cornea, the default design of a CL should incorporate progressively flatter curves in the periphery or incorporate a continuous aspheric curve. The horizontal diameter of cornea or horizontally visible iris diameter (HVID) as it is called, is 11.7–12.0 mm and vertical diameter or vertically visible iris diameter (VVID) is 10.6 –11.0 mm.

Limbal Area

Limbal area or corneoscleral junction differs from bulbar conjunctiva by presence of melanocytes, blood vessels, lymphatics and absence goblet cells. Limbal vasculature comprises terminal superficial marginal arteries (of anterior ciliary arteries origin) forming peripheral arcades called *palisades of Vogt*. These palisades of Vogt are radially oriented fibrovascular ridges analogous to fingerprints, and the term *conjunctivoglyphics/limboglyphics* has been suggested for these patterns, which are unique for an individual. Anatomical limbus, also known as *transition zone*, is racially determined and is graded from 1 to 5, with 1 being a very shallow junction and 5 a steep one.

Corneal Oxygen Requirement and Permeability

As for all tissues, cornea also requires a requisite amount of oxygen delivery to ensure vitality and function. This oxygen requirement is taken care of by tear film, aqueous humour and partly by palpebral/limbal vasculature (especially in closed eye circumstances). Corneal epithelium relies on atmospheric oxygen which has 21% oxygen at 155 mmHg partial pressure, and corneal endothelium on aqueous humour which contains 7.4% oxygen at 55 mmHg partial pressure. The fact that endothelium also relies on atmospheric oxygen is evident by occurrence of Zantos' blebs (transient endothelial changes) during closed eye condition.[5]

Corneal epithelium has high permeability to carbon dioxide with Dk value for this gas being 7 times more than for oxygen. This high CO_2 permeability helps cornea resist pH and metabolic changes. In **open eye conditions,** carbon dioxide rapidly diffuses out through tears but in **closed eye conditions,** it exits via aqueous humour. An oxygen partial pressure of 75 mmHg is essential to prevent hypoxic corneal oedema and CL material/wear must be able to deliver this critical amount of oxygen.[6] As mentioned before, oxygen exchange across a lens is proportionate to oxygen permeability of polymer and inversely related to thickness. For soft hydrogel lens, the Dk value is proportional to its water content, whereas for RGP lenses, it is proportional to silicone/fluorine content. An estimate of oxygen permeability of a lens can be made from the fact that overnight wear with conventional daily wear lenses (Dk 40) causes a 12% corneal swelling.[1]

Hypoxia causes accumulation of lactic acid and carbon dioxide, decreases pH, causes hypoxic endothelial damage manifesting as epithelial oedema/microcysts, stromal folds, corneal neovascularization, endothelial polymegathism with accompanying symptoms of pain, watering, photophobia called *overwear syndrome*.[7] Vertical striae become evident once corneal oedema causes swelling by 6% and posterior folds at 10%. Chronic hypoxia has another detrimental effect, it increases bacterial binding to corneal epithelial cells by upregulating *Pseudomonas aeruginosa* receptors and makes such corneas vulnerable to microbial keratitis.[3]

Energy Utilization

Cornea utilizes energy by both aerobic and anaerobic pathways, the end products being pyruvic acid and lactic acid (anaerobic) or carbon dioxide and water (aerobic), respectively. Glucose requirement is 38–90 mg/hour, 90% of which is contributed by aqueous humour and remaining by limbal vessels and/or tear film. The high metabolism of corneal epithelium consumes 40–66% of the supplied glucose.

During conditions of *open eye* with normal oxygen levels, aerobic metabolism prevails, generating end products of carbon dioxide and water. In *closed eye/hypoxic* conditions, anaerobic glycolytic pathway becomes more active, resulting in increased lactate production by 40–140%. Corneal epithelium has low permeability to this lactic acid which then diffuses into aqueous humour. Accumulation of lactic acid in aqueous creates increased osmotic pressure resulting in osmotically driven corneal oedema by 3–4%. The additional contributors to this oedema are reduced tear osmolarity, increased temperature and humidity. In *open eye* conditions, cornea recovers from this swelling by tear evaporation and tear hypertonicity induced osmotic deturgescence.

Corneal Repair

After any epithelial injury, re-epithelialization occurs by sliding or migration from pleuripotent limbal stem cells in 7 days, followed by laying down of basement membrane. Subsequently, release of a glycoprotein *fibronectin* by the regenerating epithelium helps in hemidesmosomal adhesion to underlying Bowman's layer. This new epithelium is friable and CL wear should be curtailed for 2 weeks after any episode of corneal abrasion.

Tear Film and Blinking Activities

Tears constitute a lacrimal river at lid margin which slowly moves towards a lacrimal lake at medial canthus with a turnover rate of 16% per minute. Tear film is composed of inner mucin layer, central aqueous layer and outermost lipid layer. The innermost mucin layer of tear film hugs the cornea and makes the hydrophobic epithelium hydrophilic. The uttermost lipid layer reduces tear evaporation and prevents tear spillover. The central aqueous layer keeps these two layers apart and delivers both nutrition and oxygen to cornea.

The act of blinking involves two main activities, that of downsweep and upsweep of upper lid generated by levator palpebrae superioris (LPS) and second, the contracture of orbicularis oculi muscle. The LPS-induced movement serves to draw aqueous component of tears over the cornea followed by spreading of lipid layer over the entire surface. Orbicularis oculi movement during lid closure creates a scissor-like lid movement towards the nose and distends the upper part of lacrimal sac, both actions serve to propel tears towards the medial canthus. Globe movement during blinking is upward, inward towards nose and backward with a well-fitted CL shadowing the globe. Rigid gas permeable (RGP) lenses on account of this movement allow for 15% tear exchange with each blink while soft lenses (SCL) with their limited movement allow only 1% exchange. This tear exchange beneath the RGP lens plays a vital role in replenishing oxygen supply and absorbing metabolic by-products of the cornea.

Normal rate of blinking is 11–12 blinks per minute which decreases during intense concentration like computer work and increases during initial period of CL wear.

Poor wetting of cornea due to presence of CL causes thinning of tear film and allows mingling of outermost oil layer with innermost mucin layer. The resultant oil mucin admixture is unable to adequately 'wet' the epithelium leading to a break-up of tear film and exacerbates pre-existing conditions of dry eye.

Adaptation to Lens Wear

During initial period of lens wear, the eye adapts to presence of foreign object in the eye by a series of anatomical, physiological and optical changes.

Anatomical: A healthy cornea adjusts to initial lens-induced hypoxia by developing hypoesthesia with an actual decrease in corneal nerve endings during the **adaptation phase.**[8]

Physiological: During initial period of CL wear, reflex tearing occurs resulting in hypotonic tears, decreased tear osmolality and subsequent corneal swelling of 2–4%. Adaptation to pre-lens value occurs within a week of continued lens wear as tear pH stabilizes. Poorly fit and cornea unfriendly material contact lenses alter corneal topography after a few weeks of wear. This results in spectacle blur, once lens wearer switches back to spectacle wear.

Optical: Habitual spectacle users wearing lenses for the first time have initial problems in depth perception and spatial perception due to a more real-sized image versus a minified or magnified image with myopic or hyperopic spectacle, respectively. This can cause the wearer to experience ocular fatigue, image distortion, swimming sensation and headache. These symptoms become more problematic in higher refractive numbers. Wearers need to be forewarned of this phenomenon and most adapt to this altered image size perception within a few weeks.

Types of Contact Lenses

Based on Material

- *Hard lens*: Lens which in its final form retains its shape without any support under normal circumstances.
- *Soft lens*: Lens which in its final form requires support to maintain its form.
- *Rigid gas permeable lens*: Hard lenses which allow sufficient oxygen to pass through its material for nourishment of cornea.

Based on Manufacturing Techniques

- *Spin cast*: This was the initial method invented by Czechoslovakian chemists Wichterle and Lim whose patent was subsequently acquired by the Bausch & Lomb Company. In this method, liquid polymer is dropped on to a rotating/spinning mould and optical power of the lens is determined by speed and centrifugal force, with higher speeds creating higher minus power. The front surface of lens is formed by surface in contact with the mould and back surface is determined by both rotation speed and polymer characteristics. This technique is used to generate high volume, standard and reproducible lenses with aspheric posterior surface.
- *Lathe cut*: In this technique, polymer in solid state (lens button) is cut with precision lathe machines. The curvature of both anterior and posterior lens surfaces is determined by curvature of the lathe. Automated lathes are used for mass production and posterior surface in this manufacturing technique is usually spheric but can be made aspheric, e.g. Silklens, Purecon.
- *Cast moulding:* Liquid polymer is placed between two moulds which determine front and back surface of the contact lens. Casting of the mould is done and finished product is polished and hydrated as required. Depending on mould surface, microscopic scars can be left on the lens.

Based on Modes of Lens Wear

- *Daily wear:* It is the term used for daily insertion and removal of a lens. Life-span of these lenses is invariably 1 year for hydrogels and 2 years for a RGP lens.
- *Extended wear:* It is the term used for overnight lens wear and has been approved by FDA from 7 to 30 nights. This terminology is used for soft lenses with examples being: Pure Vision (B&L), Focus night and day (CIBA Vision). High water content material is used for these lenses.
- *Disposable lens wear schedule:* "Disposable", as defined by FDA, means used once and discarded. It implies use of a brand new lens pair which is worn and discarded daily, e.g. Softens (B & L), Acuvue clear/moist (Johnson & Johnson), Fresh look one day (CIBA Vision), My Day (Cooper Vision).
- *Frequent replacement schedule:* Often called fortnightly/weekly/monthly disposable,

these are actually frequent or planned replacement lenses.

Color Tints

These can be divided into handling, color enhancing, cosmetic or opaque.

Handling tints: These are full diameter light tint or iris diameter tint with latter being customized, costly and more difficult to make. Full diameter tints make the lens easy to locate against a white background, e.g. lens case, sink or tablecloth, thereby the name "handling tints."

Enhancing tints: These transparent tints alter natural color of patient's eye. As expected, they are more successful in darkening a naturally light, colored iris. Hazel/blue eyes can be easily made to look light brown or grey while making a black iris to look blue is not easy using these transparent tints. Choice of color and density need to take into account occupational and safety aspects of the wearer, since darker tints can adversely affect color perception.

Cosmetic opaque: These types of lens are used by actors/detectives/criminals to alter their eye color. This category has two subtypes—incomplete coverage and complete coverage. In the *incomplete coverage*, only part of anterior surface of the CL is colored in an endeavor to impart natural depth to apparent iris color. *Complete coverage*, on the other hand, has the color on the entire anterior surface except pupil zone. Complete coverage gives an artificial look to the eye as 'color' is around 2–4 mm anterior of the expected position.

SOME OPTICAL PHENOMENA/TERMS RELATED WITH USE OF CONTACT LENSES

A contact lens differs from spectacles by having a shorter vertex distance and that tear fluid, not air is the interface between lens and eye.

Accommodation Depletion

Minus concave lenses of myopic spectacles confer a **base in prism** effect while viewing near objects. This aids convergence and reduces the need for accommodation. This accommodation advantage which is enjoyed by the bespectacled myope is lost when the patient switches thinner minus contact lenses.[9] A myope who starts to use contact lenses (CL) after many years of spectacle wear, needs to use his accommodation more, which translates into increased convergence demands due to the near reflex synkinensis. *Thus aesthenopic symptoms occur during contact lens wear.* In addition, onset of presbyopia occurs at par with emmetropic eyes, in myopes using contacts, compared to later onset for the spectacled myope.

A hypermetrope, on the other hand, using thick convex spectacles experiences a **base out prism** effect while viewing near objects and correspondingly requires increased convergence effort. This accommodative effort is reduced while switching to thinner hyperopic contact lenses leading to a reduction of aesthenopic symptoms. In a nutshell contact lenses eliminate the accommodative advantage enjoyed by spectacle wearing myope and disadvantage experienced by spectacle wearing hyperopes. Figures 3.5 and 3.6 explain this point optically.

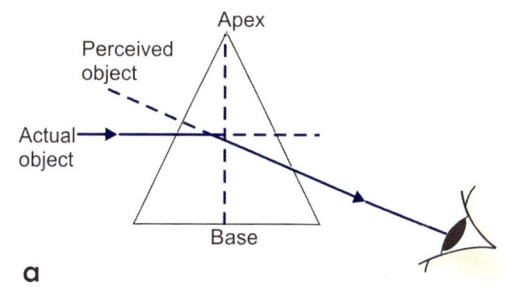

a

Fig. 3.5a: Optics of prism shows object displacement as perceived by eye to be towards the apex of prism

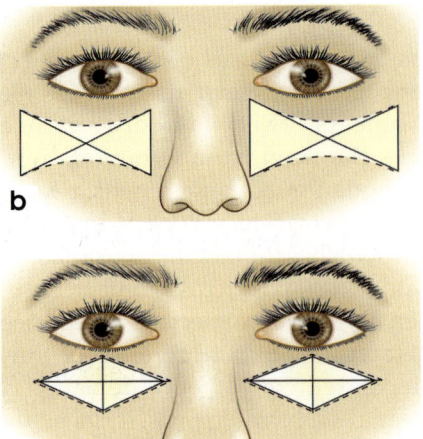

Fig. 3.5: Diagrammatic representation of: (b) Concave/minus lens as 2 prisms lying apex to apex, in front of eye thus conferring a base IN prism effect; (c) Convex/plus lens as 2 prisms lying base, to base in front of eye thus conferring a base OUT prism effect

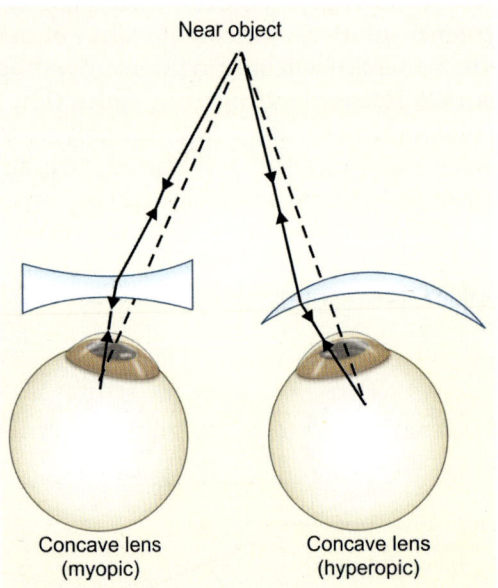

Fig. 3.6: For a near object perceived by patient wearing a **concave spectacle lens (left eye) exerts base IN prism** effect which aids convergence, whereas **convex spectacle lens (right eye) exerts base OUT** prism effect which requires patient to exert more convergence

Residual Astigmatism (RA)

When a rigid gas permeable (RGP) lens sits on the cornea, it creates a new spherical ocular surface whose curvature conforms to its central posterior curve (CPC) or base curve (BC). This occurs irrespective of original corneal topography, since the RGP lens along with entrapped tear film converts the anterior ocular surface into a spherical optical surface. Thus a rigid lens is able to neutralize both irregular and regular corneal astigmatism. Soft lenses, on the other hand, mould to the cornea and transmit refractive astigmatism of ocular surface.

Neutralization of corneal astigmatism unmasks the lenticular and other elements of refractive astigmatism, it is this exposed lenticular astigmatism which is called *residual astigmatism*. In such a scenario soft lenses provide better visual rehabilitation compared to RGP lenses.[10]

Tear Lens

Tear lens is the optics created by shape of the entrapped tear film between posterior surface of contact lens (constitutes anterior surface of tear lens) and anterior corneal surface (constitutes posterior surface of tear lens). Refractive index of this tear fluid at 1.336µ differs a little from corneal index of 1.377µ. Due to minimally dissimilar refractive indices between cornea and tear fluid, the anterior surface of fluid lens masks the optical effect of anterior corneal surface. A contact lens with spherical posterior surface like an RGP lens will create a spherical anterior surface of tear lens regardless of corneal topography.[10–12] This tear lens is the reason why RGP lenses are able to neutralize large amounts of irregular astigmatism.

Rigid back surface of RGP lens creates an anterior tear lens surface **different** from posterior tear lens surface of this tear fluid. This difference in both surfaces generates a *powered optical spherical lens*. A steep fitting lens, which vaults over central cornea, creates a *plus power tear lens* and a flat fit would create a *minus power tear lens* (Fig. 3.7a and b). The power of this tear lens has been calculated to be *0.25 D for every 0.05 mm* radius of curvature difference between base curve of lens and flat K of the cornea. The mnemonic to remember this is**: SAM FAP**, for steeper fit add minus and for flatter fit add plus, since steeper fit creates a plus tear lens requiring a minus over-correction for neutralization.

The scenario for a soft lens is different. A snugly moulding soft lens entraps minimal tear fluid with similar anterior and posterior surfaces which generates a zero *power plano tear lens.*

Spectacle Blur

This is a phenomenon associated with older PMMA lenses and with poorly fitted, cornea unfriendly RGP lenses. Long-term wear of such poorly fitted lenses cause corneal warpage, which translate into poorer vision when patient switches back to corrective spectacle wear. This effect of CL wear on corneal topography initiated the concept of programmed modification of cornea surface by CL in reducing myopia called ortho-keratology.[13]

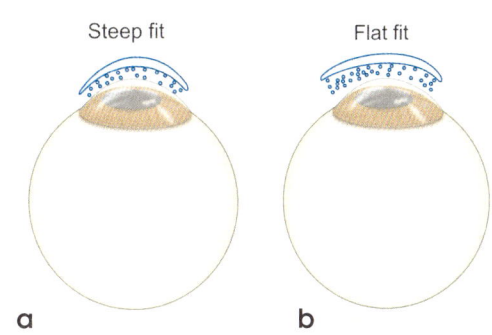

Fig. 3.7: (a) Steep fit RGP lens generates a positive tear lens optics; (b) Flat fit RGP lens generates a minus powered tear lens optics

Figures 3.8 to 3.10 depict some basic optics which would be required to understand contact lens optical aspects. They also explain about the distortion with high-powered spectacle lenses which are taken care of by contact lenses.

A brief review of astigmatism is required for understanding of contact lens properties in neutralizing this refractive error.

Astigmatism

Astigmatism is an optical error where two line foci get focused in front, behind or partly on

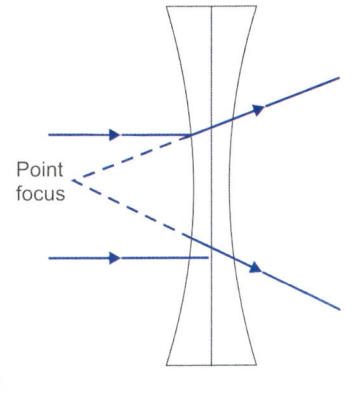
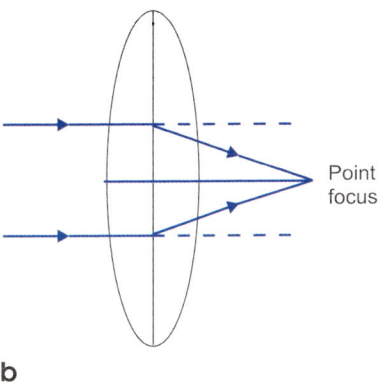

Fig. 3.8: Ray diagrams of: (a) Convergence and point focus of a convex lens; (b) Divergence and point focus of a concave lens

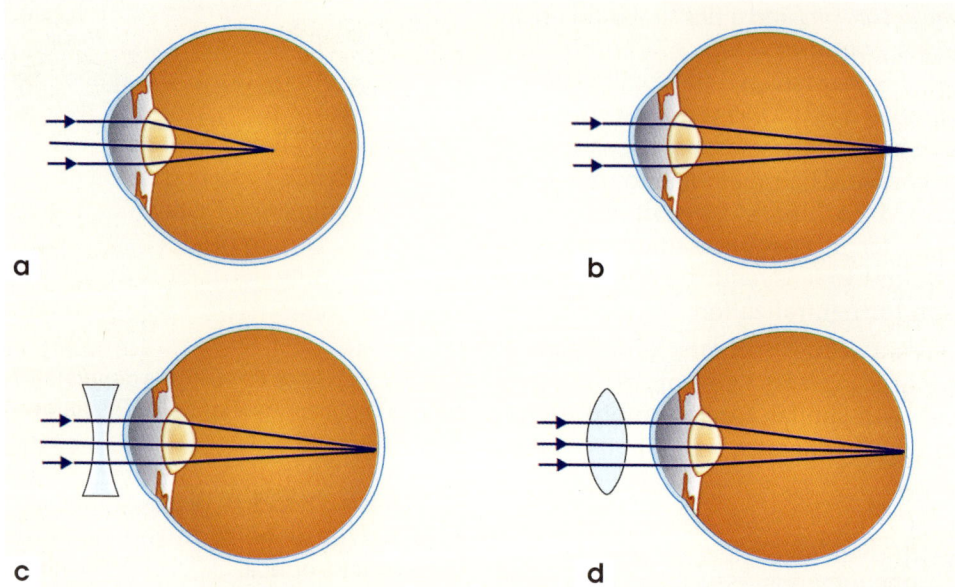

Fig. 3.9: Ray diagrams of: (a) Myopia; (b) Corrected with concave lens; (c) Hyperopia; (d) Corrected with a convex lens

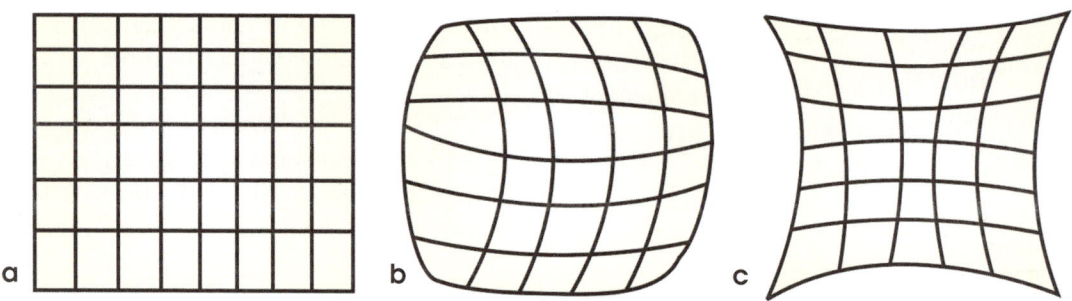

Fig. 3.10: (a) Normal grid or object; (b) Pincushion distortion with a high plus lens; (c) Barrel distortion seen with a high minus lens

the retina accordingly it is classified as simple, compound or mixed. Based on type of cylindrical correction required, astigmatism is classified as:

a. **Simple hypermetropic/hyperopic astigmatism (SHA):** One focal line falls on the retina, whereas the other is located behind the retina. The prescription would read as (+) 1.50 Dc × 180.

b. **Compound hypermetropic/hyperopic astigmatism (CHA):** Both focal lines are located behind the *retina so both principal meridians are positive.* The prescription would read as (+) 1.50/(+) 1.5 Dc × 160.

c. **Simple myopic astigmatism (SMA):** One focal line is on the retina, the other is located in front. The prescription would read as, e.g. (–) 1.50 Dc × 180

d. **Compound myopic astigmatism (CMA):** Both focal lines are located in front of the retina. *Both principal meridians are negative.* The prescription would read as, (–)1.50 Ds/(–) 2.00 Dc × 150.

e. Mixed astigmatism: One line is in front of the retina and the other is located behind the retina, *one positive, the other is negative.* The prescription would read as (+) 2.00 Ds/(−) 2.50 Dc × 120.

The cylinder can be written in plus or minus form with the latter being preferred, since lenses are ground in minus cylinder form. Thus all plus cylinder prescriptions need to be transposed to minus cylinder form before manufacture.

Correcting the astigmatic eye with *best sphere* (contact lens or spectacle form) places 'neck' of Interval of Sturm or *circle of least confusion* on the retina. Best sphere is defined as the best spherical correction (maximum plus, minimum minus) which provides optimum vision.[14]

Astigmatism Based on Aetiology

a. Corneal Astigmatism

Cornea is the main refractive component of the eye accounting for 2/3rd of total refractive power and the commonest source of astigmatism. Any change in corneal power due to alteration in curvature or opacity drastically alters the refractive milieu. Refractive interface between posterior corneal surface with aqueous humour mirrors the anterior interface between corneal surface/tear film with atmospheric air, but is much weaker and negative in power. It neutralizes 10% of anterior corneal surface astigmatism. Soft lenses by nature drape on to the cornea and transmit corneal astigmatism unlike RGP lenses which mask corneal astigmatism.[14]

b. Lenticular Astigmatism

The astigmatism which remains after correcting for corneal causes is called **residual or internal astigmatism** and is contributed by lenticular and retinal factors. The etiology of this astigmatism is meridional differences in refractive power of natural crystalline lens, different refractive index of crystalline lens, tilt and/or decentration of crystalline lens or misaligned foveal position in relation to visual axis. As mentioned before rigid lenses correct corneal and *not lenticular astigmatism.*

Astigmatism Based on Optical Type

a. Regular Astigmatism

This is the type of astigmatism where the two principal meridians are 90° apart and occurs as a result of differences in corneal curvatures. It can be further subdivided into with-the-rule, against-the-rule and oblique. It can be corrected by standard spectacle lenses or contact lenses. It must be mentioned here that axis is recorded as an angle in degrees, between 0 and 180 degrees in a counter-clockwise direction. Both 0 and 180 degrees lie on a horizontal line at level of center of pupil, and as seen by an observer, **0 lies on the right of both the eyes (Fig. 3.11).** Regular astigmatism is further subdivided into with-the-rule, against-the-rule and oblique.

> i. *With-the-rule* (WTR/direct) astigmatism occurs when refractive power of vertical (or near vertical) meridian is maximum, i.e. vertical meridian is steep. The meridian of **least refractive power is located** *horizontally* **between 180° ±30°axis**. It is seen in children due to pressure of upper lid combined with lower ocular rigidity. In other words, *axis of positive cylinder in a **pair of glasses** is oriented at 90 degrees* and *minus cylinder is placed in horizontal axis* to correct the refractive error.[15]

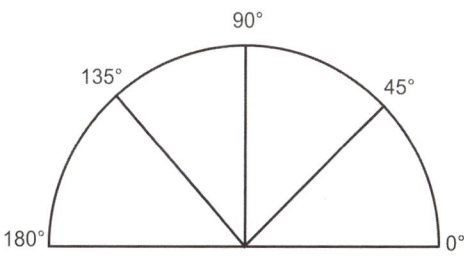

Fig. 3.11: Depiction of axis of eye

ii. *Against-the-rule* (ATR/indirect/inverse) astigmatism occurs when refractive power of horizontal (or near horizontal) meridian is maximum, i.e. horizontal meridian is steep. The **axis meridian** is, therefore, located **vertically with cylinder axis straddling axis 90° ± 30°** which means it lies between 60 and 120 degrees.[16]

Commonly seen in older individuals, it arises due to alteration in collagen structure and tension of lids during blinking causing corneal flattening around the horizontal meridian and unstable tear film.[17] In other words, *axis of plus cylinder* is *added in horizontal axis*

(or *a minus cylinder in the vertical axis*) to correct the error.

iii. *Oblique*: This is the astigmatism in which the two principal meridians lie somewhere between the axes defining either WTR or ATR astigmatism, between axis 30 to 60 and 120 to 150 degrees.

b. Irregular Astigmatism

In this type of astigmatism, meridians are not present at any identifiable axis. A result of random or irregular differences in curvature or refractive index, it is seen secondary to scarring post-trauma/keratitis or primarily due to irregular corneal surface, e.g. keratoconus.

REFERENCES

1. Holden BA, Mertz GW. Critical oxygen levels to avoid corneal oedema for daily and extended wear contact lenses. Invest Ophthalmol Vis Sci. 1984 Oct;25(10): 1161–7.

2. Bennett ESý, Weissman BA. Rigid contact lens care and application. In Cimical contact lens practice. Lippincott Williams & Wilkins, Phialdelphia 2005, 236.

3. Cavangh HD. The effects of low and hyper DK contact lenses on corneal epithelial homeostasis. Ophthalm Clinics of North America 2003,16(3):311–25.

4. Guillon M, Lydon DP, Wilson C. Corneal topography: a clinical model. Ophthalmic Physiol Opt 1986;6(1):47–56.

5. Zantos SG, Holden BA. Ocular changes associated with continuous wear of contact lenses. Aust J Optom 1978, 61: 418–26.

6. Holden BA, Sweeney DF, Sanderson G. The minimal pre-corneal oxygen tension to avoid corneal oedema. Invest Ophthalmol Vis Science 1984:25: 476.

7. Carlson KH, Bourne WM, Brubaker RF . Effect of long-term contact lens wear on corneal endothelial cell morphology and function. Invest Ophthalmol Vis Sci 1988 Feb;29(2): 185–93.

8. Millodot M. Effect of long time wear of hard contact lens on corneal sensitivity. Arch Ophthalmol 1978, 96: 1225–7.

9. Contact lenses. In: Cantor LB, Rapuano CJ, Cioffi GA. Clinical Optics; Basic and clinical Science Course. Am Academy of Ophthalmology 2015–16, 160.

10. Rosenthal Perry. Contact lenses. In: Albert DM & Miller JW Albert Jakobiec's Principles and Practice of Ophthalmology, 3rd ed., Saunders Elsevier 2008, 5279–94.

11. Kastl PR. Rigid versus soft contact lenses. International Ophthalmology Clinics: Contact lenses 1991, 31(2): 17–24.

12. White PF, Scott CA. Contact Lenses. In: Yanoff M, Duker JS. Mosby Eds. Ophthalmolgy 3rd ed., Elsevier, 2009, 71–6.

13. Rouwen AJ, Pinckers AJ, Pad Bosch AA, Punt H, Doesburg WH, Lemmens WA. Visual acuity, spectacle blur and slit-lamp biomicroscopy on asymptomatic contact-lens-wearing recruits. Graefes Arch Clin Exp Ophthalmol 1983; 221(2):73–7.

14. Rosenfield M, Logan N, Edwards KH. Subjective Refraction. In Optometry: Science, Techniques and Clinical Management. 2nd ed. Edinburgh. Butterworth Heinemann Elsevier 2009.

15. Chowdhary M. Astigmatism. In: Chowdhary M. Refraction and lens prescription for all eye care practitioners. New Delhi, CBS Publishers, 2014, 51–58.

16. Azar DT, Strauss L. Optics of the Eye. In: Albert DM, Miller JK Eds, Albert Jakobiec's Principles and Practice of Ophthalmology. 3rd ed. Saunders Elsevier 2008, 5253–55.

17. Gatinel Damien. Corneal topography and wave front analysis. In: Albert DM & Miller J W Eds Albert Jakobiec's Principles and Practice of Ophthalmology, 3rd ed., Saunders Elsevier 2008, 921–63.

Reader's Note

CHAPTER 4

Instruments used in Contact Lens Fitting

This chapter gives a brief description of the common instruments used during contact lens fitting and the different techniques of usage.

1. Torch

a. Direct torch light is used for gross examination of lids and to assess extraocular movements.

b. Oblique illumination with a flashlight illuminating the nasal canthus gives details about corneal clarity. With a contact lens in *situ*, movements and centration of lens with respect to the limbus and any foreign body trapped beneath the lens can be visualized.

2. Burton Lamp

Now supplanted by the slit lamp, this instrument allows gross simultaneous magnification and illumination. It incorporates a cobalt blue filter light for examining the fluorescein pattern in evaluating lens fit (Fig. 4.1).

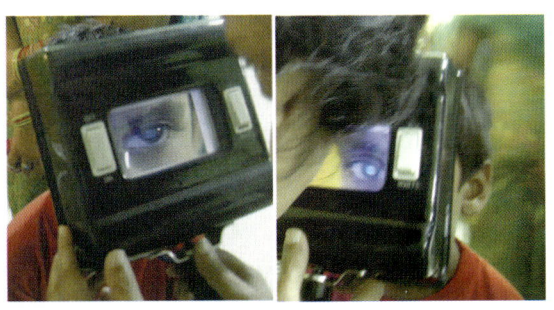

Fig. 4.1: Burton's lamp

3. Magnification Devices

These can be a direct ophthalmoscope or hand-held magnifying glass. Direct ophthalmoscope can be used to observe the conjunctiva, limbus by starting with a high plus power and adjusting both the observation distance and dialled in lens, until a clear view of the CL on eye, is obtained (Fig. 4.2). It is a very useful method to assess fit in a young child who is unable to sit at slit lamp and gets scared with the proximity of the large Burton lamp.

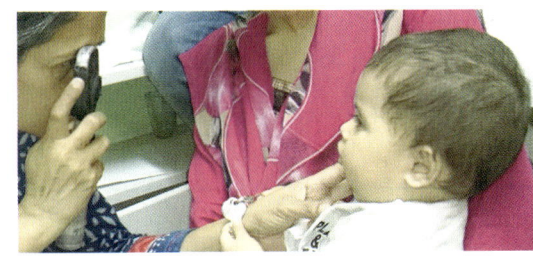

Fig. 4.2: Using a direct ophthalmoscope to view CL fit in an infant

4. Slit Lamp Biomicroscope

This ingenious device was invented by the Swedish ophthalmologist and self-taught mathematician, Allvar Gullstrand who received the Nobel Prize in 1911 for his work in optical properties of eye. An instrument essential for refined lens fitting, it combines variable magnification with controlled illumination and consists of: Mechanical support, observation and illumination system.

- *Mechanical support*: This includes forehead band, chin rest, fixation target power supply unit and locking controls.
- *Observation system*: This includes binocular eyepieces, observation tube, and magnification changer. The magnification can be varied in a stepped or continuous manner from low (7–10X) to medium (20–25X) to high (30–40X) for detailed evaluation.
- *Illumination system:* This includes lamp housing unit, slit control of width and height, filters (neutral density/cobalt blue/red-free/green), field size control, diffuser and a prism.

Structures to be evaluated during contact lens evaluation:

- *Epithelium*: Any surface irregularities, opacification, dry spots, vacuoles and microcysts need to be ruled out before deciding for lens fitting. Presence of vacuoles (20–50 mm round spaces with distinct edges) and small microcysts (collection of dead cells and metabolic by-products) signify lens induced hypoxia.
- *Stroma*: The things to be specifically looked for are striae, ghost vessels, pigment deposits and opacities. Stromal edema can be diagnosed by presence of fine, non-branching vertical striae in posterior stroma which indicate corneal swelling greater than 5–6%. Corneal folds are intersecting lines observed in direct illumination or as dark intersecting lines viewed against the endothelial mosaic in retro-illumination. Presence of corneal folds implies corneal swelling of 8–10% and indicates buckling of posterior stroma. Stromal edema and corneal folds both imply hypoxic states. Vogt's striae are fine vertical parallel lines in deep posterior stroma and Descemet's membrane in patients of keratoconus.
- *Endothelium:* The aspects to be seen in endothelium are visualized by method of "zone of specular reflection", with normal

endothelium being visible as a mosaic of fitted hexagonal cells. Abnormal structures which indicate early endothelial dysfunction, need to looked at are: Polymegethism (variable endothelial cell size), guttata (excrescences of Descemet's membrane) seen as dark spots and blebs (minute black spots in endothelium).

Examination Techniques using a Slit Lamp

These techniques are diffuse, direct, indirect, retro-illumination, specular reflection, sclerotic scatter and tangential.

Diffuse Illumination

It uses a wide open slit-width with angle of 30–45 degree between light and observation system along with a diffusing filter to reduce glare. This examination method is used to view details of anterior segment structures at a glance.

Direct Illumination

In this technique both observation and illumination systems are focused at same point. Variation in width and/or height of slit creates a parallelopiped optic section or conical beam. Parallelopiped section is used to measure corneal thickness and see details of any lesion within the corneal layers. In order to rule out corneal nerves/infiltrates or ghost vessels, high magnification is required. This is important since a patient with ghost vessels must be fitted only with a high Dk value CL to prevent hypoxia stimulated growth of this obliterated vessel.

Indirect Illumination

In this technique observation and illumination systems are not focused at the same point. Instead the focal light beam is directed adjacent to the area of observation and angle of illumination is varied by rotating body of the illumination system. It is used to view epithelial and iris details like epithelial erosions, infiltrates and microcysts.

Retro-illumination

In this method, light reflected from back of eye is used to view structures which get silhouetted in the reflected glow with objects opaque to light appearing dark, e.g. opacities, pigment, blood vessels. Angle of illumination is varied relative to observation system by rotating the body of illumination system. A moderately wide beam is used and cornea is illuminated by light reflected from iris or retina. Retroillumination can be direct, indirect or marginal and is very useful to look for epithelial edema, microcysts, limbal vessel engorgement or CL deposits.

Zone of Specular Reflection

This is used to view corneal endothelial layer. The technique is as follows: Focus slit beam on cornea and move it across cornea till a bright reflex of light filament is located in the slit beam. Increase magnification to 40X to view endothelial layer which becomes visible, adjacent and posterior to the bright reflex as a patch of dull gold with a mosaic of hezagonal cells.

Sclerotic Scatter

In this technique cornea is illumined by total internal reflection of a wide angle light source directed at limbal region. It is used to delineate localized epithelial oedema and corneal scars.

Tangential/oblique Illumination

In this method observation system is placed directly in front of eye and a large angle of 70–80 degrees subtended between illumination and observation systems. It is used to evaluate iris lesions and structures in anterior chamber.

With Filters (Cobalt Blue Filter or Wratten 47A)

A slit lamp combined with a Wratten no. 12 (yellow barrier) filter placed in front of slit lamp optics, enhances fluorescein observations of contact lens fitting. As significant light losses occur with use of filters, illumination needs to be maximum when using this technique.

Cobalt blue filter is used while studying fluorescent pattern of RGP lens fitting.

Tear Film Measures

These include measuring the tear meniscus, lacrimal river and inferior tear prism height on the slit lamp. The common ancillary tests used are-non invasive dye tests, e.g. Tear break up time (BUT) or invasive tests like Schirmer test.

5. Placido Disc

This historic device using reflective mires is the prototype on which keratometer and topography systems are based. A hand-held device, it consists of a flat disc with alternating white and black rings equidistant from one another. It has a central viewing aperture fitted with a + 5.0 D lens (Fig. 4.3).

The examiner sits 15–20 cm away from the patient and directs disc perpendicular to patient's corneal apex. An external light source positioned adjacent to patient's head is directed onto the disc. Patient is then asked to fixate on center of disc, and examiner views magnified reflection of rings on corneal surface through the central aperture. Since poor tear quality would blur the reflection, it is important to ask patient to blink just prior to final assessment. Gullstrand was the first one to photograph reflected corneal image of

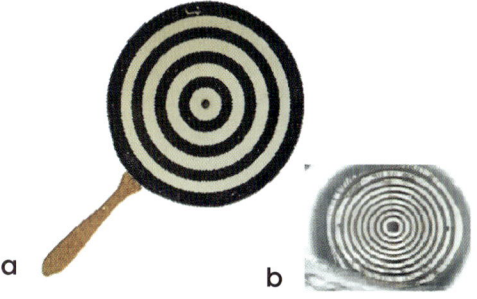

a   b

Fig. 4.3: (a) Placido disc; (b) Reflected mires of disc on corneal surface

a Placido disc and analyse its results and he interpreted the different images as the following.[1]

- Symmetrical contour/circular shape indicates a regular corneal surface.
- Regular, oval or elliptical shape indicates corneal astigmatism.
- Distorted rings indicate irregular cornea.
- Broader, larger and widely separated rings indicate the flatter meridian.
- Unequal elongation of contours in one direction and shortening in opposite direction often indicate keratoconus.

6. Keratometer/ophthalmometer

This instrument derived from Placido disc, utilizes the Scheiner principle. It was given its final form by Hermann von Helmholtz in 1851, by modification of an earlier prototype developed by Jesse Ramsden and Everard Home in 1796. It measures radius of curvature of central 3–4 mm portion (optic cap) of cornea in two meridians usually 180 and 90 degrees. These measurements called K values determine base curve (BC) of the trial contact lens. Refer to Annexure I.

The front surface of cornea acting as a convex mirror reflects illuminated mires of known linear size (object). The keratometer measures the apparent image height of these reflected mires/image (Purkinje **Sanson** image 1). This image is minified, upright, virtual and forms in front of posterior focal plane of cornea, but appears to be located within anterior chamber of the eye. To measure height of this virtual image, a short-focus telescope (long-focus microscope) is introduced in the keratometer system which converts it into a second, real, measurable image.

Doubling Principle

A doubling prism, positioned midway in the observation field, creates doubled images adjacent to one another. The doubling prism negates the deleterious effect of constant eye movements on accuracy of measurement, by ensuring simultaneous movement of both images synchronous to ocular movements. A plano prism in the system then causes a displacement proportional to distance from the objective and end point is measured once these central images are superimposed. This image height is measured and extrapolated to provide *radius of curvature in mm which in turn is converted to dioptric power (K value)*. (Annexure I)

The types of doubling systems can be fixed, variable, divided or full.

Design of keratometer has inherent flaws based on three assumptions which are:

i. Refractive index utilized is $n = 1.3375$ μ, whereas actual corneal index is 1.376 μ. Thus for a 7.80 mm cornea, dioptric power is 48.21 (assuming n of 1.376), but according to index value of 1.3375 fed into the instrument the measured dioptric power is 43.27. Thus the measured K reading is 90% of actual power. This usually does not translate in clinical error since only 90% of corneal astigmatism is eliminated by RGP lens and the keratometer's estimate of corneal astigmatism indicates this neutralizable astigmatism.

ii. Refractive index of cornea at 1.376 μ differs greatly from that of air at 1.0 μ and nominally from aqueous humor at 1.333 μ. This large air cornea difference accounts for the anterior corneal surface (ACS) bathed by air being a stronger refractive interface than posterior corneal surface (PCS) bathed by aqueous.[2] Despite this difference in refracting abilities the PCS usually mirror irregularities of ACS. In corneal astigmatism, the poorer refracting ability of the mirror image PCS neutralizes 10% of astigmatism accruing by ACS.[3]

iii. The power/location of steepest meridian and meridian 90 degrees away is based on assumption that cornea is spherocylindrical, which may not always be so.

Types of Keratometers

The two prototypes of keratometer are: One position and two position .

i. Two-position Keratometer (Haag-Streit Javal Schiotz Keratometer)

The body of this keratometer requires rotation about an axis to measure each principal meridians (Fig. 4.4a). It uses fixed doubling where two objects are placed in a circumferential track at a constant fixed distance from the eye. These objects are self-illuminated mires in the shape of a red square and a green staircase (Fig. 4.4b). The image size remains fixed while object size is adjusted to determine radius of curvature of the reflected anterior corneal surface.

ii. One-position Keratometer (Bausch & Lomb Keratometer)

This keratometer uses variable doubling devices in each corresponding meridian to produce simultaneous doubling of perpendicular pairs of mires (Fig. 4.5). Reflected rays from corneal surface pass through a disc with four apertures and image size is varied keeping the object size fixed. The presence of two prisms, aligned perpendicular to each other allows both major and minor axis powers to be measured simultaneously.

In situations where extremely flat or steep corneas beyond the measurable range of keratometer (36–52 D) are encountered, the range of this instrument can be extended by

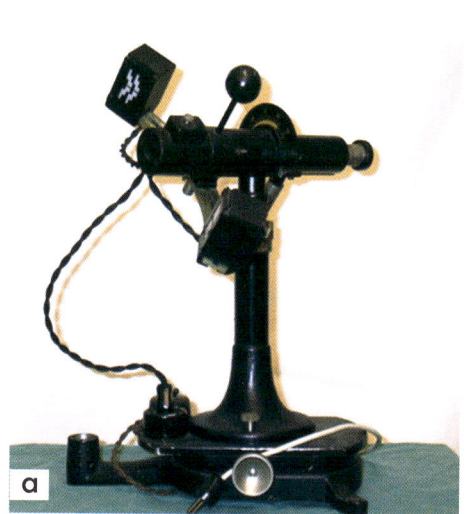

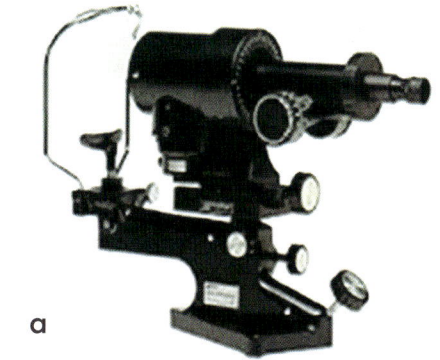

a

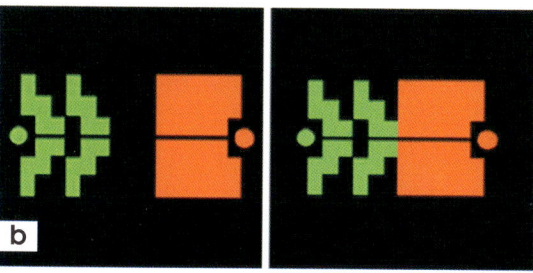

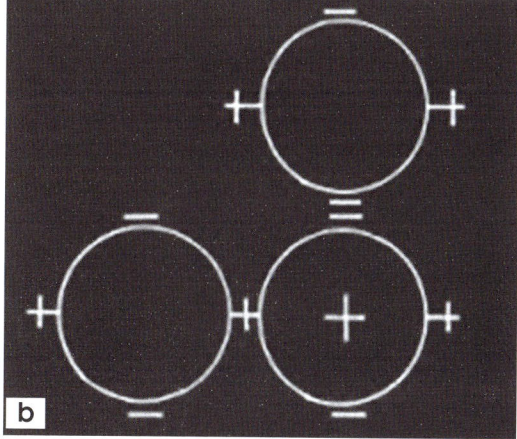

Fig. 4.4: (a) Keratometer: Haag-Streit prototype; (b) Mires seen in the Haag-Streit

Fig. 4.5: (a) Keratometer: Bausch & Lomb keratometer; (b) Mires seen in the Bausch & Lomb keratometer

an additional 9 D till 61 D, and reduced by 6 D till 30 D, by taping a (+) 1.25 D or a (–)1.00 D lens respectively in front of the objective of the instrument. This is called *extended keratometry* (Fig. 4.6).

- If +1.25 D lens is used: 9 D needs to be added to the measured K value (Fig. 4.6).
- If –1.00 D lens is placed in front of objective: 6 D needs to be subtracted from measured K value.

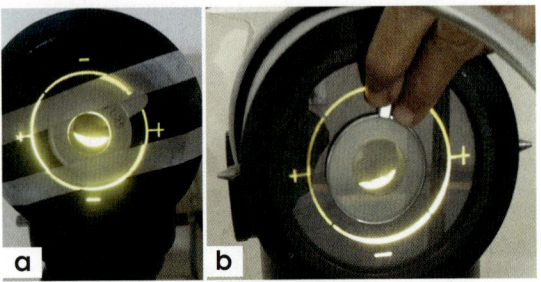

Fig. 4.6: (a) Taping of lens in front of objective end; (b) Showing (+) 1.25 D lens taped (holding of lens by hand is easier since the taping shown would distort the mires)

Calibration of the Keratometer

This is done on a frequent basis, preferably quarterly to ensure reliability of measurements. Precise polished spherical steel/glass balls of known radii are measured on the keratometer (Fig. 4.7). The formula used to measure is:

$$R = 2dh'/h$$

where R = known radius of curvature, d = image distance, h' = image height and h = mire separation

The horizontal and vertical power wheels are set at the measured radius or dioptric value of the steel ball. The steel ball is then placed in an adaptor (accessory with the instrument) and mire images are focused. If the mires do not align, eyepiece is rotated anticlockwise (maximum plus), to make the mires spring apart and then it is slowly rotated clockwise till mires re-focus and get aligned (plus signs overlap). If minus signs are not aligned, the vertical measurement knob is adjusted until they align and amount of misalignment is recorded. The difference in measure gives the error.

For example, if for a steel ball with known measurement of 46.0 by 46.0, the horizontal knob and vertical knob read 45.0 by 45.0 when mires on this steel ball become focused, then the instrument is out of calibration. When doing keratometry with this instrument 1.0 D needs to be added to both horizontal and vertical reading in order to compensate for this error.

Radii of a RGP lens can also be measured by using a prism or mirror attachment to the headrest. A 45° prism is positioned at the headrest in such a way that light reflected from contact lens surface reaches the instrument. The

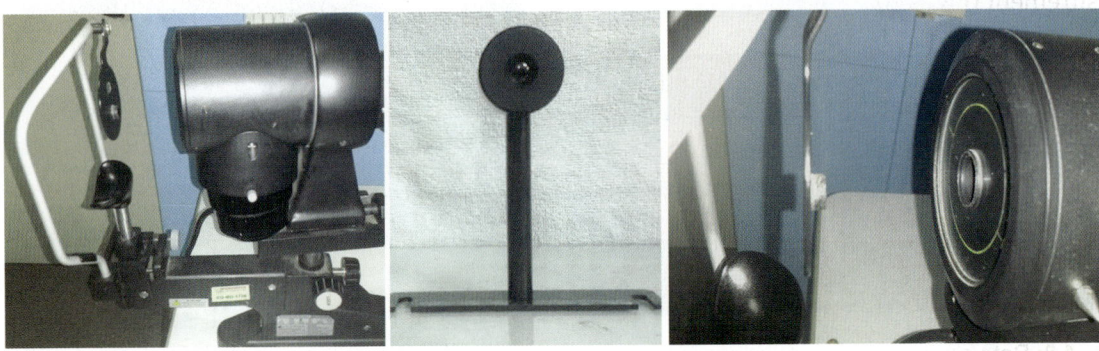

Fig. 4.7: Placement of steel ball on the adaptor in front of keratometer for calibration

keratometer readings have to be converted to equivalent mirror values using conversion tables, which are different for concave and convex side surfaces of the CL.

Procedure of Keratometry

- **Eyepiece focus:** Eyepiece is rotated *counter clockwise* and a graticule (plane sheet of paper with a bold black cross drawn using both vertical and horizontal lines) is viewed by the examiner through it keeping his BOTH eyes open. The counter-clockwise rotation blurs cross hairs and relaxes accommodation of observer. Eyepiece is then slowly rotated *clockwise* (in *plus* direction) until graticule crosshairs come to a sharp focus again. This keratometer has now been adjusted for observer's refractive error.
- **Instrument:** Chin rest is adjusted to patient's level. Outer canthus of eye should be level with eye-level mark on the headrest.
- **Patient fixation:** Patient is asked to look at the objective. He/she may be asked to look at the reflection of their own eye or at a small fixation light. Both eyes must be kept open to prevent effect of proximal accommodation by the patients. The other eye is only occluded in cases where the examined eye has poor/unsteady fixation or squint. In the latter situations if both eyes are kept open, then the better seeing or non-squinting takes up fixation and mires would be seen in a paraxial or eccentric position of examined eye leading to inaccurate measurement (Fig. 4.8).

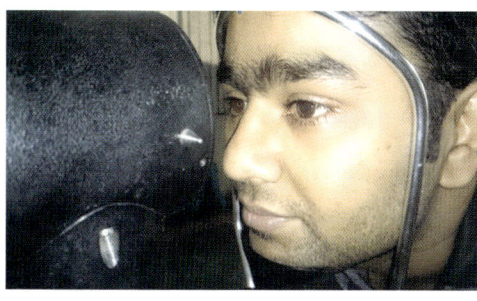

Fig. 4.8: Both eyes of the patient are open to avoid proximal accommodation

*Error due to proximal accommodation of the subject can be avoided by asking patient to keep both eyes open, and examiner by focusing the eyepiece from plus to minus.

- Keratometer is moved towards the patient until second image is seen in sharp focus on the graticule. Since the fixed test object moves along with the instrument, the object distance from first virtual image of cornea is attained simultaneously with second focal length.
- **Mires are aligned** by rotating vertical and horizontal drums to adjust the mires centrally. Image can be focused by moving the joystick (Fig. 4.9).
- **Axis location** is done next by rotating the keratometer until the axis markers on the mires are correctly aligned.

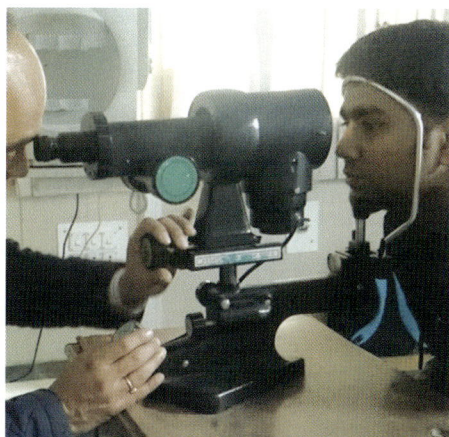

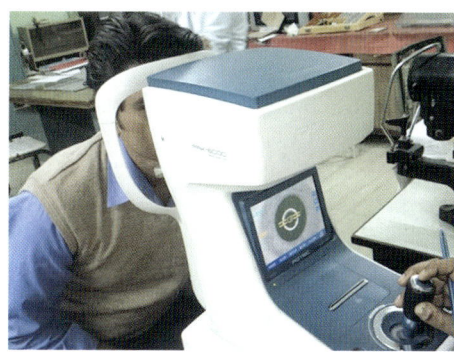

Fig. 4.9: Keratometry being performed mires are focused by moving the joystick

- **Doubling adjustment** is then done by adjusting the doubled images until the mires just touch (Fig. 4.10).
- With one position instruments, the second meridian is adjusted and aligned in a similar fashion. For two position instrument, keratometer body needs to be rotated through 90° to locate and subsequently align the second meridian.

Three readings are taken in quick succession to minimize errors due to eye movements.

Keratometry should be done on corneas free from prior lens use for at least 5–7 days. While this time interval may be sufficient for soft/RGP lens

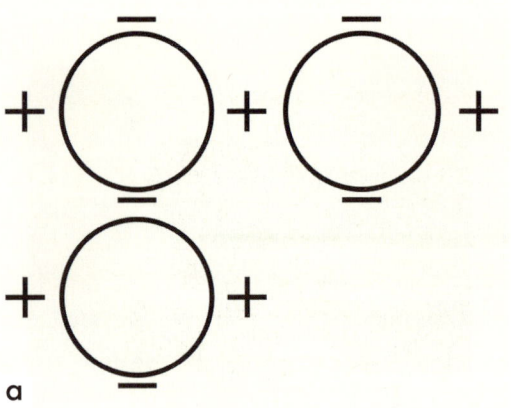

a

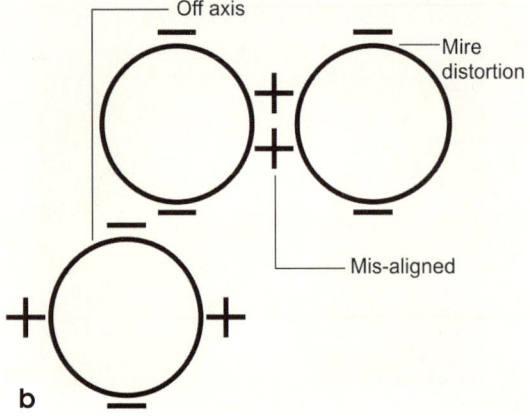

b

Fig. 4.10: (a) Mires aligned; (b) Mire-misalignment

wearer, for the older PMMA wearer's, corneal shape required weeks to recover its original shape.

7. Topographic Analysis Systems (computer-assisted elevation depression recorders)

Contact lenses are designed to fit a prolate cornea. A deviation in corneal curvature, e.g. post-refractive surgery/keratoplasty or keratoconus would lead to a poor lens fit. In such situations keratometry values are not sufficient to visualize the altered corneal surface and corneal topography is required. Topography technology uses computer-assisted algorithms to reconstruct three-dimensional view of corneal surface from images digitised by a CCD camera. Three systems are used for imaging, namely placido disc reflection, elevation-based and Scheimpflug photography.

Normal cornea is prolate in shape with steeper center which gradually slopes off to a flatter periphery. In other words, the radius of curvature increases with distance from surface apex. This is said to have a negative spherical aberration or prolate asphericity. The posterior corneal surface also has a prolate asphericity which is superior to that of the anterior cornea.[4] On elevation maps this translates into hot warm colors in center and cooling colors in the periphery, and can be remembered by the mnemonic: **Hot center, cold periphery**. Five patterns of anterior topographic shape have been enunciated by Bogan et al based on placement of hot colors as round, oval, symmetric bow tie, asymmetric bow tie and irregular.[5]

A *horizontal asymmetry* is physiological with the nasal periphery being flatter than temporal periphery. This again appears as a colder nasal side versus warmer temporal and can be remembered by the mnemonic: **Colder nose**. In young eyes radius of curvature is greater in horizontal meridian (flatter) than vertical meridian giving rise to with *the rule* *astigmatism.* This changes to against the rule in older age.[6]

In pathological conditions like pellucid and keratoconus the steep flat asymmetry occurs in vertical or oblique direction, which manifests as an *asymmetric bow tie* pattern. A shift in physiological horizontal symmetry to an inferior position may be the first evidence of forme fruste keratoconus. Increased *prolate asphericity* of both anterior and posterior corneal surface is typical of keratoconus. In corneas subjected to refractive surgery (LASIK), corneal asphericity is reversed, with curvature increasing from center to periphery, called *oblate/positive spherical* aberration and can be remembered by the mnemonic: **Hot periphery, center cold**.

The three topography imaging systems are detailed briefly.

a. **Older videokeratoscope** were based on Placido disc principle coupled with mathematical formula to provide a point to point quantitative gradient. Color coded contour map plots are generated where hot colors (red/orange) denote more curved/steeper contours and cold colors (blue/green) depict flatter or less curved contours (Fig. 4.11).

Some commonly used values of topography are:

– Sim K (**simulated** keratometry): Gives power and location of steepest and flattest meridians from a reconstructed corneal surface, analogous to K values of a keratometer.

– Surface asymmetry index (SAI): A centrally weighted summation of differences in corneal power between corresponding

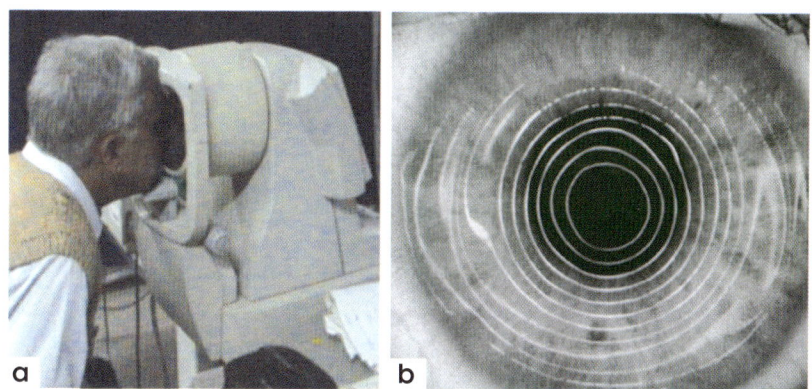

Fig. 4.11: (a) Patient on corneal topography; (b) Placido disc principle being used

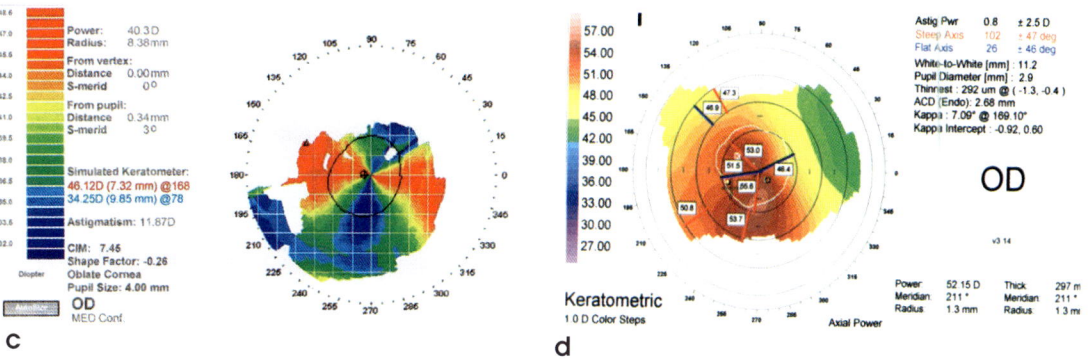

Fig. 4.11: Color coded map: (c) Horizontal bow tie pattern; (d) Keratoconus

points 180 degrees apart, on 128 equally spaced meridians crossing four central photokeratoscope mires. It approaches numeric value of zero for a perfectly spherical surface. Normal cornea is prolate with SAI values lower than 0.5.

– *Surface regularity index (SRI):* Summation of local power fluctuations along 256 equally spaced meridians, its value increases with increasing irregular astigmatism and approaches zero for a smooth corneal surface.

– *Shape Factor (SF):* A measure of corneal asphericity, a negative value implies an oblate surface (e.g. post-refractive surgery). Normal values are between 0.13 and 0.35 and borderline from 0.02 to 0.12.

– *Corneal Irregularity Measurement (CIM):* A measure of irregularity with normal range of 0.03–0.68 µm and borderline from 0.69 to 1.0 µm. Higher values denote more irregularity.

b. **Elevation-based scanning slit evaluation uses** slit scan and Placido images to give a very good composite picture for topographic analysis. Prototype is Orbscan where a series of 40 (20 from the left and 20 from the right) slit beams angled at 45° to right and left of video axis are projected onto cornea by two scanning slit lamps. A "tracking system" attempts to minimize influence of involuntary eye movement. The instrument's software analyzes 240 data points per slit (total 9600 points) and calculates the corneal thickness and posterior surface of entire cornea over a 1.5 second examination. Corneal topography is analysed using color coded contour maps of corneal power with cool colors (green, blue) representing lower corneal powers and warm colors (orange, red) representing high corneal powers (Fig. 4.12).

Analysis of Orbscan Quad map:

   i. *Top left image:* Anterior float (Elevation best fit sphere): The anterior best fit sphere (BFS) is calculated to best match the anterior corneal surface. Green is "sea level" (match with a sphere that best matches cornea). Warmer colors are above sea level, while cooler colors are below sea level.

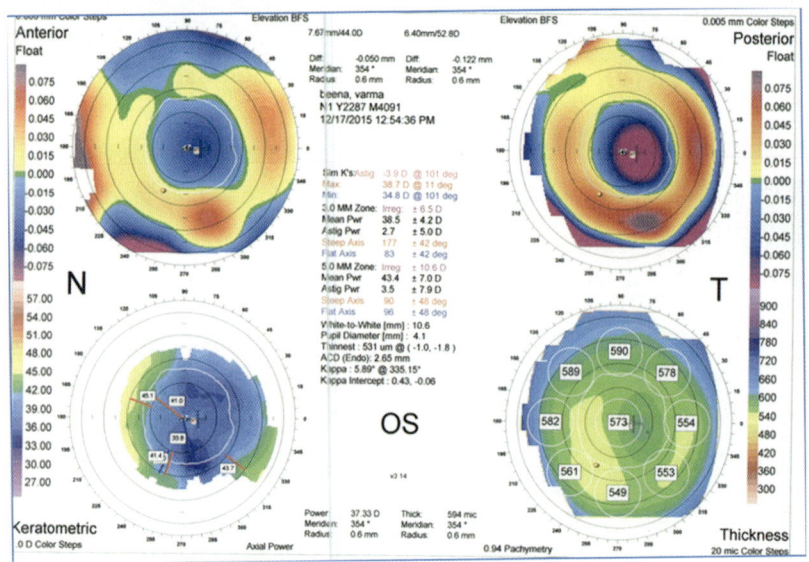

Fig. 4.12: Orbscan print out showing anterior flat and posterior floats in top row left to right, and corneal curvature map and pachymetry maps in bottom row. This is a scan of a post-radial keratotomy case

ii. *Top right image:* Posterior float (elevation best fit sphere) map: It describes back surface of the cornea using posterior corneal measurements.

iii. *Bottom left image:* Keratometric (mean power) map displays refractive power of anterior surface of cornea and translates anterior curvature into corneal power.

iv. *Bottom left:* Thickness (pachymetry) map demonstrates corneal thickness of entire cornea as well as thinnest point of the cornea. Warm colors indicate thinner cornea while cooler colors indicate thicker corneas. Figure 4.13 shows some prototype Orbscan printouts of conditions of keratoconus, pellucid degeneration.

c. **Scheimpflug principle based system** is represented by Pentacam scanner. This measures pachymetry, corneal topography, anterior and posterior corneal curvature and astigmatism. Two cameras capture corneal image from 0 to 180° and unlike slit-scanning devices, central cornea data points of center can be more precisely measured. Elevation data is independent of axis, orientation and position. This modality is currently being used for keratoconus screening with certain guidelines for anterior and posterior elevation. Elevations of more than 15 μ for anterior float and more than 20 μ for posterior float indicate pathology. Risk of keratoconus is given by certain indices, namely index of surface variance (ISV) ≥41, index of vertical asymmetry (IVA) ≥0.32, keratoconus index (KI) >1.07, central keratoconus index (CKI) ≥1.03, radii minimum (Rmin) <6.71, index of height asymmetry (IHA) ≥21, index of height decentration (IHD) ≥0.016 and aberration coefficient (ABR) ≥1.0.

Pachymetry measures include pachymetry map (corneal thickness), and pachymetric indices. Corneal thickness is measured from top of epithelium to anterior surface of endothelium, excluding tear film. It is measured both at apex and at thinnest point (TP) including location and distance of thinnest point versus apex and converts into color coded map.

Newer pentacam models incorporate contact lens fitting software which provide an automatic power calculation for contact lens with pre-programmed recommendations for rigid and soft contact lenses. In addition use of real fluorescein image simulation on the cornea, helps in providing best possible contact lens fit to the patient.

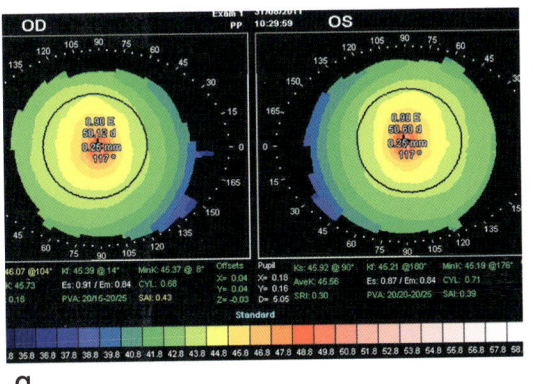

a

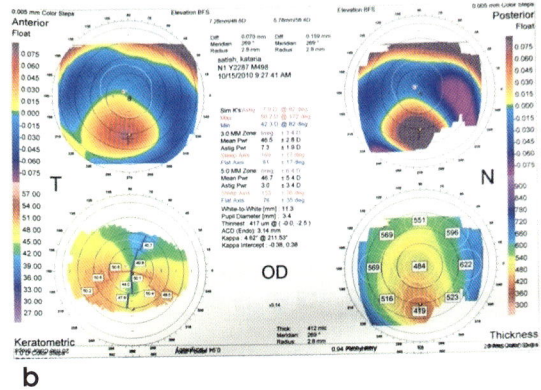

b

Fig. 4.13: Orbscan showing (a) Keratoconus; (b) Crab claw/kissing birds appearance of-pellucid marginal degeneration (PMD)

A few differences between Orbscan and pentacam are given below. Orbscan takes vertical image slices, separated from one another with no common point, whereas pentacam maintains central point of each meridian by re-registering for any eye movement. The rotating Scheimpflug imaging process of pentacam also provides for correction of eye movements, easy fixation and reduced examination time. Since pentacam calculates power of anterior and posterior corneal surface separately, therefore, map of corneal power differs significantly from Placido disc based topographic values with posterior surface elevation bring more reproducible in former.

8. Corneal Thickness Measurement Techniques

- **Ultrasonic pachymeter** (A-scan or time amplitude): A transducer of 20 MHz. Frequency is used to define corneal boundaries. Measurement is based on time taken for sound wave to travel from probe tip to cornea, anterior chamber interface and back. For correct values the ultrasonic beam needs to be aligned with the visual axis.
Time interval between anterior and posterior corneal surfaces is measured in microseconds, which is converted into millimetres taking into account speed of sound in cornea. Margin of error is minimal to the tune of 0.1 to 0.2 mm.
- **Optical pachometer:** This older instrument consists of a beam-splitting device which can be attached to the slit lamp. A doubling prism allows two corneal images in the optical section to be juxtaposed. The distance between the opposing corneal surfaces is measured as the corneal thickness.

9. Radiuscope (Microspherometer)

It is an instrument which measures radius of curvature of anterior and posterior surface of a CL by using Drysdale method (Fig. 4.14a).

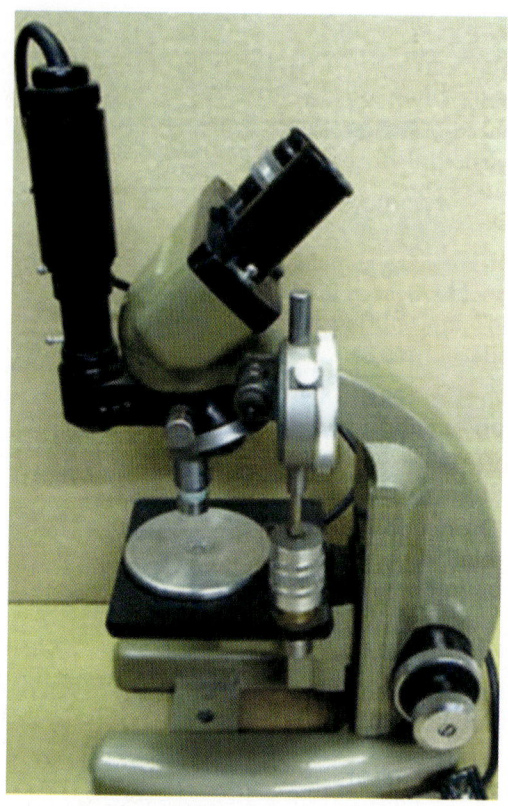

Fig. 4.14a: The radiuscope

Measurement is made after putting drop of water on the CL placed convex side down on a special mount. A spot of light is centered in lens middle and microscope is raised to maximum height. Subsequently radiuscope is focused downward until a spoke pattern becomes clear. This "aerial image" representing reflection from lens posterior surface dictates setting of pointer scale to zero (first position). The microscope body is made to continue its downward journey till image of the **bulb filament** becomes clear (second position). If microscope is made to move further down a third image or second **spoke pattern** is focused (third position) (Fig. 4.14b). This represents lens surface and the scale reading gives radius of curvature of lens surface in millimeters.

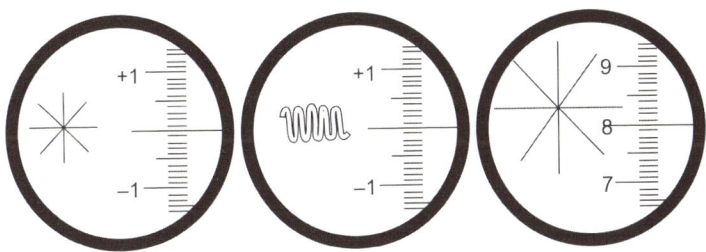

Fig. 4.14b: Sequential images 1st, 2nd, 3rd seen in downward flousing journey of a radiuscope

10. Ultrasonic Cleaner

This is used to clean debris and deposits from soft and RGP lens. It is an ancillary cleaning method in addition to the regular cleaning protocol of lens disinfection used by wearer (Fig. 4.15).

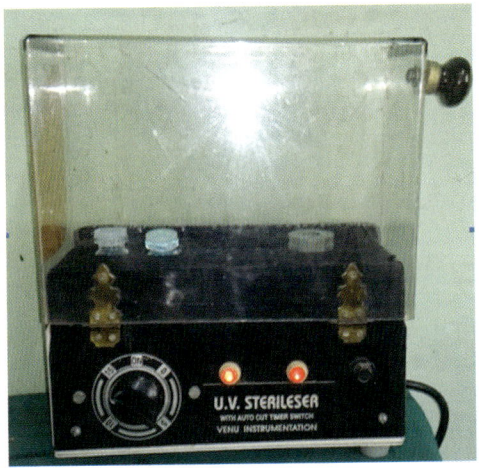

Fig. 4.15: Ultrasonic cleaner with a soft lens inside the well for cleaning

REFERENCES

1. Gullstrand A. Photographic ophthalmometric and clinical investigation of corneal refraction. Am J Optom Arch Am Acad Optom 1966: 43:143–214.
2. Azar DT and Strauss L. Geometric Optics. Pages 5241–51 in Albert Jakobiec's Principles and Practice of Ophthalmology 3rd ed. Eds: Alber D, Miller J. Philadelphia. Saunders Elsevier 2008.
3. Bennett and Rabbetts, Clinical Visual Optics. Butterworths, London, UK, 1984, 420–1.
4. Patel S, Marshal J, Fitzke F. Shape and radius of posterior corneal surface. Refract Corn Surg 1993;9:173–81.
5. Bogan SJ, Waring GO III, Ibrahim O et al. Classification of normal corneal topography based on computer assisted videokeratography. Arch Ophthalmol 1990;108:945–9.
6. Gatinel Damien. Corneal topography and wave front analysis. Pages 921–63 in Albert Jakobiec's Principles and Practice of Ophthalmology 3rd ed. Eds: Albert DM and Miller J W. Saunders Elsevier 2008.
7. Ambrosio R Jr, Alonso RS, Luz A, Coca Velarde LG. Corneal thickness spatial profile and corneal volume distribution: tomographic indices to detect keratoconus. J cataract Refract Surg. 2006; 32(11): 1851–9.

Reader's Note

CHAPTER 5

Fitting Methodology

This chapter details the indications of contact lens usage with a brief description of optical advantages enjoyed by them. It also discusses the methodology of fitting a contact lens.

INDICATIONS AND OPTICAL ADVANTAGES OF CONTACT LENSES

A. Optical

i. Refractive errors: Myopia, hyperopia, regular astigmatism. Optical advantages of lens over spectacles in these situations are:

- Object size is more consistent with 'real-world' size (that is, less minification or magnification) since corrective lenses are closer to center of rotation.[1]
- Dynamic vision: Lenses ensure stable vision during intense ocular movements, as they remain centered while *in situ* placement on the eye.
- Field of vision is enhanced by 15–20% since lenses are closer to nodal point of eye. In addition, field restrictions due to spectacle frames are avoided.[1]
- Reduces peripheral distortion inherent to optics of high-powered spectacles: A high-minus power lens has decreasing magnification or increasing minification towards lens periphery. While viewing an elongated object, images of peripheral parts of this object get magnified less than those closer to center, resulting in a "barrel" distortion of the image.[2] A plus-power spectacle lens by nature creates spherical aberration with resultant "pincushion" distortion. The patient complaint is of rectangular/square objects like door frames appearing bent, curved in at the middle leaving a small aperture insufficient for the spectacled person to pass through inside giving an impression of *closing in* onto the approaching person. A graphic description on use of aphakic glasses by an ophthalmologist further states that *on actually passing through the door these curves recede gracefully.*[3]

ii. Aphakia: In both monocular and binocular aphakia, lenses do away with the cumbersome, unsightly, heavy spectacles. They also reduce magnification induced by the aphakic glasses (25%) to acceptable limits so that spatial perception and depth perception is almost normalized. Lenses enlarge and enhance field of vision by removing prismatic aberration of high plus glasses (roving ring scotoma, Jack in box phenomenon) (Refer to Chapter 11, page 143). This ensures that the aphakic patient can use his eye movements and not depend on head movements to scan the entire field (required during aphakic spectacle wear). During use of these head movements magnification and distortion effects of aphakic spectacles very often cause a swimming sensation to the patient.[3] Use of contacts thus rids the patient of these troublesome symptoms, are more comfortable to use and socially more acceptable. In patients of uniocular aphakia, contact lenses minimize aniseikonia and improve functional level of binocular vision, since no relative spectacle magnification (RSM) is induced by the contact lens.[4] Most patients tolerate up to 3% magnification difference between two eyes, differences greater than this need to corrected by use of a contact lens.

iii. Oblique/irregular astigmatism like keratoconus, postkeratoplasty, regression of myopia postrefractive surgery and corneal scars. Contact lenses are extremely beneficial in visual rehabilitation of these cases as regular astigmatism induced in such situations, cannot be fully corrected by spectacles which often provide suboptimal vision.[5-8]

iv. In anisometropia of refractive origin, contact lenses paint a more accurate, 'real-world' image size on the brain. In axial anisometropia, however, spectacles optics are superior due to aspect of relative spectacle magnification (RSM).

v. Aniseikonia correction: Contact lenses minimize aniseikonia of refractive origin, whereas spectacles minimize aniseikonia of axial length origin. Wearers with retinal image problems subsequent to aniseikonia and/or anisometropia are benefited with use of contact lenses.

B. Therapeutic

- Albinism/Aniridia: These patients face incapacitating glare which hampers daily life activities. Tinted contact lenses with a central clear optics help by cutting off peripheral rays of light and by allowing only the central rays to pass through, thereby providing functional vision.

- Nystagmus: Tinted lenses reduce peripheral aberrations and enhance visual field which may reduce both amplitude and frequency of nystagmus. Sometimes contact lenses may be detrimental in these cases by making the nystagmus more prominent or evident as the concealing effect of spectacles is lost. In addition, to place a contact lens accurately in an eye with nystagmus may not always be possible. Each case thus needs to be evaluated on an individual basis before prescribing lenses.

- Bandage lens: These lenses are used to aid healing of epithelial defects, both iatrogenic and pathological. They may be further modified by impregnation with antimicrobial drugs (drug eluting CL).

C. Cosmetic

Prosthetic/cosmetic shells are used in disfiguring scars and unsightly eyes. In the former, prosthetic CL with central clear pupil are employed and for the latter opaque pupil lenses are used to hide the scarred non seeing eye.

D. In Sports

- In sporting activities contact lenses allow a more unrestricted field of vision with reduced peripheral/spatial distortion. As mentioned before lenses enhance peripheral field by 15–20%, which in turn translates into better body awareness and enhanced eye hand/body/foot coordination.

- *Object size is more consistent with 'real-world'* size (that is, less minification or magnification).

- *Stable vision* is provided during precise ocular movements in dynamic conditions. Many sports involve physical contact with co-players and accurate awareness of immediate environment. In such situations CL help in retaining good vision by remaining *in situ* on the eye. Spectacles, on the other hand, are liable to fall off, slip down the nose, get fogged/steamed up or broken. The latter causes injury from shards of broken spectacles and is one reason why myopes do not venture into sports involving dynamic body movements.

- Improved *spatial localization, depth perception* and peripheral awareness leads to better placement of field players, evaluation of ball motion, racket/bat/oar movements.
- In bright sunlight sports like water or winter sports, lenses *reduce glare* by obviating spectacle lens reflections and aberrations. In addition, protective eyewear can be more easily worn over lenses than over unwieldy spectacles.

APPROACH TO A PATIENT WHILE FITTING A CONTACT LENS

I. Relevant History

Before deciding feasibility of lens wear and type of contact lens to be prescribed a basic estimate should be made of wearer's daily activities, educational and occupational needs, recreational activities, place of residence and socioeconomic background.

In addition, *ocular and systemic co-morbidities* need to be looked into before prescribing lenses. A prior ocular surgery especially glaucoma filtering surgery like trabeculectomy is a contraindication for any lens usage especially a soft lens whose diameter straddles limbus and compress/impairs functioning of the trabeculectomy bleb. Compromised corneas subsequent to complicated cataract surgery, corneal perforation repair or inflammatory event would warrant use of specialized lenses with enhanced oxygen transmission and extremely good tear clearance for continued corneal health. Systemic co morbidities like diabetes, thyroid disease, atopy, sinusitis or excoriative/pustular skin conditions adversely affect lens care/safety.

Relevant drug history with special attention to use of topical steroids and anti-glaucoma drugs should be taken as they can interfere with physical and optical properties, of lens. For example, systemic use of anti-histaminics contribute to a dry eye, oral contraceptives modify corneal hydration and subsequently its curvature, immune suppressive/antineoplastic drugs impair natural defence mechanism of the cornea and tear film. Contact lens parameters and its usage may alter, if and when such drugs are used by the wearer. By the same connotation conditions like diabetes, pregnancy would alter lens fitting on a day-to-day basis and may necessitate changes in lens power and dimensions. *Annexure III* is the proforma used in our clinic incorporates the relevant history taking points.

The ambient environment of the wearer also needs to be assessed since persons exposed to chemical fumes, dry and dusty environment, temperature extremes would have problems with high water content soft lenses which require an optimum environment, to retain their hydration and therefore optical properties. Lower water content hydrogels or the more robust RGP lenses may be a more viable option for such patients.

II. Ocular Examination

The ocular parameters to be evaluated before prescribing contact lens are:

a. *Ocular and head movements*: Ocular examination must include fixation preference and ocular motility. Abnormal ocular movements like nystagmus and strabismus, frequent accompaniments of poor vision acquired in childhood would impair the ability of the wearer to insert a lens. Such movements would contribute to decentration of contact lens especially in end gazes. Rigid lenses are more vulnerable to decentration in such situations.

Head/hand tremors and upper limb incoordination, frequent in the elderly also need review, as they often make lens insertion and handling difficult.

b. *Visual acuity*: This needs to be recorded under both high and low contrast conditions. Both distance and near vision need to be taken in order to gauge the visual requirement of lens wearer. For pseudophakes, aphakes and children near correction assumes equal, if not more importance than distance correction.

For children and hyperopes a cycloplegic refraction and postmydriatic test is mandatory, whereas for myopes and adults dry refraction suffices. This spectacle refraction would dictate power of trial lens to be selected. In the trial method the lens closest in base curve and spherical power to the refraction is selected, with BC proximity taking precedence. Closer the back vertex power of trial lens is to patient's final prescription, better is the adaptation and perceived optical benefits.

c. *Palpebral aperture and lid characteristics:* Lid position, lid tone and margin position need to be noted as they determine lens fit and diameter especially of a RGP lens. A sharp inner lid margin helps retain a RGP lens *in situ*. Lid tone is graded subjectively on eversion as loose, average or tight. A normal lid tone causes the lid to snap back on pulling it away from the globe. A very floppy lid would not be able to hold the lens in contact with the cornea and a tight lid would dislodge the lens from its resting position during blinking (Fig. 5.1).

The skin of eyelids is evaluated for any excoriation, scales, crusting, discharge dryness, erythema or swelling. Lens wear can traumatize corneal epithelium and in presence of smoldering lid infection the responsible organisms could cause corneal lesions (Fig. 5.2). In addition, abnormal lid milieu would foster defective tear resurfacing and subsequently lens deposits.

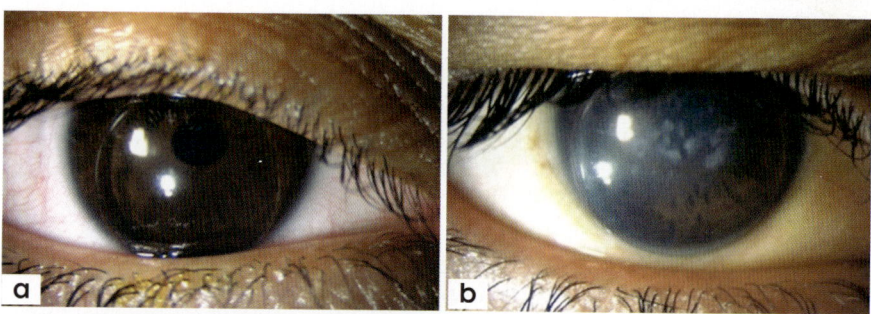

Fig. 5.1: RGP lens in eye with: (a) A tight lid; (b) A flaccid lid

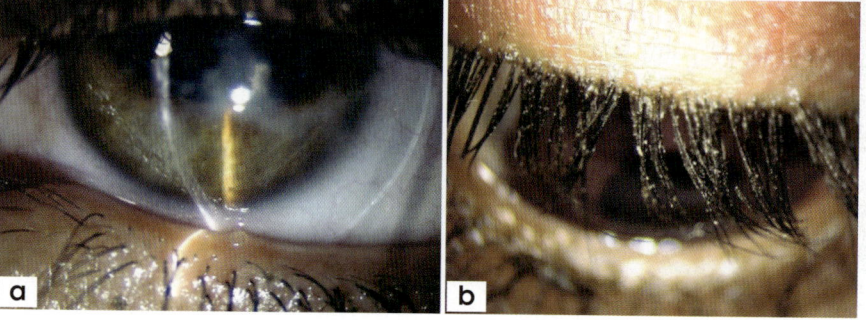

Fig. 5.2: Soft lens worn in a patient with: (a) Meibomianitis; (b) Squamous blepharitis

d. *Conjunctiva:* All three parts of the conjunctiva, namely bulbar, limbal and palpebral need to be checked. The upper lid must be everted to evaluate any pathology in 5 specific areas of tarsal plate, namely upper, central, lower, nasal and temporal junctional tarsal areas as shown in Fig. 5.3. Abnormal findings of erythema, papillae, follicles, pannus or concretions need to be noted. Contact of lens edge with lid undersurface during lid blinking causes microtrauma and these pre-existing conditions responsible for altered surface get exacerbated. Any tear debris or poor lens fitting also enhance this trauma and initiates a cascade of inflammation culminating in giant papillary conjunctivitis, with subsequent lens intolerance.

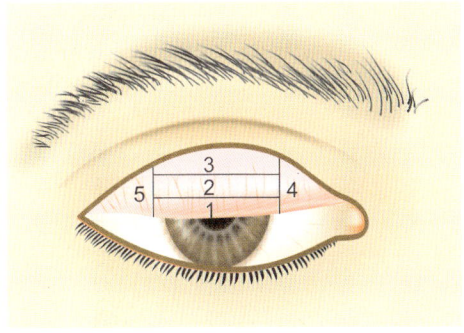

Fig. 5.3: Palpebral conjunctiva is divided into 5 zones and presence of any abnormal structures like papillae, follicles are noted for each zone

e. *Cornea with special reference to limbus*: Size, transparency, corneal topography all are important to determine contact lens type and dimensions. Any limbal irregularity like pingecula, dellen or ischemia would hamper tear flow beneath a rigid lens and fitting of a limbus encompassing soft lens (Fig. 5.4). Three and nine o' clock staining and lens intolerance could ensue, if this aspect is not taken care of.

f. *Iris:* Horizontal visible iris diameter (HVID) and vertical visible iris diameter (VVID) are measured by placing a transparent plastic millimeter scale in front of eye in primary gaze, while avoiding parallax. For a RGP lens, total diameter of lens should be 2.0–2.5 mm less than HVID, whereas for a soft lens, it is 2.5–3.0 mm more than HVID. Many soft CL are prefabricated in diameters of 13–13.5 mm, thus alterations are not always feasible. In case of children lens diameter needs to be customized to size of HVID.

g. *Tear film*: This is assessed by tear meniscus (tear film along the lower lid margin), tear debris, tear break up time (BUT) and Schirmer test. Break up time is assessed after staining tear film with 1% fluorescein and asking patient to look ahead without blinking. Appearance of multiple random 'dry spots' indicate tear thinning and denote BUT. Normal BUT is greater than 10 seconds and random dry spots occurring before 10 seconds indicate a mucin deficiency.

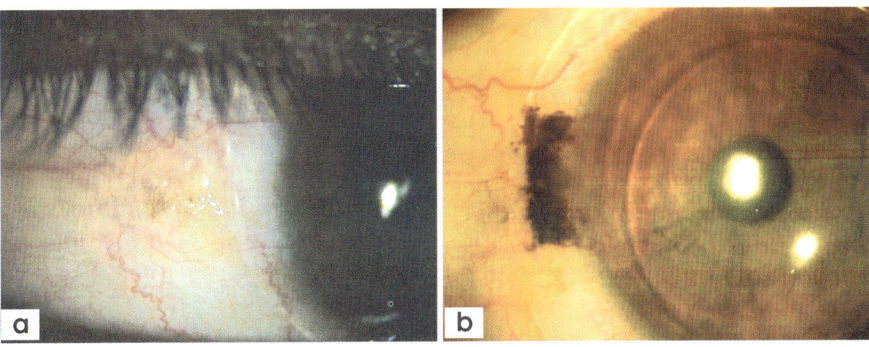

Fig. 5.4: (a) Pingecula beyond margin of soft lens; (b) Conjunctival melanosis within the soft lens diameter

Schirmer test, on the other hand, evaluates aqueous content of tears and is used to quantify dry eyes. A sterile 41 filter paper of 5 mm width and 35 mm length is placed in the eye without instilling any topical anaesthesia. Ten mm or more of wetting of the strip in a 5 minutes time span is taken as normal.

h. *Lacrimal status*: Lacrimal sac health also needs to be evaluated to rule out any lingering infection or tear stasis. Both have the potential to cause corneal infiltration with a contact lens *in situ*.

i. *Pupil diameter:* Normal pupil size in adults varies from 2.0–4.0 mm in bright light to 4.0–8.0 mm in dark. Pupil diameter needs to be measured in a brightly lit room with drapes drawn, to simulate photopic conditions (approximately 200 lux) and in mesopic conditions of low illumination of <100 lux. Scotopic or night time pupil measures are difficult to assess.

Small optic zones in the lens which do not entirely straddle a scotopic pupil, cause incapacitating visual phenomenon like blurring, image jump, and ghosting. Inadequate lens centration is another aspect which causes problems during scotopic and mesopic viewing conditions. For high powered lenticular lenses where optic zone differs significantly from peripheral carrier zone, edge flare and glare are common complaints of scotopic viewing conditions (Fig. 5.5). This occurs due to the fact that refractive correction is present only in the optic zone with peripheral carrier zone having no power. Thus when light rays emanating from image, traverse from edge of optic zone into the pupil, blurring and ghosting occurs. This aspect is very important while fitting lenses on postrefractive surgery cases where ablated zone margins, especially if decentered, can further confound night time vision. Use of 1% brimonidine drops has been reported to stabilize

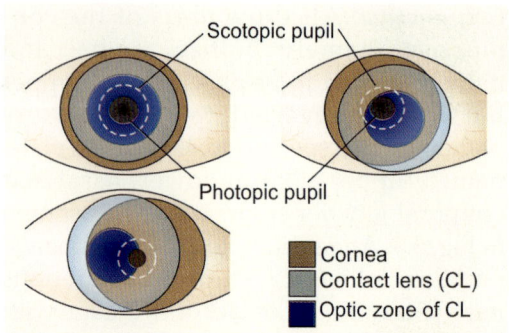

Fig. 5.5: Optic zone centration over photopic and scotopic pupil

pupil in this situation and reduce edge glare and flare. An infrequent but important cause may be distorted pupil subsequent to trauma or colobomat (Fig. 5.6).

j. *Intra-ocular pressure (IOP)*: Baseline measurement of IOP is important for older patients and those with conditions predisposed for glaucoma like uveitis, pigment dispersion syndrome and aniridia. Pressure measures through a contact lens are fallacious, with IOP underestimation occurring when measurement is done over minus lens. It is thus advisable to remove CL prior to measuring IOP.[9] Recent studies have, however, found that non-contact tonometry performed through a soft hydrogel may not alter actual IOP measures.[10, 11]

k. *Retinal examination:* While fitting high/moderate myopes a baseline indirect ophthalmoscopic examination with indentation is advisable to rule out any treatable peripheral retinal pathology, which if diagnosed should be lasered before commencing with contact lens use. This examination has to be performed on an annual basis in moderate/high myopes when they come for a CL change.

l. Specific contact lens related tests include slit lamp biomicroscopy, keratometry, corneal topography, details of trial lenses

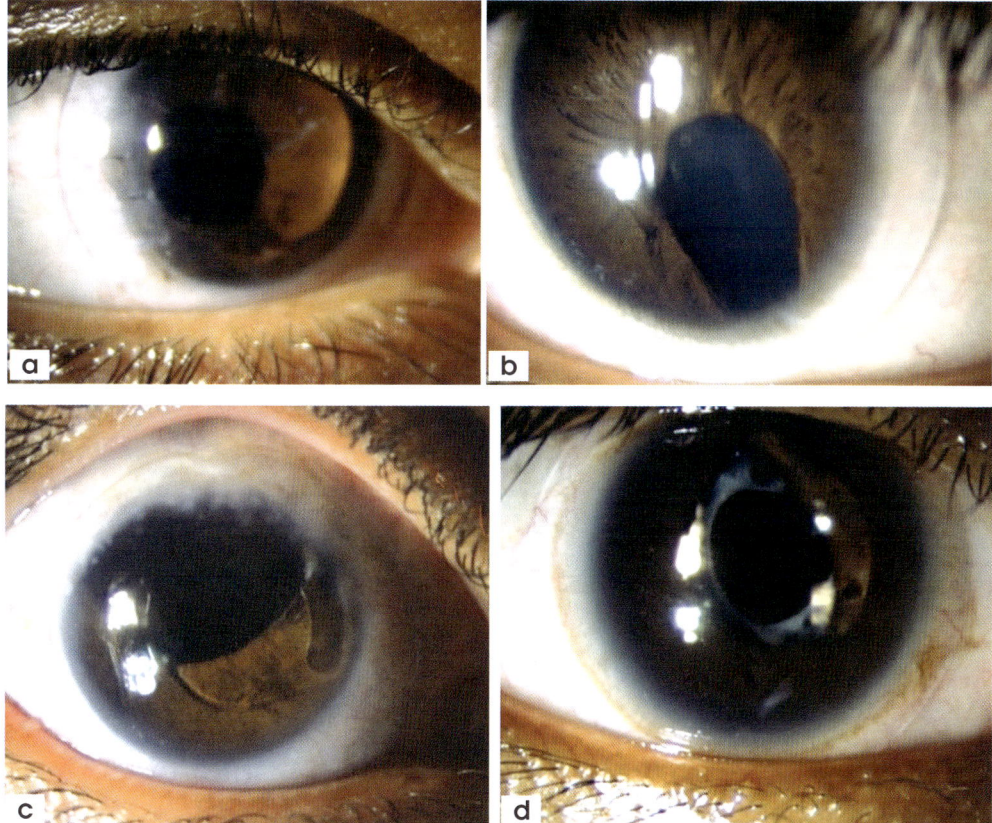

Fig. 5.6: Eccentric pupil conditions: (a) Aphakic lens over repaired corneal perforation; (b) Colobomatous eye with high myopia; (c and d) Over pediatric IOL surprise

used, parameters of final lenses prescribed are described in the following chapter on RGP/soft lens fitting.

m. *Follow-up information*: These include basics of stability and crispness of vision, hours of lens usage, lens health, corneal and lid health and complaints, if any. Frequency of follow-up and aftercare visits need to be spelt out to the wearer and a chart of the same be given. In our set up the contact lens proforma includes the follow up information (Annexure III).

REFERENCES

1. Wong ACM. Optics of Intraocular lens in Albert Jakobiec's Principles and Practice of Ophthalmology. 3rd ed. Eds Albert DM, Miller JK, Saunders Elsevier, 2008; 5295–315.
2. Chowdhary M. Aberrations of the Eye. In: Chowdhary M. Refraction and lens prescription for all eye care practitioners. New Delhi, CBS Publishers, 2014:17.
3. Woods AC. Communications. Patient reactions to disability. The adjustment to aphakia. Br J Ophthal 1964: 48, 349.
4. Mc Mohan T, Szczotka Flynn L. Fitting the abnormal cornea. In Eds Krachmer JH, Mannis MJ, Holland EJ. Cornea. Fundamentals, diagnosis and management Vol 1. 2nd ed. Elsevier Mosby, Philadelphia, 1313–24.

5. Opaciæ KC. Correction of astigmatism with contact lenses. Acta Clin Croat. 2012 Jun; 51(2):305–7.

6. Galindo-Ferreiro A, Galindo-Alonso J, Sánchez-Tocino H, Palencia-Ercilla J. Contact lens fitting in 133 eyes with irregular astigmatism. Arch Soc Esp Oftalmol. 2007 Dec;82(12):747–51.

7. Titiyal JS, Sinha R, Sharma N, Sreenivas V, Vajpayee RB. Contact lens rehabilitation following repaired corneal perforations. BMC Ophthalmol. 2006 Mar 14;6:11.

8. Jupiter DG, Katz HR. Management of irregular astigmatism with rigid gas permeable contact lenses. CLAO J. 2000 Jan;26(1):14–7.

9. Liu YC, Huang JY, Wang IJ, Hu FR, Hou YC. Intraocular pressure measurement with the noncontact tonometer through soft contact lenses. J Glaucoma. 2011 Mar;20(3):179–82.

10. P G Fýrat, C Cankaya, S Doganay, M Cavdar, S Duman,E Ozsoy, and B Koc. The influence of soft contact lenses on the intraocular pressure measurement . Eye (Lond). 2012 Feb; 26(2): 278–82.

11. Allen RJ, Dev Borman A, Saleh GM Applanation tonometry in silicone hydrogel contact lens wearers. Cont Lens Anterior Eye. 2007 Dec;30(5):267–9.

Reader's Note

Reader's Note

CHAPTER 6

Fitting a Rigid Contact Lens

Rigid gas permeable lenses convert an astigmatic cornea into a smooth, spherical refractive surface which is provided by anterior surface of the contact lens. In addition, posterior lens surface neutralizes irregularities of the front surface of cornea by generating a malleable *tear lens*. This property makes these lenses ideal in correcting both regular and irregular corneal astigmatism. Older, rigid hard lenses, were also capable of neutralizing astigmatism but poor oxygen permeability of their PMMA material made them cornea unfriendly. Current era rigid gas permeable (RGP) lenses score over earlier PMMA predecessors by their high oxygen permeability conferred by their silicone and fluorine polymer content.

Rigid gas permeable lenses are more robust and durable compared to more friable, fragile soft lenses (Fig. 6.1). The compact material of these lenses prevents absorption of vapors,

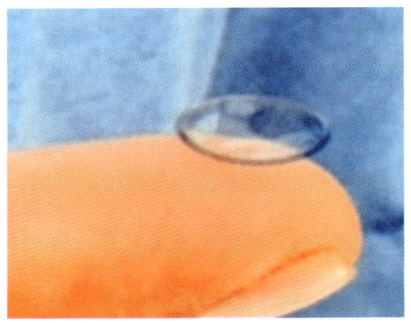

Fig. 6.1: A RGP lens

fumes, chemicals and makes them a more viable option for patients working in such environments and for those requiring frequent ocular medications. The compact material also makes these lenses resistant to microbial adherence and invasion. In advent of lens deposit or scratches, polishing with special devices can be done to rejuvenate the lens, thus enhancing life span.

Rigid Lens Properties and Design Parameters: Physiological and Optical Effects

Let us take a look of various aspects of RGP lens and understand how alterations in them change lens fit.

A. **Center of gravity (CG):** Center of gravity dictates both lens stability and centration. It is influenced by lens diameter, central lens thickness and back vertex power. Of these variables, diameter change has the greatest impact with a diameter change of 0.1 mm having a 7-fold greater effect on CG versus a 0.01 mm change in lens central thickness.[1]

   i. *Diameter*: For small diameter lenses, CG is displaced anteriorly. An anteriorly placed CG causes CL to undergo greater rotational moment induced by gravity and enhances lid interaction. Both these aspects translate into excessive lens movement and serve to destabilize the lens. This is the reason of poor fit with small lenses. Large diameter lenses, on the other hand, have a posteriorly (inwards) displaced CG which makes them less vulnerable to decentration during ocular movements.

ii. *Center thickness:* A thicker lens has a more anteriorly placed CG versus a thinner lens leading to decreased *on eye* stability.[2]

iii. *Back vertex power*: A concave (minus) lens has a more posteriorly placed CG than a convex (plus) lens, thus alterations in OD have a lesser effect on CG of minus lenses compared with plus power lenses.[3]

iv. *Fit*: A steep fitting lens has a more posteriorly placed CG than a flat fit (Fig. 6.2).

B. **Back surface of lens:** Posterior surface of a RGP lens is designed to perform four functions: Provide adequate edge lift in periphery, allow free tear exchange, distribute compression pressure of lens over a wide corneal area so as to minimize physical stress and facilitate smooth lens movement. Since it is this surface which comes into contact with cornea, any disturbance in it would directly affect corneal health. The parameters determining back surface fitting are back optic zone diameter, back vertex power, midperiphery and back surface design.

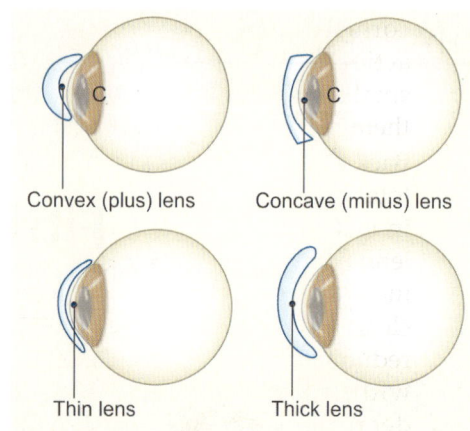

Convex (plus) lens   Concave (minus) lens

Thin lens   Thick lens

Fig. 6.2: Centre of gravity alterations with thickness and power of lens

i. *Back optic zone diameter* **(BOZD):** Back optic zone diameter dimensions are dictated both by pupil size and by optical considerations. This diameter should at all times be greater than mesopic pupil. If BOZD is smaller than mesopic pupil, it would cause refraction to occur simultaneously at optic zone, first curve junction and lens periphery resulting in ghosting of image, reduction of contrast and image quality. Excessive increase in BOZD, on the other hand, would increase lens sag resulting in increased tear lens thickness (TLT) leading to a tight/steep fit (Fig. 6.3). Decrease in BOZD minimizes lens movements and is sometimes utilized to fit steeper

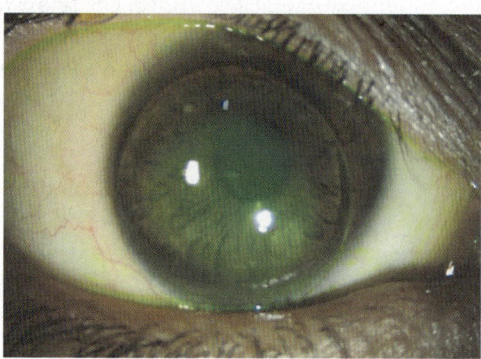
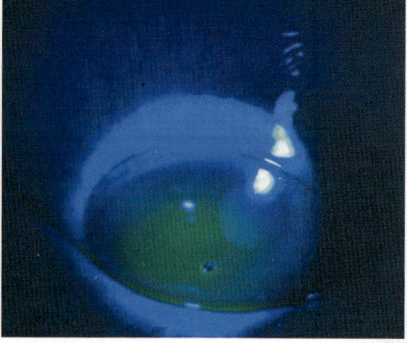

Fig. 6.3: Increasing the OD makes lens fit steeper

corneas. However, increased inter-action of lids and gravity on these small diameter lenses tend to make them more liable to decentration.[4]

Back optic zone diameter (BOZD) and total diameter (TD) need to be altered in synchronization to ensure similar lens fit. For a lens with constant TD, increased BOZD would reduce edge clearance.[5] If, on the other hand, TD is reduced without altering BOZD, edge width and edge clearance would decrease leading to poor tear ex-change. This would cause arcuate staining of peripheral cornea, tear instability and lens intolerance. *For each 0.05 mm increase in BOZR (flatter fit), the BOZD must be increased by 0.7 mm to maintain same sagittal relationship and TLT constant at optimal 22 microns.*[6]

Increasing the front optical zone diameter narrows the front peripheral width. In a lens with a thick edge (minus power lens), this creates a minus carrier and causes a high riding lens (lid attachment fit).

ii. *Back vertex power (BVP):* Back vertex power compensation is also required for any changes in BOZR. An increase in BOZR (lens flattening) by 0.05 mm would cause *tear lens* power to increase by –0.25 D, which would affect over-refraction. In cases of significant corneal astigmatism of > 1.50 Dc, a 0.05 mm decrease in BOZR is required for each 0.50 D increase in corneal astigmatism

iii. *Back mid-periphery:* Back mid-peri-phery is visualized as a 360° band of contact adjacent to central pooling of fluorescein in a steep fit and a circular band of clearance in a flat fit (Fig. 6.4). The clearance zone created under it allows tear exchange, distributes lens weight equitably on the cornea and influences stability of CL. A steep mid-periphery seals off tear exchange and creates localized zone of bearing resulting in decreased lens movement and corneal hypoxia.

iv. *Back surface design:* Peripheral curves are ground on posterior lens surface to allow optimal lens fitting for an aspheric cornea. These curves help to circulate tears and maintain corneal health. Lens design incorporates these progressively flattened, blended spherical curves or has a continuous aspheric curve (ellipsoid). The design of these peripheral curves, which

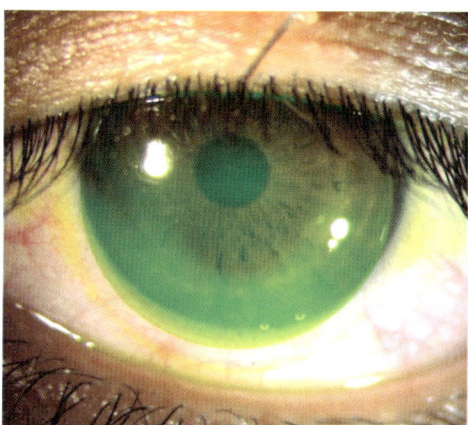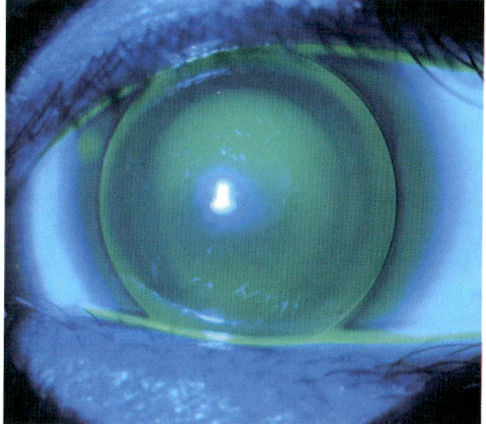

Fig. 6.4: Back mid-periphery visualized as band of contact (steep fit) or band of clearance (flat fit)

differs in different lenses, makes it critical in allowing axial edge clearance or tear flow. This axial edge clearance (AEC) is dependent on width and radius of peripheral curve with width having a greater contribution. Good fit aims at achieving axial edge clearance (AEC) of 0.08 to 0.10 mm.[7] Any decrease in peripheral curve radius (PCR) requires an increase in OD in order to maintain the same AEC.

The two main types of inadequate back surface periphery fit are too flat or too steep configuration, consequences of which are detailed below:

• *Excessive edge clearance/ stand-off the lens*: A wide peripheral edge, increases stored tear volume in edge reservoir, alters surface tension forces and adversely affects lens stability. It causes excess lens motility, poor centration (superior dentration being more common), increased lens mislocation (onto conjunctiva) and/or lens ejection due to increased lid interaction. Tear exchange process generated by act of blinking create bubbles which absorb and dissolve on their own. In cases with defective edge clearance, these bubbles remain entrapped, the process being named as *dimple veiling*. These entrapped bubbles along with thinning of tear film next to lens edge, cause epithelial surface desiccation, dellen formation and 3 and 9 o' clock staining (Fig. 6.5).

• *Inadequate edge clearance*: This causes poor tear exchange and reduced lens movement. A thinned viscous tear film ensues which further impedes lens movement, leading to epithelial desiccation and corneal indentation (Fig. 6.6). It can also cause dimple

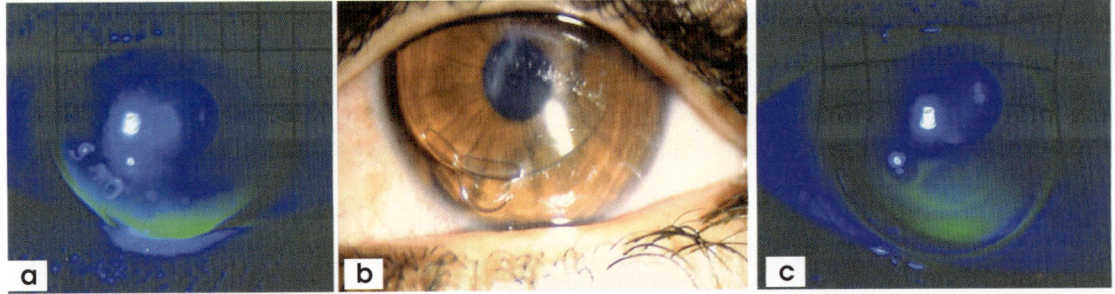

Fig. 6.5: (a) Excessive edge clearance; (b) with dimple veiling, excessive at 7 o'clock; (c) inferior arcuate staining

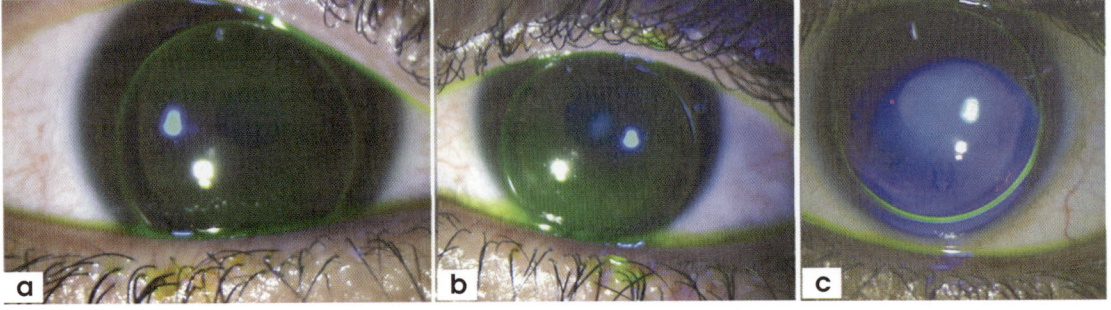

Fig. 6.6: Inadequate edge clearance

veiling (Fig. 6.7). Visible after lens removal, this phenomenon occurs due to bearing pressure applied by the tight lens edge, exacerbated by blinking (Fig. 6.8). Since most lens removal methods involve enga-gement of lid margins at lens edge, lens removal becomes difficult if edge lift is minimal. Prolonged use of such a lens results in hypoxia due to inadequate tear circulation and 3 and 9 o'clock staining.

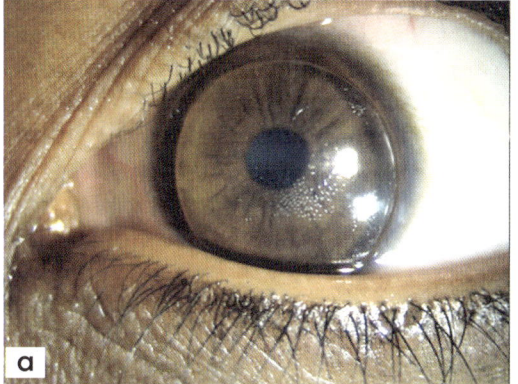

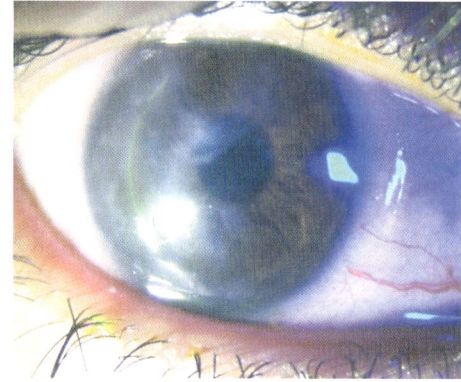

Fig. 6.8: Steep back mid-periphery causing arcuate indentation on cornea postlens removal

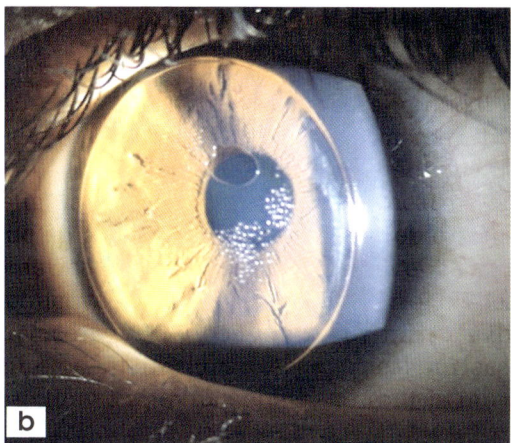

- *3 and 9 o'clock staining:* The pheno-menon occurs due to both excessive lens edge thickness/edge clearance and due to insufficient edge clear-ance/lens movement causing lens edge "stand-off". This results in inadequate bridging of corneal epithelium by lids while resting on lens edge at 3 and 9 o'clock positions of peripheral cornea (horizontal meridian), causing tear film thin-ning and epithelial desiccation. Once inner mucin layer of tear film (both beneath and above lens edge) gets disrupted, tears are unable to wet the epithelium sufficiently. Minimal tear exchange, appearance of dry spots and epithelial desic-cation ensue, resulting in 3 and 9 o'clock staining (Fig. 6.9). Red-ucing central and edge thickness, smoothening lens edge, blinking exercises and using lubricating drops are some modalities used to treat this condition.

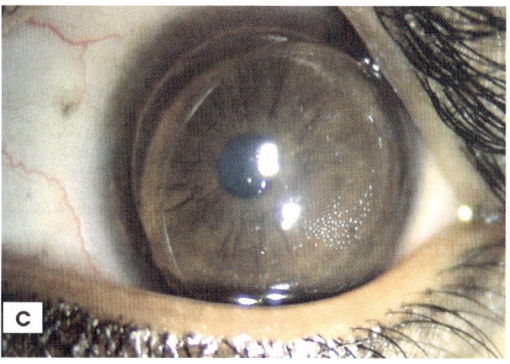

Fig. 6.7: Dimple veiling due to inadequate lens clearance

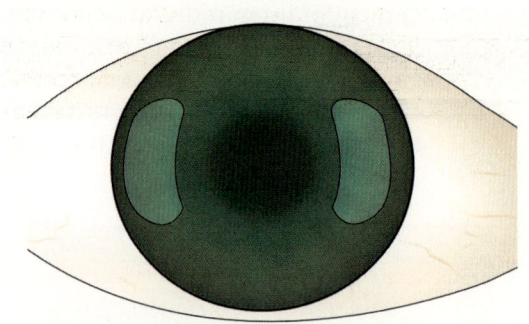

Fig. 6.9: Showing 3 and 9 o'clock staining

C. Lens thickness:

i. *Central thickness (Tc)*: Changing central thickness of a RGP lens affects lens fitting by altering front surface profile, edge profile, CG and oxygen permeability. Increased lens thickness shifts the CG anteriorly which results in increased lens movement, increased lens-lid interaction resulting in lens instability. Conversely, thinning of a lens causes an inward shift of the CG which translates into improved lens stability. An inverse relationship exists between oxygen permeability and lens thickness, otherwise known by ratio Dk/t or oxygen transmissibility. As evident by this ratio, oxygen transmission can be increased by reducing center thickness (Tc).

The conclusion from above facts is that a thinner lens has better stability along with better oxygen transmissibility. However, this reduction is limited by aspect of lens durability, lens handling and thickness of less than 0.16 mm leads to contact lens deformation/flexure with ensuing visual fluctuations.[8] Very thin lenses, lesser than 0.08 mm can also become uncomfortable as these very flexible lenses are prone to blink induced deformation.[1]

ii. *Junction thickness*: Increased junction thickness allows lens to position in central or slightly high up location. Thinning of junction thickness improves comfort; minimizes upper lid interaction but positions lens lower down (due to reduced lid attachment).

D. **Edge profile:** Edge design depends on BVP, lens design, material properties, and manufacturing technique. Lens edge determines comfort, tear meniscus and physiological changes like 3 and 9 o'clock staining. An anteriorly rounded, thin, smooth edge decreases lid interaction and enhances comfort. A thick edge causes more lid interaction especially in vertical meridian resulting in either low riding lens (if upper lid engages more with thicker edge and pushes lens down) or high riding lens (if upper lid carries the lens). A minus powered lens (concave lens) has a larger unfinished edge thickness and a plus lens (convex lens) a smaller one, thus lid attachment fit is easier accomplished with minus powered lenses. An edge thickness of about 0.12–0.14 mm is optimal for comfort and durability.

E. **Residual astigmatism:** Normally a spherical back surface RGP lens adequately corrects low to moderate corneal astigmatism, due to tear lens neutralizing approximately 90% of corneal astigmatism. This, in turn, unmasks lenticular or retinal component of astigmatism which is known as *residual astigmatism.*

F. **Corneal shape:** Prolate shape can be fit with a standard, spherical or aspherical RGP lens but for oblate shape specialized lenses, especially those with reverse geometry design are usually required.

G. **Vertex distance:** This is the distance from back surface of spectacle lens to anterior surface of eye. The standard vertex distance is about 12 mm and it affects *effective power* of lens for power greater than 4.0 Ds. This is due to the fact that lens power at *corneal plane* differs from that required at *spectacle plane*. For power ranging from 0.25 to 4.0 D, the change is so minuscule that it can be ignored. But for powers >4.0 D the conversion table needs to be used so as to be *vertex* the spectacle power to corneal plane.

Compensated power

$$= \frac{F \text{ (Spectacle sphere power)}}{1 - d \text{ (vertex distance)} \times F \text{ (spectacle sphere power)}}$$

The way to remember is: A plus lens moving away from eye, becomes stronger and a minus lens becomes weaker.

Refer to Annexure II: Vertex conversion table.

H. Lens flexure: This is the term given to alteration in shape of RGP lens fitted onto an astigmatic cornea, over a period of time, as a result of capillary attraction of tears and pressure exerted by blinking movements. A sufficiently thick contact lens would resist these forces and retain its shape, but in clinical situations lens thickness is never thick enough to withstand such forces on a long-term basis.

Amount of flexure depends on lens material, thickness, fitting relationship and BVP. Lens flexures in turn, alters both lens and tear *lens* optics, induces a plus cylinder with axis aligned to flat K which ultimately partially corrects residual astigmatism. This is partly, the reason, why a patient is often more comfortable with his old lens than a new lens of similar dimensions and shape.

I. Tear lens optics: Tear film trapped between back surface of a RGP lens and front surface of cornea contributes its *tear lens optics* to those of the RGP lens. A steep lens with a greater sagittal height is able to trap more tear film under it and form a "plus" tear lens due to its convex dimensions. This tear lens adds to plus power of a convex lens applied to correct a hypermetropic error or subtracts from minus power of a

concave lens applied to correct a myopic error. A flat fit, on the other hand, creates minimal tear film entrapment at its center and more at its periphery, thereby generating a concave "minus" tear lens (Fig. 6.10).

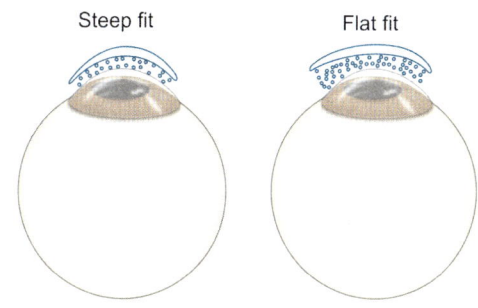

Fig. 6.10: Steep fit generates a plus tear lens, and flat fit a minus tear lens

Example:

A *trial lens* with a base curve 9.2 and *power + 3 Ds* is applied on a patient with +7 D *hypermetropia*. On performing over refraction the wearer requires a +3.5 *Ds add* over trial lens for patient to read 20/20. Thus prescription of final lens to be ordered would be +3 D *plus + 3.5 D = 6.5 Ds*. But for this patient who has a +7 D *hypermetropia,* the required lens should have been *after* vertex distance correction +7.6. Thus the discrepancy is of 7.6–6.5 = 1.1 D. This dioptric difference is due to a positive power of positive tear fluid lens created by steep fit of the trial lens, adding a +1 D due to a plus tear lens. On re-evaluating fit and refitting with a well-fitted lens of BC 9.4/ power +4.5 D, the over refraction now comes to +4.5 D. This makes lens prescription to be +3 plus +4.5 = 7.5 D which is close to actual figure extrapolated from patient's refractive data.

To restate this, steep lens with its addition of a **"plus" fluid tear lens** OR a flat lens with it accompanying **"minus" fluid tear lens** would give a refractive surprise. The power of this tear lens amounts to 0.25 D for every

0.05 mm radius of curvature difference between base curve of lens and flat K of the cornea. The **SAM FAP** rule can be applied, which states that in fitting *steeper* than K, *add* the same amount of *minus* to the prescription, whereas if fitting *flatter, add* the same amount of *plus* to the prescription.

The whole art of fitting a contact lens on the eye is thus about balancing different optical and physical phenomenon to reach the Goldilocks zone of what is best for the wearer's eye.

Indications of RGP Lens

- Regular astigmatism >1.5 Dc, where toric soft lenses are not an option.
- Regular astigmatism >5.0 Dc powers, where toric soft lenses are not easily available.
- Irregular astigmatism as in keratoconus, healed keratitis, postkeratoplasty and marginal degenerations, e.g. pellucid marginal degenerations.[9]
- In residual refractive error, post-refractive surgery
- Recalcitrant allergy with soft lenses, e.g. recurrent giant papillary conjunctivitis
- Complications like neovascularisation, solution toxicity with SCL
- Certain occupational environments involving exposure to excess heat, fumes and chemicals.
- Severe dry eyes

Advantages over SCL

- Crisper vision due to better optics. This is due to the fact that a RGP lens resurfaces and replaces corneal surface, whereas a soft lens mirrors underlying corneal irregularities. Soft lens give a softer vision since light is slightly diffused as it passes through larger quantities of water contained in the SCL material.
- Creates a liquid tear lens between posterior lens surface and anterior surface of cornea, which corrects most of corneal astigmatism.
- Good tear exchange helps in maintaining corneal physiology and reduces chances of debris build up and corneal infection.
- Good oxygen permeability makes it a safer lens for corneal health.
- Can be modified (peripheral curves blended) and polished (superficial scratches erased) over time. This enhances life span of a RGP lens to almost double that of a soft lens.
- Lesser incidence of allergies and deposits.

Disadvantages with a RGP Lens

- Patient comfort with a RGP lens is much less than a SCL, especially in the initial few weeks of wear.
- Smaller dimensions of a RGP lens vs SCL can cause ghosting if light enters the pupil through peripheral curves or lens edge in scotopic viewing conditions.
- Lens drop out in extremes of gazes is common with a poorly fitted lens.
- Technique of insertion and removal is more difficult compared to a SCL, so repeated demonstrations are required.
- Gradual build up wearing time is required thus this lens does not provide instant uninterrupted vision, during early days of wear.
- Adaptation is more time consuming, watering and foreign body sensation experienced by wearer is significant. Some patients with sensitive lids may never be able to wear these lenses.
- Hydrophobic polymer attracts lipids and can cause foggy vision.
- Learning curve to fit such lenses is steep for the fitter.

Fitting Technique of a RGP Lens

Following is the detailing of lens fitting method.

Step I. Trial Lens Selection Parameters

i. **Back optic zone radius (BOZR):** The **BOZR** chosen is within +/−0.10 mm of the flat K value. In cases of regular astigmatism of >3 Dc, 1/3rd of difference between corneal radius is added to flat K value to arrive at the final K.

Example: Keratometric readings of 44 D axis 180° and 50 D axis 90°, Final K = flat K (which is this case = 44) + 1/3 of 6 (difference between flat and step K 50–44) = 44 + 2 = 46. Trial lens selected should thus have K of 46 D +/− 0.10.

Amount of corneal astigmatism assessed by keratometer can also determine choice of BOZR.[8]

- In astigmatism <0.75 Dc, fit on flat K
- Astigmatism between 0.50 and 1.0 Dc, fit on flat K or 0.05 steeper
- Astigmatism between 1.0 and 2.5 Dc, fit on flat K or 0.05–1.0 steeper.
- Astigmatism > 2.5 Dc. Toric back optic zone is preferred.

ii. **Total diameter (TD/OD):** This has to be determined from corneal size or horizontal visible iris diameter (HVID). Usually, an RGP lens whose diameter is 2 mm smaller than HVID is chosen as the first trial lens. A simple way to calculate the lens diameter is given below:

- For HVID of <11.0 mm, a small diameter lens (8.5–8.8 mm) is used.
- For HVID between 11.0–11.9 mm, medium diameter lens (9.0–9.2 mm) is used.
- For HVID of >12.0 mm, large diameter lens (9.5–9.6 mm) is used.

The game changers for this simplistic rule are corneal curvature, pupil size and width of palpebral aperture. Corneal curvature may change this equation with small diameter lenses required for fitting corneas steeper than 46 D and large diameter lens being used for better centering on corneas flatter than 42 D.

iii. **Back optic zone diameter (BOZD):** The BOZD should be at least 1.0 mm larger than average pupil size in normal room light to avoid edge flare.[8] A small BOZD is defined as less than 7.20 mm; medium as 7.20–7.90 mm, large greater than or equal to 8.00 mm. Large BOZD gather a larger tear pool beneath it which translates into a steeper lens fit. Thus BOZR would require proportionate flattening in situations where a large BOZD has to be ordered. Lens periphery in larger BOZD also would require adjustments to the rapidly flattening peripheral curves.

iv. **Lid/lid aperture:** Patients with wider palpebral aperture, lax lids and/or excessive lens movement benefit from being fitted with larger diameter lens.

v. **Lens power:** The BVP of diagnostic lens should be as close as possible to patient's spectacle prescription so as to provide vision as close to normal and minimize potential alterations in lens fitting arising from variations in power.[8] Since CG of plus powered lens differs from minus powered lenses and lens fit for the two types is very different, it goes without saying that myopes should always be assessed with minus power trial lenses and hyperopes with plus trial lenses.

High back vertex power lenses of > 8.0 D need to be made larger than average, to allow for adequate lenticulation of front peripheral design. High power convex lens normally *rides low* due to its weight and to ensure that it is lifted sufficiently high to enable OZ to straddle mesopic pupil, it has to be fitted a little steep.

High power **convex lenses** also have a naturally thin peripheral edge. This thin edge is neither properly picked up nor retained well by the upper lid leading to an abrupt drop of CL post blink. This again contributes to low riding of the lens. High power **concave lenses**, on the other hand, have a relatively thicker lens edge, which is easily grasped and retained by upper lid leading to high riding (lid attachment) fit. In high minus lens, center of gravity lies posterior to corneal apex which also enhances pick up action of upper lid.

Step II: Trial Lens Placement and Evaluation

Reflex tearing usually follows any lens application and must be allowed to abate before assessing fluorescein pattern and dynamic lens fitting characteristics. This usually takes around 5–10 minutes. If fluorescein is instilled during this time, the excessive tearing would wash out the dye and assessment of pattern would be misleading (Fig. 6.11). In addition, excessive lacrimation would lead to greater lens excursion, which would cause fluctuations in vision and give erroneous results in dynamic fitting. Patients can be advised to maintain inferior direction of gaze while blinking, to minimize lens edge feel during initial adaptation phase.[8] Once tearing has subsided, the lens fit is evaluated keeping in mind the following factors.

i. **Centration of a lens:** Lens requires to be centered in primary gaze, lateral gaze and down gaze. Good centration is a result of balance of forces acting on the lens. These forces are: Surface tension at lens edge,

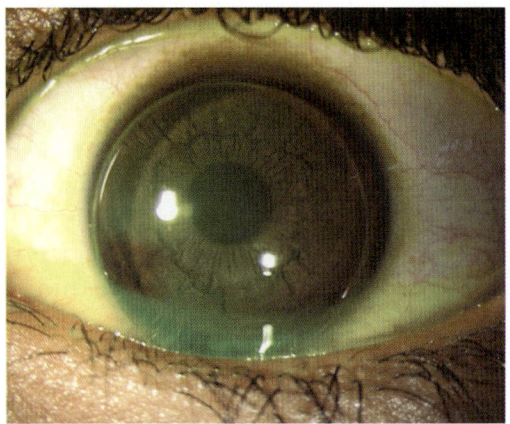

Fig. 6.11: Washing out of fluorescein dye due to excessive tearing

reaction pressure profile under the lens counteracting the surface tension, lens weight, viscous resistance, lid pressure and pre-lens tear film meniscus.[10] High minus power concave lenses with thick periphery hook onto the upper lid and depict lid attachment during movement. This effect can be utilized in high plus power convex lenses with thin periphery, by making a negative peripheral carrier to permit *lid attachment* for this, otherwise heavy, low riding lens. As long as the optic zone covers pupil in scotopic/mesopic illumination and lens edge does not cause limbal compression, minor amounts of decentration are accepted by wearers (Fig. 6.12).[8]

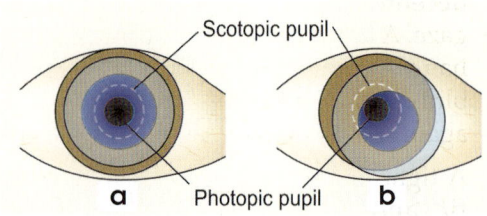

Fig. 6.12: Effect on decentration of lens on vision. Stippled are demarcated optic zone; (a) Centered on pupil: Both scotopic and photopic pupil well covered by optic zone; (b) Lens decentered downwards: Optic zone bisects scotopic pupil, thereby leading to ghosting in dim light

ii. Entry of tear fluid from periphery and edge meniscus serves to increase post-lens tear film volume and decenter a RGP lens. This same maneuver is taught to wearers for lens removal by allowing influx of tears, by lifting edge of lens.

iii. **Lid tone/plapebral aperture:** Lid tone is assessed either by inspection and/or *pinch test*. Normal lid position in primary gaze places lower lid margin next to limbus at 6 o'clock visible iris portion, and upper lid margin crossing iris at 10 and 2 o'clock position, creating a palpebral width of 9.5 mm (Fig. 6.13).

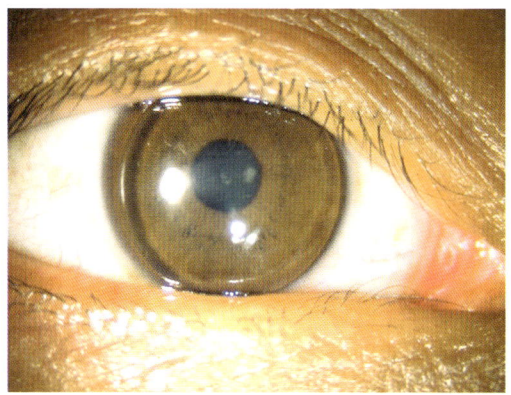

Fig. 6.13: Normal lid position with contact lens in eye

Lower lid helps in supporting and centring the lens. A low riding, flaccid lower lid is unable to provide this support and leads to low riding lens which can decenter in primary or reading/down gaze. A lax/flaccid upper lid, on the other hand, is unable to pick up lens during blinking and center it adequately which again results in low riding of a lens.

A tight upper lid causes a *lid attachment* fit and is diagnosed by the lens maintaining a high riding position in-between blinks (Fig. 6.14). For wider palpebral apertures and tight lids overall diameter of lens would need to be reduced, whereas for loose, flaccid lids a lens with larger total diameter would center better.

It must be remembered that initial foreign body and increased lid sensation after insertion of trial lens often causes lid spasm, which can masquerade as a tight lid. Thus a waiting time of 10–15 minutes should be given in an eye fitted with RGP lens before evaluating fit and commenting on lid tone.

Step III: Assessment of Fit

This is done by two methods—dynamic fit and static fit, the former studies lens movements and the latter uses fluoroscein dye.

1. DYNAMIC FITTING ASSESSMENT METHOD

Dynamic fit is dependent on **lid movements**. Lens fit is initially observed in primary gaze where its centration and stability are checked. Subsequently it is assessed during blinking and in different gazes, primarily lateral and down gaze. Lens lag is measured horizontally and vertically in mm and influence of both upper and lower lid is assessed. This fit is best observed on slit lamp.

i. **Primary gaze**
- **Decentration:** Decentration is assessed by comparing center of lens with geometrical center of cornea. Accurate

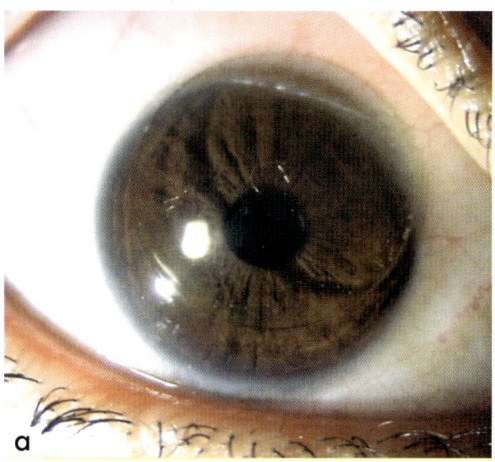
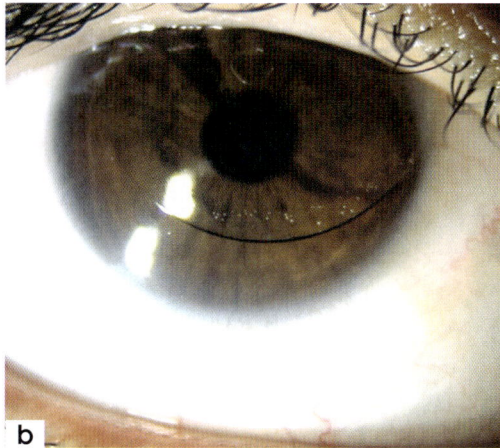

Fig. 6.14: (a) Steep fit; (b) Minimal fall back in up gaze (upriding)

centration of a RGP lens is difficult to achieve and most patients accept a slightly decentered lens. Excessive decentration, however, causes blurring of vision, conjunctival irritation, lens instability/intolerance.

- **Stability:** Stability is defined by position of rest assumed by lens after reflex watering has subsided.

ii. **Blink induced lens movement:** Lens movement is assessed during a soft blink. During *down sweep* of upper lid the lens gets pulled up due to Bell's phenomenon, subsequently during *up sweep* lens drops down and recenters in *post-blink phase* (Fig. 6.15).

- **Extent/path/speed:** Post-blink re-centration is measured by assessing highest point reached on cornea by inferior lens edge. Then the extent of downward excursion made by lens to regain its pre-blink position is assessed. A 1.5–3.0 mm vertical smooth movement across corneal surface with and following each blink is aimed for, as it provides stable vision with adequate tear exchange. The path taken by the CL can be vertical or oblique (temporal-nasal), with a near vertical direction synchronous with blinking being desirable.
- **Type:** Movement is categorized as smooth or rocky, apical rotation or lid attachment and reflects fitting relationship between lens back surface and anterior surface of cornea. The *movements* typify a condition, a few of which are listed below:

- *Smooth movement* implies alignment fit.
- *Rotational movement* about corneal apex from superior to an inferior position implies a central corneal touch (flat fit). In this condition central BC is flatter than corneal apex, so path of least resistance for lens movement is around corneal apex (nasal or temporal side). It must be remembered that a lens invariably settles on steepest part of cornea or apex (Fig. 6.16).[11]
- *Small rocking* movement about flatter meridian is seen in a steep fit over a toric cornea.
- *Lid attachment* movement is seen when lens rides high between blinks with very little post-blink movement. Such lid influence becomes more relevant in distorted cornea like keratoconus or post keratoplasty cases.
- *Erratic excessive movement (drunken lens)* is seen in cases of high corneal toricity and is a feature of unstable lens.

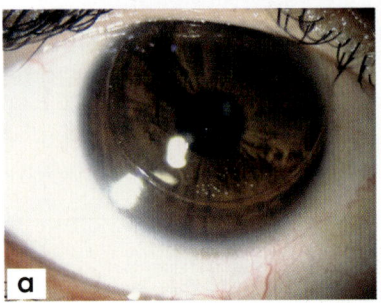 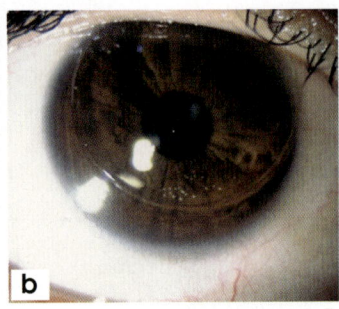 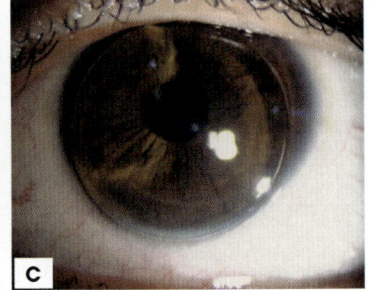

Fig. 6.15: Sequential lens movement: (a) Initial process of dropping down post-lid blink (b and c) Lens drops down to settle in position c

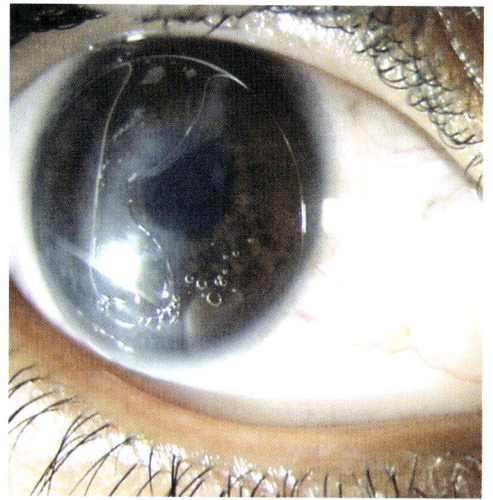

Fig. 6.16: Lens rotation around apex of a scarred cornea

iii. Gaze induced lens movement: Lens movement is assessed during lateral and vertical gazes. Minimal movement is a characteristic of steep fit and excessive of a flat fit (Fig. 6.17).

2. STATIC FITTING ASSESSMENT BY FLUORESCEIN APPLICATION

Static fit is independent of lid action and is thus valuable in evaluating different lens designs or alterations in fit over time. To evaluate this fit fluorescein dye is used to fill the tear film between back surface of lens and front surface of corneal. The dye then spreads across the globe due to tear film movement initiated by lid blinking. Fit is assessed in three zones, central, mid peripheral and peripheral.

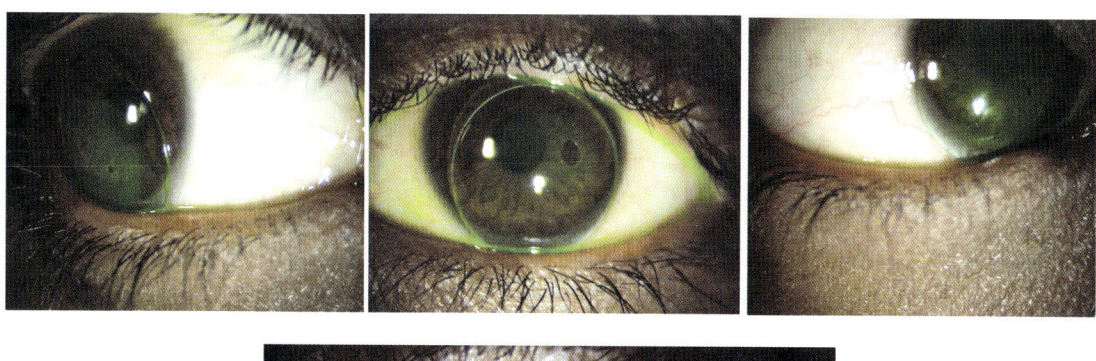

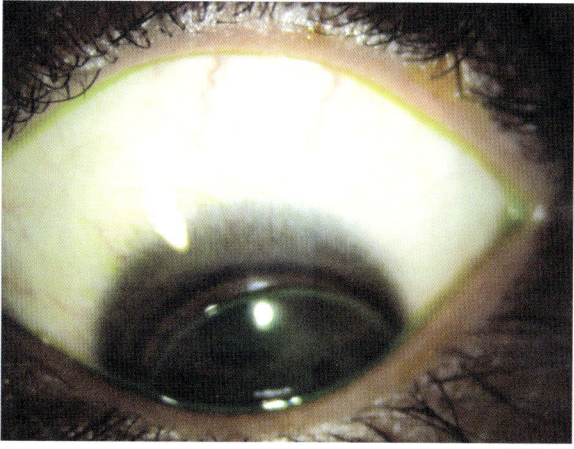

Fig. 6.17: Static and dynamic fit of "steep fit". Note minimal lens lag on lateral and downward eye movement

Fit is labeled as **steep** (central pooling), aligned or **flat** (central touch or dark zone, with no dye). Width of pooling and touch zone is assessed along the horizontal meridian.

Technique of application: Fluorescein dye is applied by wetting a sterile strip with lubricant drop and touching it to inferior tear meniscus. The fluorescein strip should never be wet with topical anesthetic solution as that would *quench* the property of fluorescence. Excess fluid is removed by shaking the paper prior to ocular instillation. Another way to apply is to pull up the upper lid, ask patient to look down and touch the strip gently to the superior bulbar conjunctiva (Fig. 6.18). The fit is then evaluated using cobalt blue filter (on the slit lamp), which turns the fluorescein stained tear film bright green due to emitted fluorescence. Using a yellow barrier filter over the slit lamp eyepiece increases the green fluorescence.

Different types of lens fit defined by both static and dynamic assessment are detailed below:

i. Steep or tight fit:

  a. *Signs on Static assessment*: For ease of understanding we may divide this evaluation by dividing the lens into three parts, central, midperipheral and peripheral.

   – **Central zone:** Steep fit is diagnosed by seeing an apical pool of fluorescein stained green tear film which indicates excessive central clearance

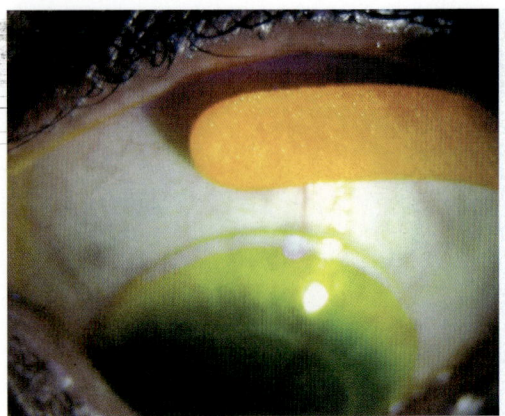

Fig. 6.18: Technique of fluorescein staining

or vault by the back surface of lens. (Fig. 6.19). Trapped air bubbles under the lens, blue heavy touch at mid-peripheral transition region, with minimal lens edge clearance are other signs. Remedy is to make BOZR larger or increase BC.

   – **Mid-periphery:** This term is used for an undefined zone within optical zone of the back surface and not the actual midpoint between lens center and edge. Mid-periphery is the contact zone in case of steep fit and lack of contact in a flat fit. As evident in Fig. 6.20 a *band of contact* is observed adjacent to the zone of pooling. This bearing area may be present in entire 360° or be localized to a few clock hours and are known as heavy or light bearing respectively.

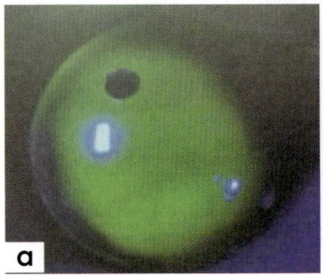
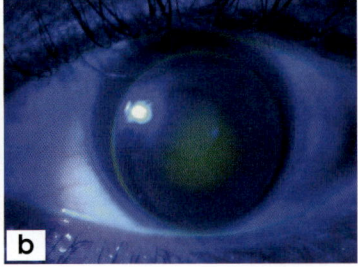
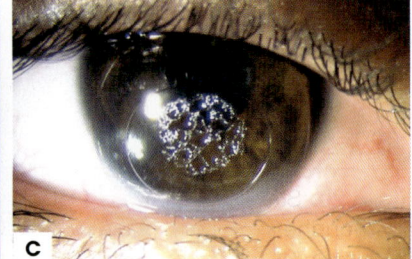

Fig. 6.19a to c: (a) Steep fit; (b) Steep with poor edge clearance; (c) Extremely steep fit with retained air bubbles

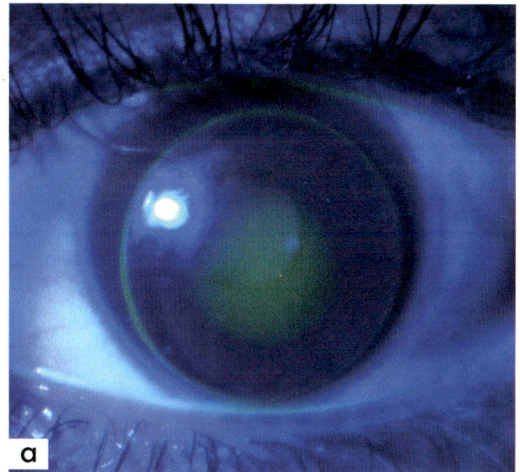

Fig. 6.20a: Steep fit: Central optic zone (clearance /pooling of fluorescein), mid-periphery and periphery (touch), edge clearance (0.05 mm)

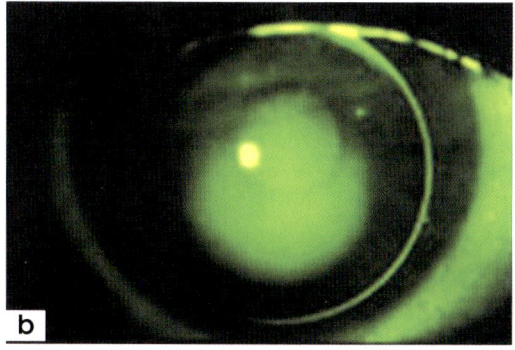

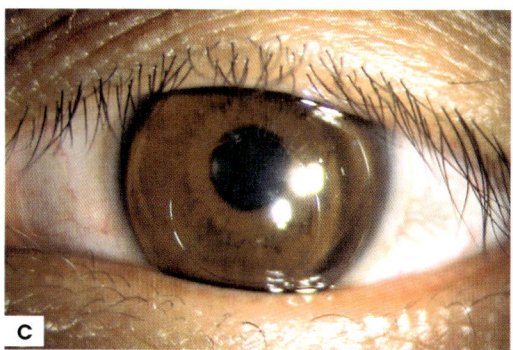

Fig. 6.20: Steep fit. (b) Note the central pool with mid-periphery peripheral contact, minimal edge clearance. (c) Excessively steep fit with entrapped air bubble in centre

– **Peripheral zone:** This zone is important for evaluating peripheral lens clearance. In a steep fit the peripheral zone shows reduced edge clearance depicted by a narrow edge width (less dye seen). Corneal epithelial indentation by lens edge signifies extreme steepness and implies a very *tight peripheral curve*. In case of a flat fit or in excessive edge lift this zone is very wide (excess dye seen). The grading of fit has been very lucidly explained in Table 6.1 by Guillon.[12]

b. *Signs on dynamic assessment*

– **Sluggish movement (laggard lens):** A tight fit is diagnosed by well centered or slightly inferior, but stable lens. A steep lens hugs the cornea and impedes free tear flow, thereby causing tear thinning and exposure of more viscous, deeper mucin layer of tear film. The lens when it rests on this viscous layer experiences an increased viscous drag, which translates into a *poor lens movement (less than 1.0 mm)*. The lens movement remains sluggish despite pushing of lens through the lid.

The solution is to replace with a lens with either larger BOZR, flatter peripheral curves, smaller BOZD or a smaller overall lens diameter. An increase of 0.05 mm in BOZR would require a concomitant increase of 0.50 mm in BOZD to maintain an equivalent fit.

ii. **Flat or loose fit:**

a. *Signs on static assessment*

– **Central zone:** There is a limited zone of central corneal touch (dark zone). This occurs with lenses of larger BOZR (flatter) where central back surface of lens rests against relatively steeper central cornea. It

Table 6.1: Guillon grading of fit of RGP Lens					
Guillon has advocated a grading scale for types of fit[12]					
Grades	+2	+ 1	0	–1	–2
General fit	Excessively steep	Slightly steep	Alignment	Slightly flat	Excessively flat
Peripheral fit – Width	Excessively wide (0.4 mm)	Slightly wide (0.3 – 0.4 mm)	Optimal (0.2– 0.3 mm)	Slightly narrow (0.1– 0.2 mm)	Extremely narrow (< 0.1 mm)
– Height	Excessive	More than optimal	Optimal	Less than optimal	Insufficient
Mid-peripheral fit	Hard, well defined contact	Poorly defined contact	No contact		

manifests as *apical touch* (blue zone with absence of fluorescein seen as black area), with excess fluorescein in mid-periphery and peripheral zone. This needs to be differentiated from a very tight lens, where there would be an entire absence of green glow of fluorescein stained tears, as the dye is unable to travel beneath an extremely steep lens (Fig. 6.21a).

– **Mid-peripheral zone:** The mid-periphery exhibits clearance from the cornea, evident as fluorescein stained tear film (bright green)

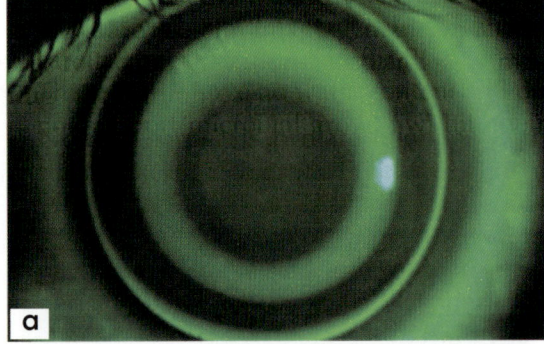

Fig. 6.21a: Flat fit : Central optic zone (touch), mid-periphery (clearance), periphery (feather touch), edge clearance (0.1 mm) *Courtesy:* Abhilekh Aneja

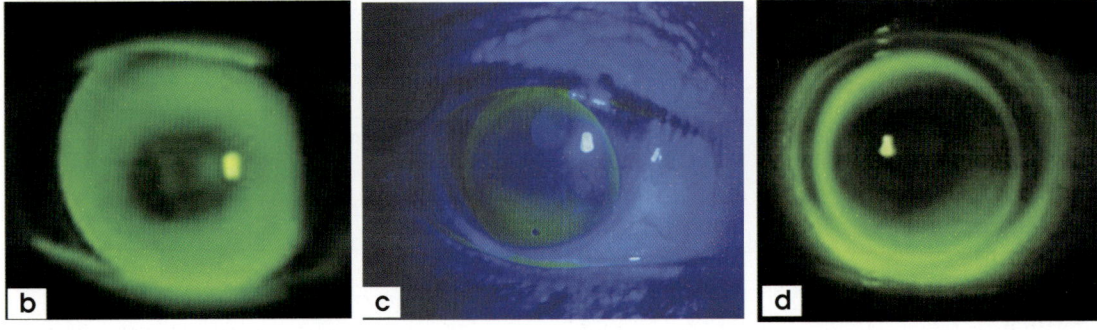

Fig. 6.21 (b, c, d): Flat fit. Note the apical touch and excessive pooling of fluorescein in the intermediate and peripheral zones

– **Peripheral zone:** Excessive edge clearance with excessive amount of fluorescein dye (Fig. 6.21b to d).

b. *Signs on dynamic assessment*:

– **Excessive movement (drunken lens):** During dynamic assessment a loose fit lens displays excessive excursion of >2.0 mm, resulting in high or lateral riding position. Due to inadequate centering forces, lens is left to vagaries of lid and ocular movements. High riding is a consequence of upper lid forces pulling up the lens. When the lid is unable to retain of lens, it falls slowly to an inferior location on the cornea. Thus resting position of lens is inconsistent and it rotates around corneal apex on either nasal or *temporal* side, while returning to a low resting position on the cornea. This occurs because BC of lens being flatter than corneal apex, makes path of least resistance to be around the apex. A flat/loose lens often shows a considerable lag in its movement following any change in gaze, leading to physical discomfort and visual blur. The remedy is to fit a steeper curve lens (smaller BC), larger BOZD for a deeper central tear depth or larger OD permitting lid attachment.

A lens continually decentered to one side implies altered corneal topography, against the rule astigmatism or is a flat/small lens.

iii. **Apical alignment fit:** This pattern shows alignment or slight apical clearance over central 7.00 mm region, mid-peripheral touch and edge clearance of about 0.50 mm width, with upper edge of lens fitting under upper eyelid. It should also include centered OZ over pupil, adequate lens movement and tear exchange with each blink and adequate edge lift

providing 360° clearance. This fit is an optimal fit (Fig. 6.22).

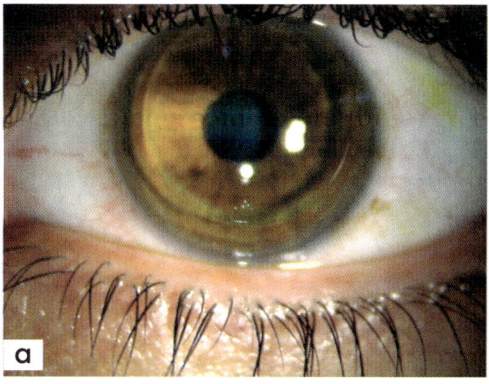

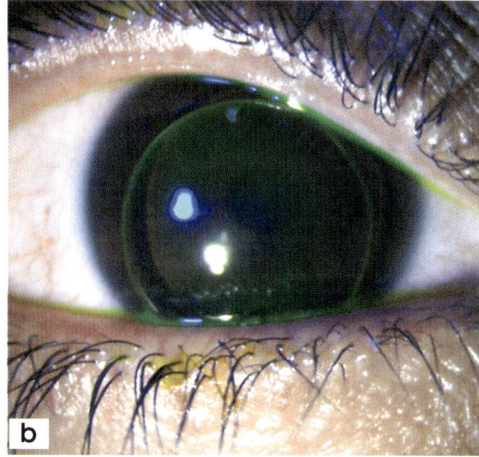

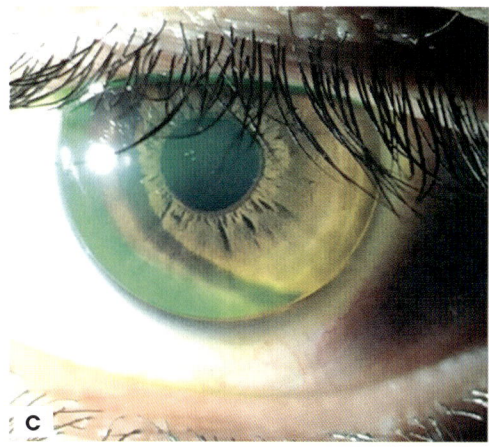

Fig. 6.22: Apical alignment fit: (a) Well-aligned in primary gaze; (b) Diffuse feather clearance; (c) Adequate edge clearance

iv. **Lid attachment fit:** In this fit, lens maintains a high riding position in between blinks. It is seen into tight lids or in high minus lens (with increased peripheral thickness), which gets picked up by the lid. This fit is comfortable, as upper lid margin sensation to lens edge is avoided during blinking. Such a fit is also seen with a flat periphery, large diameter and/or with the rule astigmatism. The solution is obvious in first two causes and the last cause requires fitting of a lens with back surface toric design.

v. **Low riding lens fit:** Low riding lens, showing rapid dropping post-blink implies a small diameter, a thick/heavy high plus lens or lack of lid attachment (Fig. 6.23a). The solution is evident in first two causes with the last cause requiring a negative peripheral carrier to be added. In this fit the upper edge of lens is exposed to margin of descending lid with constant impact causing discomfort and reducing blink rate. This in turn increases lens drying, 3 and 9 o' clock staining and lens intolerance. This fit is also seen in lenses fit over ectatic corneas (Fig. 6.23b).

vi. **Astigmatism:** In with-the-rule astigmatism, a greater pooling of fluorescein occurs along the steeper, vertical meridian (vertical dumbbell), whereas for against the rule it is along the horizontal configuration (horizontal dumbbell) (Fig. 6.24).

Characteristics of an Ideal Fit

- Slight central pooling (apical clearance) with peripheral edge clearance on fluorescein staining.

- Well-centered lens on primary gaze. Minimal downriding or lateral decentration is acceptable in patients with high astigmatism.

- Good visual acuity with comfort.

- Adequate excursion of >1.5 mm while blinking. This is essential, for constant replenishment of underlying tear film. Atmospheric oxygen is no longer freely available to cornea since oxygen diffusion is limited through the thick RGP lens, therefore cornea underneath a rigid lens depends on oxygen mixed in tear film for its nutrition. In case of soft lenses situation is reversed, with significant amount of oxygen diffusing through the thin hydrogel material and tear oxygen being unavailable due to snug fitting SCL (not allowing generation of an adequate *post-lens* tear film.)

- Normal facial appearance (head posture).

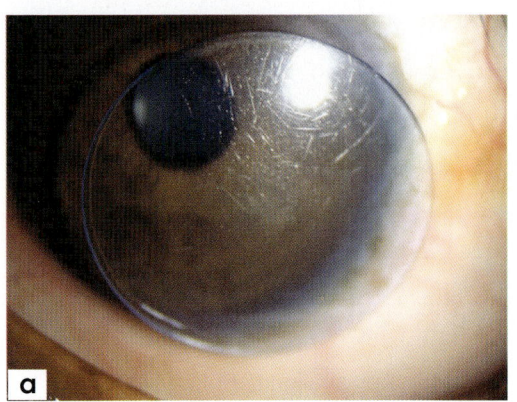 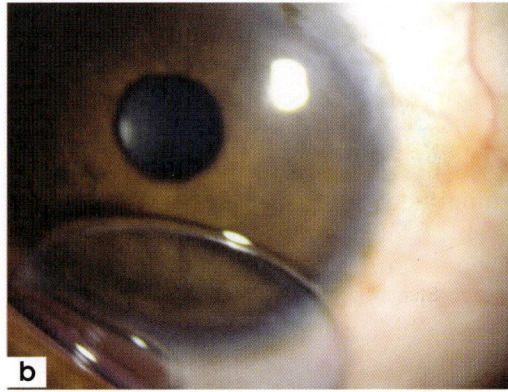

Fig. 6.23: (a) Low riding lens; (b) Lens expulsion in a keratoconus case

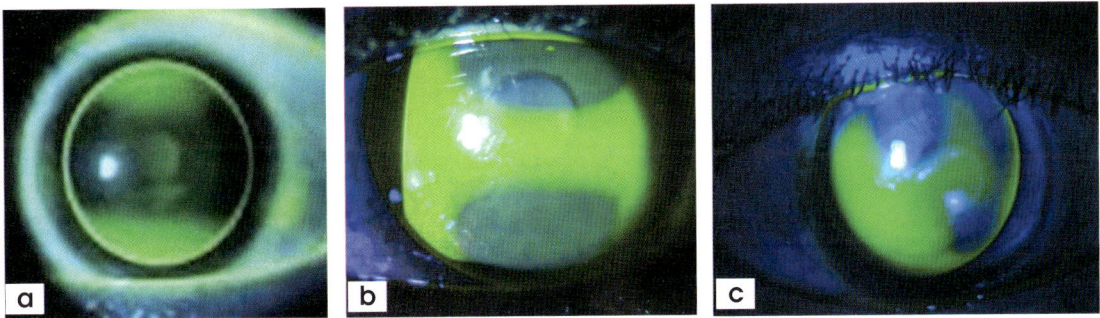

Fig. 6.24: Static fit depicting (a) With the rule astigmatism; (b) Against the rule astigmatism; (c) Oblique astigmatism

Figure 6.25 diagrammatically represents different types of static fit.

Step IV: Power Finalization

Once lens fit has stabilized and optimal fit has settled, lens power is finalized by performing **over-refraction**. Over-refraction involves performing retinoscopy over the lens *in situ*, to determine BVP. It is to be done in steps of +/−1.0 D steps initially and refined with 0.50 D and 0.25 D steps. If the over-refraction is greater than ±4.00 D, the vertex distance compensation should be performed as mentioned in *Annexure II*.

Remember lens power determines both lens thickness and front surface shape, which in turn determines lens excursion, position or in other words the *lens fit*. Thus for an accurate assessment of fit it is advisable if the power of the trial lens be within a few diopters of the ordered lens, so that during over refraction, no power surprises arise.

If the BOZR of prescribed lens is same as trial lens, final power would be the sum of trial

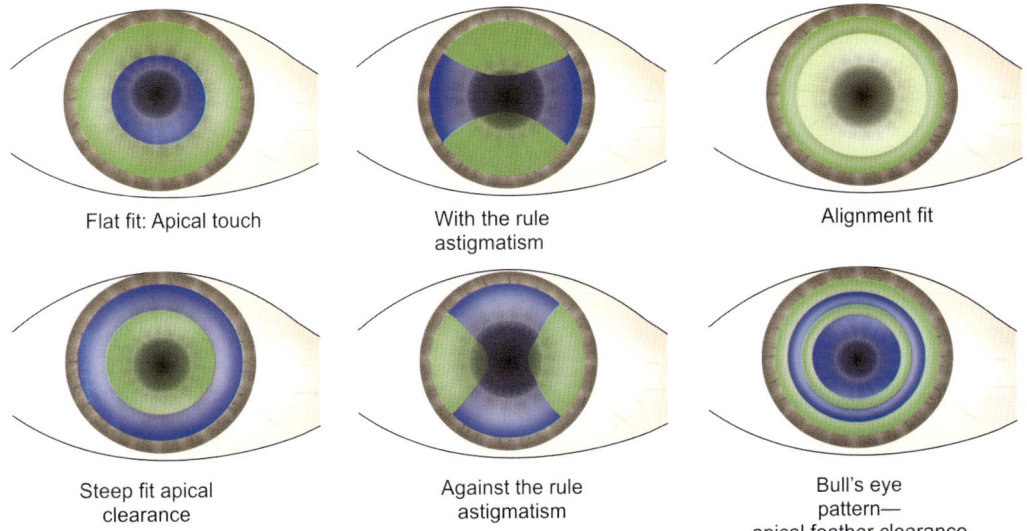

Flat fit: Apical touch

With the rule astigmatism

Alignment fit

Steep fit apical clearance

Against the rule astigmatism

Bull's eye pattern—apical feather clearance

Fig. 6.25: Pictorial representation of various types of fluorescein patterns on static fit, green color implies fluorescein stained fears are present

lens power + compensated over-refraction. If base curve ordered is steeper or flatter than that of the trial lens, tear lens effect needs to be considered (SAMFAP rule).

Lens Inventory

A requisite for successful RGP lens fitting is to have a large inventory of trial lenses. This makes it possible to fit a lens appropriate for different types of eyes.

Trial set for RGP lens fitting should have two diameters for each BVP, usually diameters of 9.2 and 9.60 mm suffice for majority of patients. Back optic zone radius need to range from 7.00 to 8.40 mm in 0.1 mm steps and from 7.60 to 8.00 mm in 0.05 mm steps. Recommended BVP selection is – 3.00 D for low minus and – 6.00 D for higher minus powers.

Follow up Protocol

After prescription, lens wearing time is stepped up in phases starting from 2 to 3 hours of wear on the first day. Subsequently one hour is added for each following day till by the end of 1 week the patient is able to wear the lens for 8–9 hours.

At follow up visits:

- Visual acuity with CL *in situ* is checked.
- Fluorescein staining and dynamic fit is done to re-evaluate the fit.
- Lens is checked for any deposits/scratches under high magnification.
- Patient should be asked to demonstrate lens insertion and removal to ensure adequacy of technique.
- Lens case should be checked for cleanliness.

REFERENCES

1. Cornish R, Sulaiman S. Do thinner rigid gas permeable contact lenses provide superior initial comfort? Optom Vis Sci. 1996 Mar;73 (3):139–43.

2. Bennett ES, Sorbara L. Lens design, fitting and evaluation. Rigid gas permeable lens. In Bennett ES, Henry VA. Eds. 2nd ed Clinical manual of contact lenses. Philadelphia: Lippincott Williams & Wilkins. Butterworth Heineman 2000, 96.

3. Philips AJ. Rigid gas permeable and hard contact lens fitting. In Phllips AJ & Stone J. Eds 3rd ed. Contact lenses. New Delhi. Jaypee Publishers. 1994: 337–8.

4. Tuong C, Jackson JM. Optical Zone Size Changes and GP Lens Performance. GP Insights. *Contact Lens Spectrum*, Volume 30, Issue: August 2015, 15.

5. Theodoroff CD, Lowther GE. Quantitative effect of optic zone diameter changes on rigid gas permeable lens movement and centration. International Contact Lens Clinic.1990; 17 (3–4): 92–5.

6. Atkinson TCO. A re-appraisal of the concept of fitting rigid lenses by the tear layer and edge

clearance techniques. J Br Contact Lens Ass 1984: 7: 106–110.

7. Atkinson TCO. A computer assisted and clinical assessment of current trends in gas permeable lens designs. Optician 1985 Jan: 16–22.

8. Veys J, Meyler J, Davies I. Rigid contact lens fitting . In Essential Contact Lens Practice; A practical guide. Mumbai. Johnson & Johnson Vision Care Institute, 2002, 61–78.

9. Ichijima H, Cavanagh HD. How rigid gas-permeable lenses supply more oxygen to the cornea than silicone hydrogels: a new model. Eye Contact Lens. 2007 Sep;33(5):216–23.

10. Hayashi TT, Fatt I. Forces retaining a contact lens on the eye between blinks. Am J Optom Physiol Opt. 1980 Aug;57(8):485–507.

11. Mc Mohan T, Szczotka Flynn L. Fitting the abnormal cornea . In Eds Krachmer JH, Mannis MJ, Holland EJ. Cornea. Fundamentals, diagnosis and management Vol 1. 2nd ed., Elsevier Mosby, Philadelphia. 1313–24.

12. Guillon M. Basic contact lens fitting in Rubin M & Guillon M (eds). Contact lens practice. Chapman Hall Medical 1994, 587–622.

Reader's Note

Reader's Note

CHAPTER 7

Fitting a Soft Contact Lens

Of the worldwide estimated number of contact lens wearers beyond 140 million, almost 90% use soft lenses or hydrogels.[1–3] As the term implies soft lens moulds or drapes over the anterior ocular surface and conforms to corneal shape. To achieve this effect, its diameter has to be larger than the cornea and the BOZR flatter than the cornea. A well-fitted lens moves adequately with ocular movements and should cover entire cornea in all cardinal positions. Stable vision, instant comfort, ease of insertion by wearer and ease of evaluating fit by fitter are the major benefits of a soft contact lens (SCL).

Soft Lens Properties and Design Parameters: Physiological and Optical Effects

A. **Lenticular lens:** This lens is made in such a way that the front surface incorporates optical portion in the center surrounded by a peripheral skirt (carrier). The radius of curvature of peripheral carrier is flatter than the central optical portion and this flat skirt helps in stabilizing the lens. Such a design is especially useful in high refractive errors. For high plus lens this lenticular design serves to reduce weight of the lens, prevents downriding of lens, thereby aiding centration. For a high minus lens lenticular design reduces the edge thickness, prevents up riding of lens and again helps in lens centration.

Another advantage of lenticular lens is that since only the center carries the optical portion, lens periphery does not suffer from side effects of a concave (minus) lens, namely increased edge thickness. This reduction in edge thickness for a high minus lens power to a thin periphery reduces lens edge feel and enhances comfort. For a high plus power lens the reduced peripheral mass reduces lens bulk, enhances stability and comfort (Fig. 7.1).

B. **Lens rigidity:** Lens rigidity is the major determinant of lens position and motility. Less rigid lens hug the eye, generates a thin post lens tear film which increases viscous drag resulting in reduced lens movement. More rigid lenses permit thicker post lens tear film, thereby allowing increased lens movements. Rigidity in turn is determined both by material and manufacturing technique with spin cast lenses being less rigid; more elastic compared to lathe cut lenses.

C. **Wetting angle:** A low wetting angle means that water easily spreads over entire lens surface and a high wetting angle implies coalescing of water into a drop on the lens surface. Lower wetting angles where the tear film clings evenly onto the CL translate into increased comfort and crisper optics. (Refer to Chapter 3 page 12)

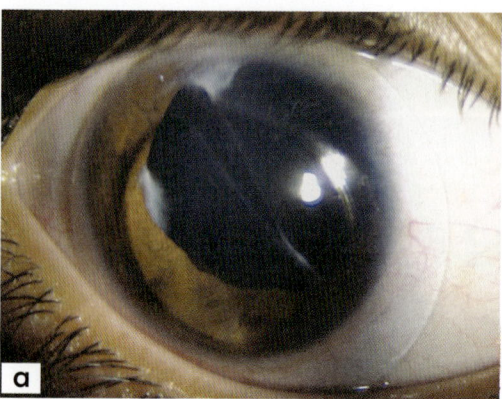 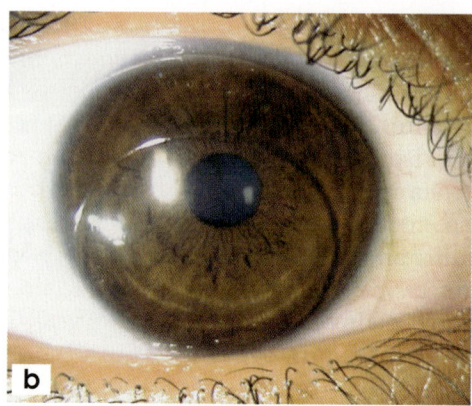

Fig. 7.1: Lenticular lens fit: (a) Aphakia (high hyperopia); (b) High myopia

D. Water content: Water content of hydrogels ranges from 38 to 75% (by weight) and they are categorized depending on water content as: Low water content with <40% water, medium water content with 50–60% water and high water content with >60% water. Altering water content of a lens, changes its "on eye" fitting, by changing its rigidity.[4]

High water content lenses are thicker, less rigid, have higher oxygen transmissibility and are more susceptible to changes in ambient temperature or humidity. These low rigidity lenses confirm better over ocular surface and generate a thin post-lens tear film. For a given prescription, a shift to higher water content material, leads to *increased thickness* which offsets some of rigidity loss and causes increased lens-lid interaction. Better oxygen permeability offsets disadvantage accruing due to this increased lens thickness.

Low water content lenses are more durable, less affected by vagaries of climate and easier to handle/insert. The greater rigidity and durability of low water materials make them a better option for use in lower powers since reduced thickness diminishes its effect on cornea lid physiology.

The capacity of soft lenses to absorb preservatives from care system also depends on its water content. Higher water content, increases propensity of lens to accumulate protein deposits on its surfaces and promotes allergy.

E. Surface charge: The surface charge of a soft lens influence propensity and rapidity for protein build up. Hydrogels are classified as ionic or non-ionic with former having a negatively charged surface. Non-ionic hydrogels are treated to reduce this negative surface charge so as to decrease protein deposition.[4]

The four categories of FDA in classifying soft lens materials based on surface charge are:

Category 1 = low water, non-ionic,
Category 2 = high water, non-ionic
Category 3 = low water, ionic
Category 4 = high water, ionic

F. Sagittal depth/height/ sag: Sagittal height is the term given to area beneath a contact lenses while on the cornea. Factors which govern sagittal height of anterior eye are: corneal diameter, degree of corneal asphericity, central corneal curvature, and curvature of the paralimbal sclera/conjunctiva, in order of contribution.[5] Sagittal depth of a lens is the perpendicular distance from central posterior portion of lens to an imaginary line depicting lens diameter. Relationship between sagittal height of lens and anterior curvature of cornea determines lens fit with good fit requiring inner sag of lens to be more than that of anterior eye. A balance needs to be drawn since increasing lens sag makes the fit *tight*, whereas reducing sagittal height *loosens* the lens fit (Fig. 7.2). This is the reason of altered lens fit subsequent to changes in BC or CPC. Alteration in lens diameter and/or base curve changes the sagittal depth in the following manner:

a. As BC increases in mm, the sagittal depth decreases leading to a flatter fit. As BC decreases in mm the sagittal depth increases leading to a steeper fit.

b. As overall diameter increases in mm, the sagittal depth increases leading to a steeper fit. Conversely, as overall diameter decreases in mm the sagittal depth decreases leading to a flatter fit.

G. **Overall diameter/total diameter (OD/ TD):** This is the dimension in millimetres from one edge of lens to the other edge. It is a major parameter in determining lens centration both during primary position and secondary eye movements. An increase in lens diameter tightens lens as sagittal height is increased, whereas a decrease in diameter will loosen the fit. To retain the same fit while altering OD, a concomitant change is required in BOZR, e.g. if overall diameter is increased, then BOZR also needs to be concomitantly increased to offset effect of diameter change on ratio of sagittal height to OD.[6] *An increase in diameter by 0.5 mm would require BOZR to be increased by 0.3 mm, to retain the same fitting characteristics.* For example: For a lens with BOZR = 9.1 mm and OD = 13.5 mm, an increase of OD to 14 mm would cause tightening/ steepening of lens. Thus BOZR would need to be changed to 9.4 mm to ensure an equivalent 'flattening' in order to retain original ratio of sagittal height/total diameter. This rule is not applicable for *aspheric* lenses, where back surface curvature alteration and not overall diameter alteration alone influence fitting.

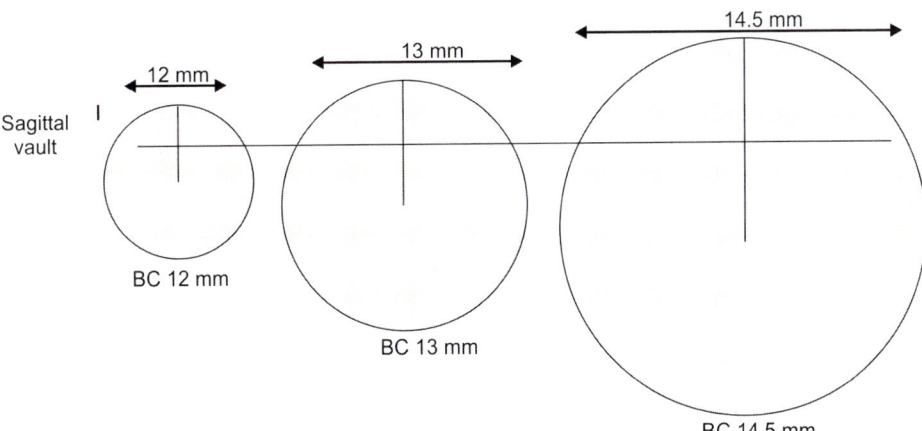

Fig. 7.2: As overall diameter increases, sagittal depth/sag of a lens increases, which causes fit to become steeper

H. Back surface design: Back surface design properties determine *in situ* lens behavior and vary with different lens makes. Thus two lenses of different makes with similar power, similar total diameter would behave differently on the wearer's eye. This occurs due to difference in material, number of peripheral curves, radii, widths, thicknesses in different lens series. **Thus the lens ordered must be of *same make* whose trial lens had been used**.

I. Base curve (BC): This is the name given to radius of curvature of central posterior surface. This part of lens moulds onto anterior curvature of cornea and is held to it by capillary action of tear film. Measured in mm, it is converted to dioptres by taking the reciprocal of radius. This curve aligns the lens onto the cornea and is measured by the *radiuscope*.

J. Optic zone (OZ): The optic zone occupies entire front surface of a single cut lens but only central part of a lenticular lens. On back surface of lens it encompasses total area minus peripheral and intermediate curves. As the name implies it carries the optical correction and art of good fitting requires this zone to be kept in front of pupil during all gazes especially primary gaze. The OZ is specified in mm and can be verified by an instrument—the *lensometer.*

K. Intermediate and peripheral curves (IPC): These are a series of sequentially flatter curves ground onto back surface of lens, starting from edge of base curve and finishing at lens end. The peripheral curves are usually one to two in number. Since natural shape of cornea is aspheric with a steeper center and flatter periphery, peripheral curves are also made flatter to central BC so as to simulate corneal contour. These curves are designed to aid centration, allow adequate tear film flow and thus help in maintaining corneal vitality. Poorly ground peripheral curves cause 3 and 9 o'clock staining, lens intolerance and visual blur over a period of hours. These curves can be verified with a magnification loupe or *hand held magnifier.*

L. Blend: Blend is the name given to smooth junction between central base curve, peripheral or intermediate curves, depending on lens type (bicurve or multicurve).

M. Lens edge: This is the most important determinant of comfort with both shape and thickness playing a role. Sharp lens edges dig into the cornea, traumatize under surface of lid during blinking and are best avoided. Blunt or rounded edges also called *deal pattern* are preferred. Edge shape can be verified using a *profile analyzer.*

N. Lens thickness (L/Tc): Lens thickness is distance between anterior and posterior surface at its geometric center. Measured in mm it is determined by lens power and can be verified by the *thickness gauge*. As evident, concave/ minus lens would have a thinner **Tc** than a convex/plus lens. The minimum thickness of a high minus lens is limited only by dimensional stability of the polymer used. Lens thickness and lens profile/design significantly influence lens movement. This was understood after pioneering work by Hayashi et al who found displacing force required to shear a lens to be proportional to inverse of post-lens tear film thickness.[7,8] Thin lenses mould closely to anterior eye and create a very thin post-lens tear film which makes lens movement difficult. Thin lenses and those with thin edges, thus exhibit minimal movement during blinking and center better. This is the reason why thin/ very thin lenses require fewer fitting parameters (increments), as steps which cause clinically significant differences would poduce minimal alteration in 'on-eye' behavior. Thicker lenses, on the other hand, mould less on the cornea, interact more with lids, generate a thicker post-lens tear film and thus exhibit greater movement with blinking. Thick *edge profile* lens seen in high minus lens also causes more movement for the same reason. Thicker lens or lenses with thick edge profile are thus more prone to decentration. Thickness of conventional soft lenses is in the range of 0.10–0.18 mm, *hyper-thin* lenses being 0.07 to 0.035 mm thick.[9]

O. **Lens power:** The lens power is focal length of the contact lens in air. It is the difference between power of central anterior and posterior curves. Specified in dioptres, it is measured by a *lensometer*. Measurement is performed keeping anterior convex surface facing away from optical end of lensometer. To measure a soft lens, a special graticule with option of holding soft lens in solution is required.

P. **Manufacturing technique:** Basic material of a SCL is polymer HEMA with same cross-linking agent. It is the *varying rates* of cross-linking within the polymer which dictate change in lens properties and lens fit. Spin-cast manufacturing delivers the least rigid and most elastic variant and lathe cut delivers more rigid, inelastic material.

Q. **Lens centration:** This is conventionally denoted by Cartesian *coordinates*. However, due to inconsistency of horizontal co-ordinates, e.g. +x for right eye indicates nasal decentration, whereas for left eye +x would imply a temporal decentration, this system has not gained universal acceptance. *Binasal system* describes nasal decentration as positive (+ve) regardless of any eye. Vertical coordinates are depicted by +ve for up and –ve for down. The simplest method is *literal description*, e.g. 1.0 mm nasal decentration OU or 1.0 mm down riding OD, as this avoids any confusion.

Advantages of Soft Lenses

- Lenses of first choice for spherical refractive errors with astigmatism less than 0.75 D cylinder.
- Preferred lenses for high refractive errors including aphakia. In such powers RGP lenses are bulky and difficult to fit /center.
- Patients with significant astigmatism who are intolerant to RGP lenses.
- Where comfort and cosmesis are primary objectives of lens wear.
- Occasional/social wear. Soft lenses are easy to fit, convenient to use and require little re-adaptation each time spectacle wear is substituted for lens wear, and are therefore ideal in such situations. Disposable lenses are preferred hydrogel options in this scenario as they do away with requirements of storage and cleaning in between the infrequent usage.

Disadvantages of Soft Lenses

- Inadequate correction of regular astigmatism >1.5 D. In cases with high refractive errors like aphakia or high myopia with mild corneal astigmatism, the spherical equivalent is used as the final power of SCL. In such situations *4 to 1 rule* is applied, wherein corneal cylinder lesser than 25% of spherical component can be left uncorrected. Thicker soft lenses are more effective in masking corneal astigmatism.
- Poor correction in cases with irregular astigmatism.
- Lenses are inherently fragile, deposit prone, requiring meticulous care.
- Lenses require a stringent disinfection protocol since risk of infective keratitis is high otherwise.
- Allergy and giant papillary conjunctivitis is more frequent.
- Not suitable for dry, dusty, windy climates which alter optical properties of these high water content lenses.

Contraindications for Soft Lens

Absolute

- Corneal hypoaesthesia.
- Poor hygiene and adherence of lens wearer to cleaning protocols.

Relative

- Dry eyes.
- Pregnancy/hormonal imbalance.
- Uncontrolled diabetes.
- Occupations with exposure to chemicals/ fumes/dust. Soft lens dimensions alter with changes in environmental humidity. This causes alteration in optical properties and thereby vision quality. Hydrogels absorb fluids, ambient fumes and colors. Thus their use during festivals like Diwali and Holi where powdered colors and firecracker generated smoke can cause corneal toxicity. It is therefore recommended that SCLs are not worn during these festivals.

Temporary

- Active infection or inflammation of lids/ lacrimal sac/cornea

Variables Affecting Lens Fit

A. Lens related

- *Total diameter*: An increase in OD usually increases lens "sag" and tightens fit. However, an increased diameter by covering more of a cornea with disturbed topography and/ or a displaced apex could sometimes improve corneal coverage and vision.
- *BOZR:* An increased BOZR causes increased lens movement and decrease in BOZR decreases lens movement. However, this equation may always not be so predictable, thus a dynamic fit needs to be assessed independent to BOZR changes.[10]
- *Peripheral lens design:* The peripheral design dictated by relationship between front and back peripheral curves significantly affects lens fit.

B. Eye related

- *Ocular sag:* This requires a trial lens fitting for assessment as sag depends on corneal and scleral shape (radius and diameter).
- *Corneal apex:* Displaced corneal apex causes lens displacement *as a contact lens centers over steepest part of the cornea.* Increase in total diameter of lens expands corneal coverage and is often resorted to in patients with displaced apex.
- *Lid pressure:* Tight lids cause lens to ride high and loose lids lead to decreased lens movement. Tightness of lids exerts more effect on lens fit than flaccid lids.
- *Tear morphology:* A reduction in tear pH causes steepening of lens by affecting its ionic contents primarily. This assumes relevance in situations of unsatisfactory fit wherein altering type and make of lens with same numerical coordinates could allow a better fit.[10]

TECHNIQUE OF FITTING A SOFT LENS

There are two ways to fit a SCL: Inventory method and Diagnostic method.

I. Inventory method/Empirical Prescribing

This prescribes final lenses based on HVID and keratometric readings, without subjecting wearer to a trial fit. It requires a large inventory of lenses and lens confirming best to individual eye is selected. Chair time required is less as lens dispensing is immediate. However, keeping large enough inventories is not logistically feasible option for most practitioners. Secondly, the fit may fall short of best fit as it relies only on keratometer (which only estimates central 3.0 mm of cornea). Fitting a trial lens, on the other hand, gives an estimate of pattern of entire corneal coverage and takes into account lens sag. Thirdly, over-refraction on a CL *in situ* gives an accurate assessment of final refraction.

For these reasons empirical method of fitting is not the preferred modality.

II. Diagnostic/Trial Lens Method

The lens of nearest BOZR is selected from trial set. Common range stocked in most trial sets is BOZR 7.90–9.30 mm with those utilizing less rigid materials, containing fewer increments in steps of 0.4 mm and those using relatively rigid lenses, containing more increments in steps of 0.2 mm. The back vertex power is selected as close as possible to patient's prescription so as to allow accurate assessment of visual benefits. The following paragraphs detail step by step algorithm in fitting SCL by trial lens method.

Step I: Back optic zone radius (BOZR) / Base curve (BC) selection

The corneal curvature is measured in two meridians at 90 degrees to each other by the keratometer. In case of spherical refractive errors both meridians would have the same value, and for regular astigmatism one meridian would be steeper and other flatter. The K value required to calculate BC is based on *Flat K (flatter meridian value)*.

When fitting a soft lens a value of 0.6 or 0.8 is added to this flat K to arrive at initial trial lens BOZR. For soft lenses of less flexible lens material (thicker, low water content) 0.8 mm is added and for more flexible material (thinner, high water content) 0.6 mm is added to flat K to arrive at BOZR. A trial lens of this BC is selected from fitting set.[11] *In fitting of spin cast lenses, keratometry has a little role as the posterior surface of such lenses is aspheric.*

After placing trial lens in the patient's eye, fit is reviewed after a settling time to allow lens to equilibrate with ocular environment. *Factors influencing settling time are*:
– High water content and high powered lenses take longer to equilibrate due to greater water volume, thus fit needs to be reassessed only after 15–30 minutes.

– Sensitive lids, abnormal curvature require a longer settling time.
– High power lenses may have thicker edges (high minus) or thicker center (high plus) which again require more time to equilibrate.

The factors to be considered while finalizing the BC are lens centration/lens movement, lid profile and visual acuity:

i. *Lens centration /movement*: For adequate centration a 1 mm symmetric overlap of limbus, in primary and other gaze positions is desirable. The optic zone of CL should cover both mesopic and scotopic dimensions of pupil in **primary gaze** and preferably in horizontal gaze too. Centration has to be checked in **x and y** axis with the former being most important as it is used in daily activities like reading and latter axis assumes more relevance in occupations like sports, land survey, acting. Decentration or lens lag is defined as the amount by which lens trails behind eye movements. *In primary gaze*, lens should not decenter more than 0.2–0.75 mm (Fig. 7.3).

Centration and lens movement are also checked on *blinking* with eye in primary position. Adequate lens movement with blinking is essential since it ensures tear exchange beneath lens and flushes out waste debris. A well-centered lens lags by 0.5 mm and re-centers quickly on lateral and up gaze. Excess lag of >1.5 mm indicates flat fit, whereas no lag implies a steep fit (Fig. 7.4).

Lower lid "push up" test: This test is done in primary gaze for final confirmation of lens centration. The lens is deliberately unsettled with a finger pushing inferior edge of SCL through the lower lid. This pressure is then released and subsequent journey of lens back to its original position is noted. In this maneuver, ease of lens movement from its resting position, speed and quality of re-centration following intentional

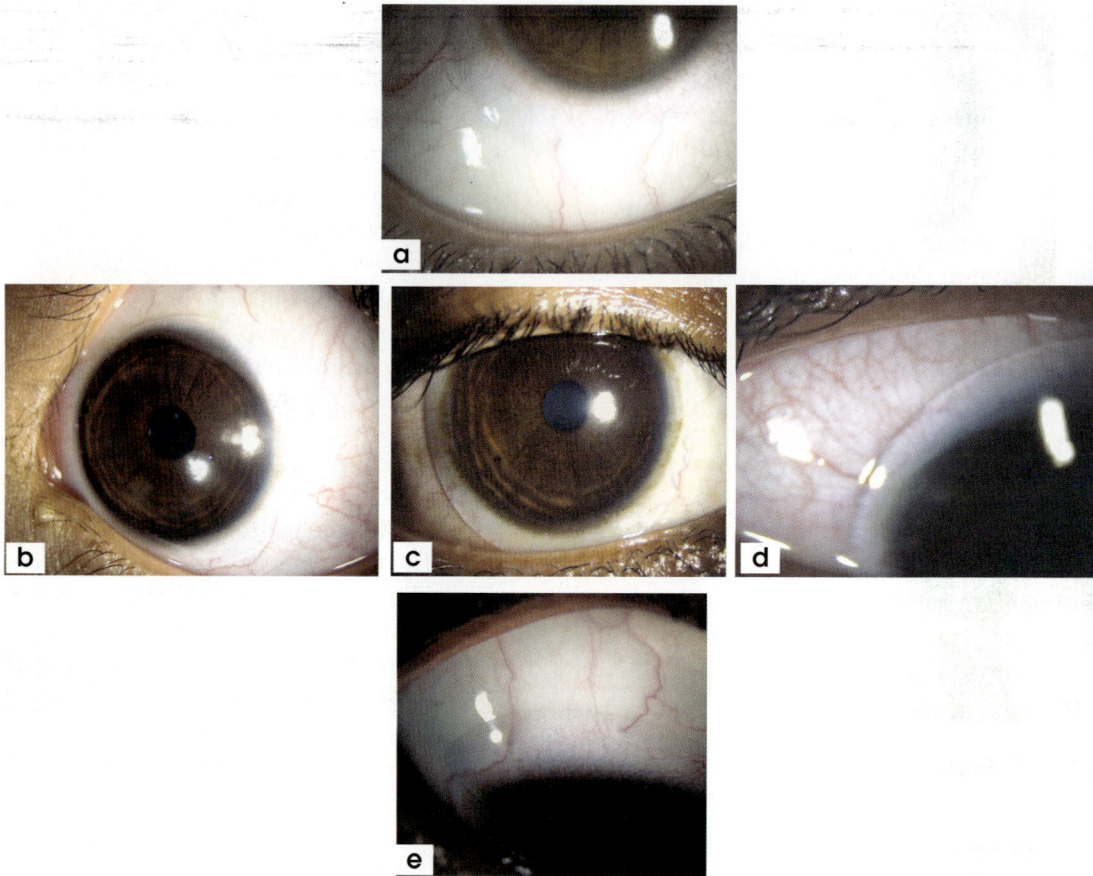

Fig. 7.3: Soft contact lens optimal fit in primary gazes and x and y axis.

displacement is observed. The rationale behind this is: Squeeze pressure generated by push up test initiates fluid movement behind the lens and a loosely fit lens with greater reservoir of fluid beneath it, will generate more movement.[12] A steep fit lens will not move much and a flat one will move too much, the latter taking more time to resettle back onto primary position (Fig. 7.5).

A decentered lens provides suboptimal optical performance and produce localized thinning of *post-lens tear film* in regions of heaviest touch (greatest bearing pressure). This causes tear film disturbance, microtrauma, discomfort and lens intolerance. By exposing parts of cornea, a decentered lens also con-tributes to corneal dessication and dellen formation.

ii. *Lens movement:* Lens movement also depends on lens **type** (convex, concave, high or low power, lenticulated or full aperture), lens thickness, back surface design (aspheric, monocurve, bicurve), **lens material**, and manufacturing technique (spin cast or lathe cut).

Thinner spin cast lenses move less, optimal movement being 0.5 mm. Thicker lathe cut lenses move more with optimal movement being 1.0 mm. Since tear exchange is minimal under a soft lens, oxygen demand of cornea is met through diffusion from the atmosphere. Thus lens movement is not as critical for a hydrogel lens as it is for a RGP lens.

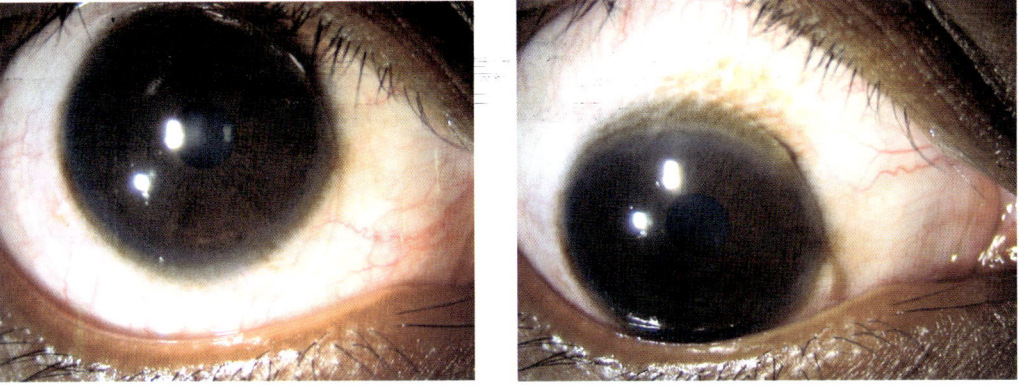

Fig. 7.4: Flat fitting lens: Note excess lag on upward and downward gaze

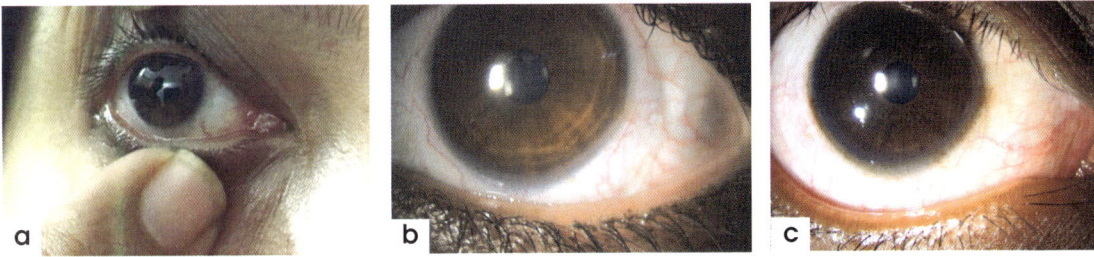

Fig. 7.5: Push up test: (a) Being performed (b) Does not move (steep fit) (c) Moves excessively (flat fit)

Easily displaced lens, increased lag and very fast to recenter lens usually implies a flat fit, whereas difficult to displace, lethargic/jerky movement, tendency to stay in an eccentric position once displaced, are signs of a steep/tight fit. If the lens fails to return at all, then the fit is *very tight*.

Alteration in lens profile also needs to be observed during these movements. Any **edge buckling** or **fluting** (lifting away from the eye) indicates an excessively flat lens, or an inside out lens. Ingress and entrapment of air bubbles in areas of edge lift-off in regular corneas also indicate a flat fit (Fig. 7.6).

iii. **Lid profile**: This also influences lens movement to a certain extent. Changes in lid occur due to anatomical (ethnic) and physiological (age change) differences. Different sizing of interpalpebral aperture and upper lid anatomy occur in Indian, Caucasian, Oriental races, with the latter having smaller palpebral apertures and short lids. Younger people especially children have smaller interpalpebral apertures and tight lids, whereas the elderly have lax lids. Tight lids contribute to upriding lens and poor movement in primary gaze (Fig. 7.7).

iv. **Changes in visual acuity:** Comfort and stable vision post-blink are surrogate indicators of fit.

• *Steep fit:* Vision clears *immediately* after a blink followed by a quick degradation. This occurs due to lid pressure during blinking forcing lens to conform to central cornea, leading to a transient improvement in vision quality. However, in inter-blink period,

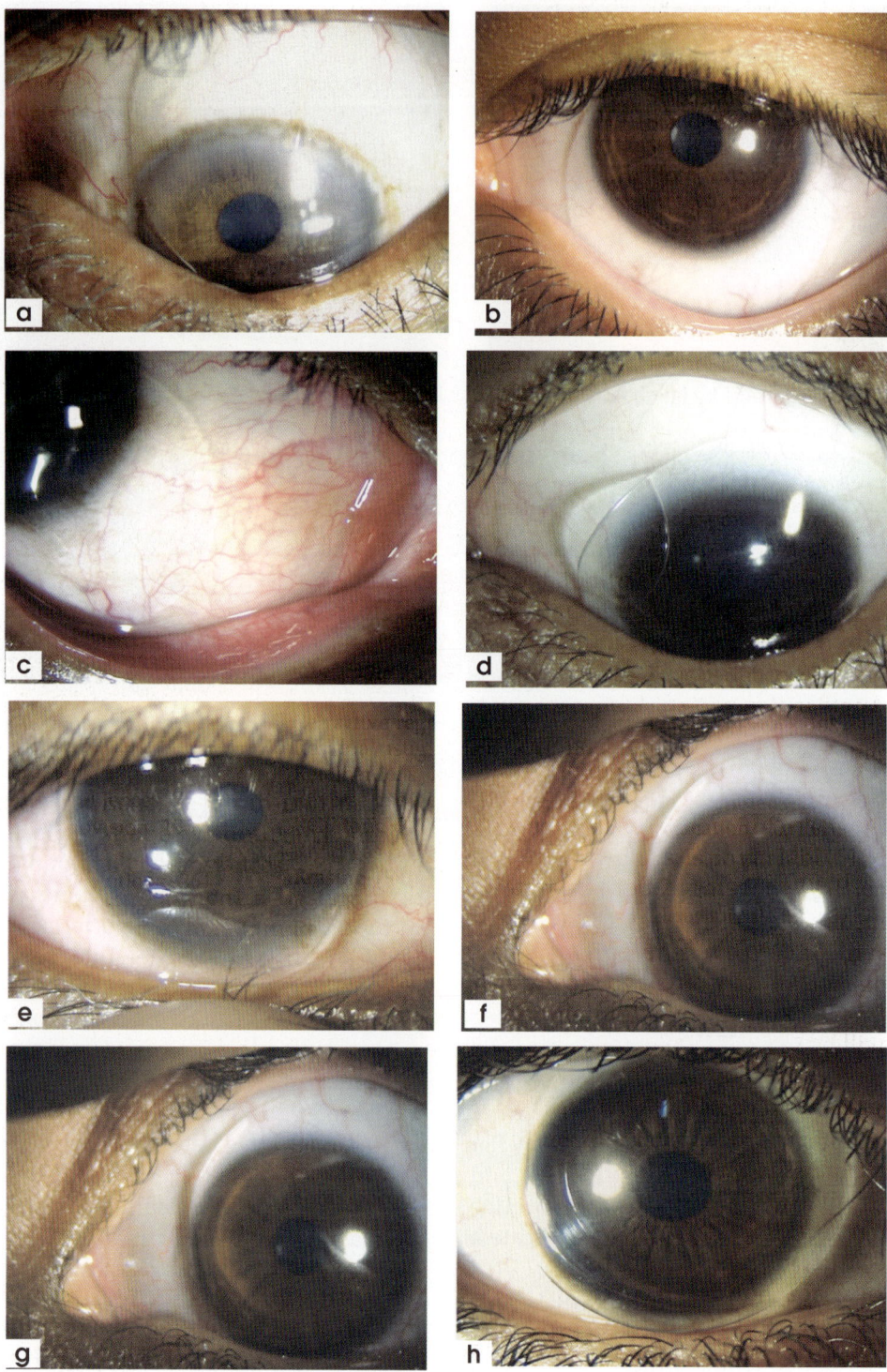

Fig. 7.6: Manifestations of flat fit: (a to c) Excessive movement in down gaze, primary and lateral gaze; (d to f) Edge fluting and buckling; (g and h) Inside out lens

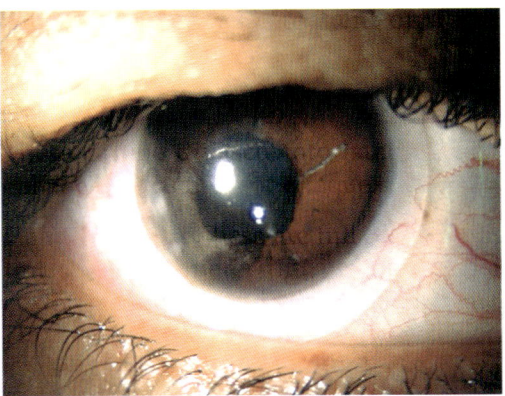

Fig. 7.7: Tight upper lid

the lens returns to its 'stand off' position due to its inherent visco-elastic property, and assumes an irregular aspheric shape leading to visual deterioration. The classical symptoms of such a fit are : initial crisp vision, followed by a feeling of hotness, pain in eye and vision blur.

Another sign of tight fit is *crimping* of perilimbal vessels under lens periphery. This is diagnosed by constriction, blanching of blood vessel and/or any apparent 'step' in blood vessel calibre coinciding with lens edge. It is also known as limbal or peri-limbal 'scuffing' (Fig. 7.8). If left untreated tight fit causes conjunctival vessel engorgement with corneal edema. Vision with patient's own spectacles will be hazy for a few hours post-lens removal, as a consequence of corneal edema. In extremely steep fit cases *conjunctival indentation* occurs due to lens edge digging onto the perilimbal conjunctiva. Rarely low grade anterior chamber inflammation can occur.

The eye can usually withstand around 40–60% lens tightness. For high water content, thin lenses around 60% tightness are acceptable, whereas for lower water content lens with a lower DK value up to 40% tightness is tolerated.

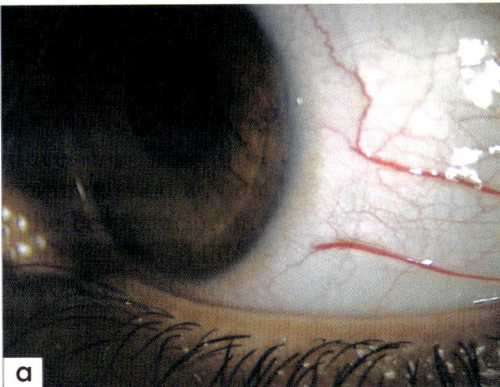

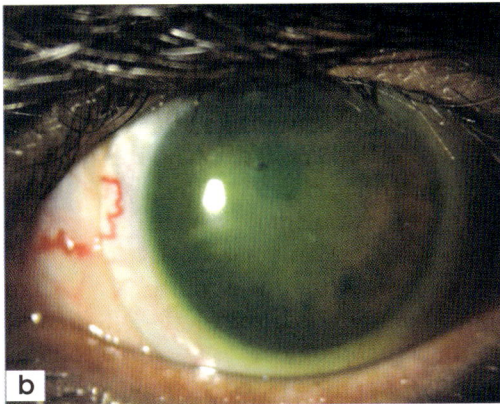

Fig. 7.8: Tight fit: (a) Mild-blood vessel (b) Engorgement but no step beneath lens edge. Severe: Patient presents with diffuse corneal edema and decrease in vision, after a few hours of wear. Note engorged vessel and step on nasal side at 9 o'clock.

It must be kept in mind that hydrogels tend to lose water when placed on the eye, leading to an *'on-eye tightening'*. *For this reason the final prescription should be dispensed only after evaluating fit in situ after 15–20 minutes of wear.*

• *Flat fit*: The visual clues for a flat fit are clear vision in primary gaze position which *blurs immediately after a blink*. Excessive lens movement often leads to decentration of lens, which regardless of direction of decentration is forced to mould to shape of anterior eye. Such acquired shape is both optically incorrect and confers distortion to area of eye it rests on. This further exaggerates optical ill effects of decentration and gives rise to fluctuating vision. Lens edge curling/wrinkling, edge stand-off (fluting) are other signs of flat fitting of lens. An inferior lens lag in primary eye position and feeling of discomfort by wearer due to excessive lens mobility also indicate a loose fit. Table 7.1 depicts the differences in tight and flat fit.

Table 7.1: Differences in steep and flat fitting of a soft contact lens		
	Steep/tight fit	Flat/ loose fit
Lens movement on blinking	Poor < 1 mm	Excessive
Lower lid push up test	Immobile lens	Too much movement
Lens edge effect on limbal blood vessels	Blood vessel crimping/conjunctival compression	No effect
Refractive surprise	Contributory optics of the tear lens come into play	Fluctuating vision
Visual acuity	Initial crisp vision	Blurred vision
Lens drop out	Minimal/none	Possible
Side effects	Hot angry eye after some time as a consequence of hypoxia	Excessive watering and *feeling of the lens* in the eye

Figure 7.9 depicts the prototypes of flat, optimal and steep fit.

Step II: Calculating back vertex power (BVP) for spherical SCLs

After allowing for a requisite settling time of 5–10 minutes for the optimal fit lens, an **over-refraction** is performed. This adaptation time permits patient comfort to occur and for lens to equilibrate to eye environment. Over refraction detects any residual refractive error. It should be done with a retinoscope and never with an autorefractometer. Refraction needs to be finalized in minus cylinder form and any residual spherical error is added to the power of trial lens. For any residual cylindrical error the following **4:1 Rule** is adopted: If spherical component of an astigmatic prescription is 4 times more than cylindrical component, vision with the prescription' best sphere will be acceptable. For patients whose cylinder component exceeds ≥ 1.50 Dc, soft toric lenses (incorporating cylindrical correction) would need to be tried, since spherical soft lenses do not mask astigmatism >1.5 Dc.

Final BVP should be close to spectacle prescription taking into account the vertex distance correction. Tear film dynamics play a *nominal role* in ordering final BVP unlike RGP lens situation as the insignificant tear volume underneath a well-draped SCL does not contribute an optical component. Thus a final BVP of contact lens to be ordered differs a little from the ocular Rx. The contact lens power arrived at after overreaction and correction of vertex distance must be confirmed with the original refraction.

Although a reduced visual acuity may be acceptable for social/occupational and other occasional wear situations, it may not be sufficient for certain occupations with stringent visual needs, e.g. architects, surgeons and pilots. The personality of the patient also plays a role in this aspect as certain patients have higher demands and expectations of aided vision.

Step III: A "walkabout trial" allows the wearer to appreciate lens feel, alteration in vision, comfort and difference in spatial orientation.[10] In other words, a real time feel can be given before finalizing lens parameters. Patients with higher refractive errors may observe some peripheral distortions or lack of it after years of spectacle wear. The initial difficulty in judging distances on switching to CL wear from spectacles may impair some real world activities transiently.

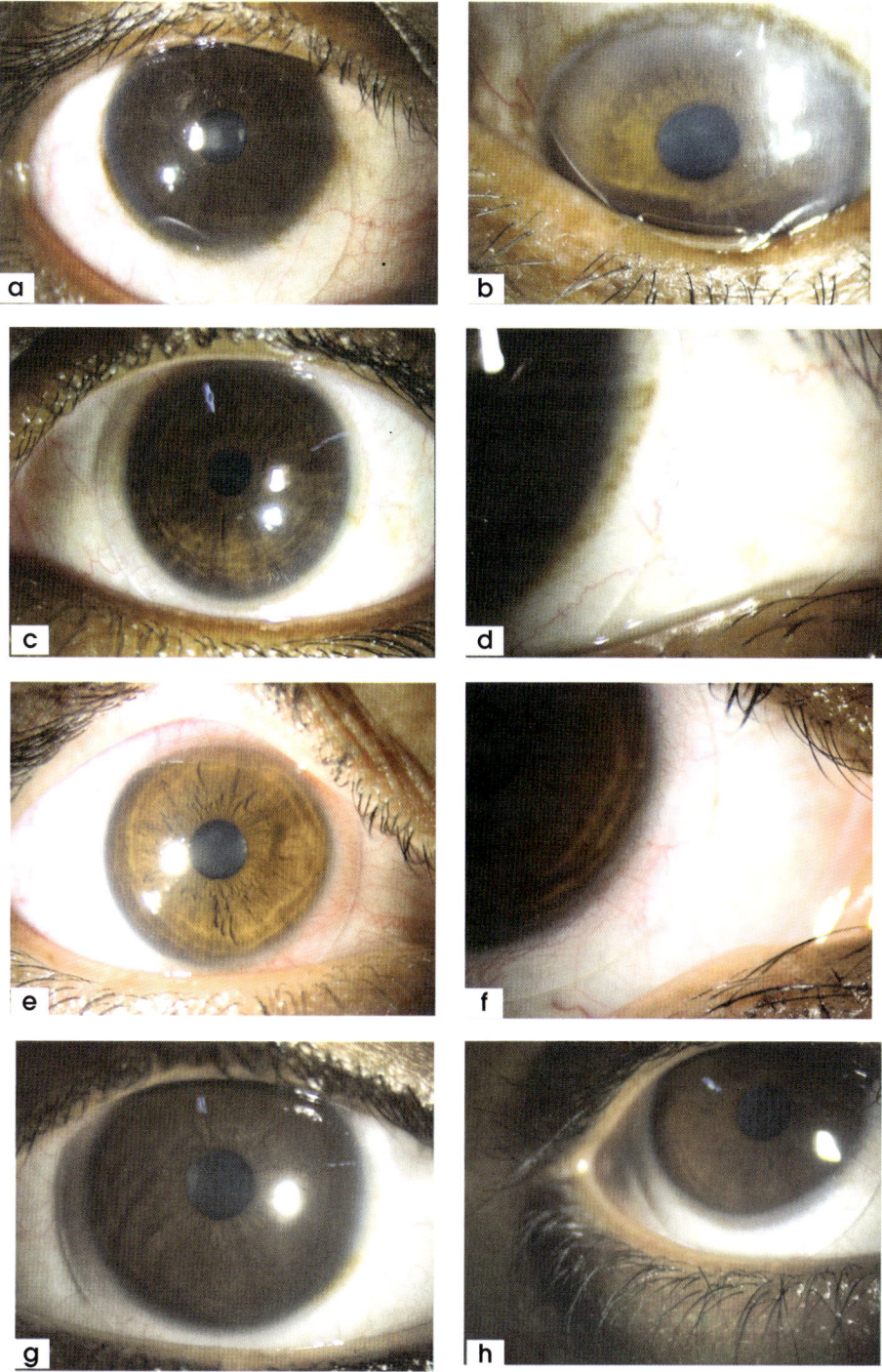

Fig. 7.9: *Flat fit:* (a) Excessively motile lens post-blink; (b) Edge lift in down gaze. *Optimal fit:* (c) Primary gaze; (d) No vessel impingement. *Steep fit:* (e and f) Note tight fit with crimping of blood vessels and (g, h) lack of movement

After prescribing the final lens, patient is reviewed again with contact lens in the eye. The first follow up visit is scheduled after 1 week of lens wear. At this follow up, patient is asked to come wearing the lenses for at least 2–3 hours prior to appointment time. Specific questions about comfort and vision quality are asked. Examination is performed for vision, lens centration and movement in primary gaze, lateral gaze and down gaze. Any problems with insertion and removal are specifically asked for and rectified. In order to clarify this, patient may be asked to insert and remove lens in front of the fitter. Technique of lens cleaning and status of lens container can also be checked at this stage.

REFERENCES

1. Stapleton F, Keay L, Jalbert I, Cole N. The epidemiology of contact lens related infiltrates. Optometry and vision science. American Academy of Ooptom 2007; (84) : 4, 257–72.

2. Contact Lens Wearer Demographics and Risk Behaviors for Contact Lens—Related Eye Infections — United States, 2014 CDC. Center for disease control and prevention, August 21, 2015/64 (32); 865–70.

3. Key JE Development of contact lenses and their worldwide use. Eye Contact Lens. 2007 Nov;33 (6 Pt 2):343–5.; discussion 362–3.

4. American Academy of Ophthalmology. Contact lens. In Clinical Optics. Basic and clinical science course 2015–16. Section 3. 151–93.

5. Young G, Holden B, Cooke G. Influence of soft contact lens design on clinical performance. Optom Vis Sci. 1993 May; 70(5):394–403.

6. Gasson A, ý Morris J A . Soft Lens design and fitting. The Contact Lens Manual. A practical guide to fitting. Eds 4th ed. Butterwort, Heinemann, Elsevier 2010.

7. Hayashi T, Fatt I. Forces retaining a contact lens on the eye between blinks. Am J Optom Physiol Opt. 1980 Aug;57(8): 485–507.

8. Hayashi T, Fatt I. A lubrication theory model of tear exchange under a soft contact lens. Am J Optom Physiol Opt. 1976 Mar;53(3):101–3.

9. Snyder AC, Schoessler JP. Corneal thickness changes associated with daily and extended contact lens wear. Am J Optom Physiol Opt. 1983 Oct;60(10):830–8.

10. Veys J, Meyler J, Davies I. Soft contact Lens fitting. In Essential Contact Lens Practice. A practical guide. Johnson & Johnson Vision care book. 2002, 49–60.

11. Harold A. Stein, Raymond M. Stein, Melvin I. Freeman. Soft contact len, Chapter 14. In The Ophthalmic Assistant: A Text for Allied and Associated Ophthalmic Personnel. 9th ed. 2013, Elsevier Saunders.

12. Martin D, Holden B. Forces developing beneath hydrogel contact lens due to squeeze pressure. Phys Med Bio 1986;30: 635–49.

Reader's Note

Reader's Note

Reader's Note

CHAPTER 8

Fitting a Toric Lens

A **toric lens** is a lens with different optical power and focal length in two orientations perpendicular to each other which is used to correct regular astigmatism.

Astigmatism is defined as that optical defect of the eye where due to variable refractive power of different meridians, a point focus of light cannot be formed on the retina.[1] A 'toric' surface is the name given to a refracting surface with two regular radii, one smaller than the other.

Physiological and Optical Concepts Relating to Toric Lens Fitting

a. **Lid movement/tension:** During blinking the upper lid pushes against superior edge of a contact lens, creates a rotational force which moves the lens medially and inferiorly or *down and nasal*. A toric lens design with differential thickness is more vulnerable to this nasal rotation. Due to greater mass of upper lid, versus lower lid, the former prevails and is the main destabilizing/stabilizing component for a toric lens. Lower lid, however, assumes an important role in cases of prism ballasted or truncated toric lens by holding and aligning the inferior lens edge and laxity or ectropion of lower lid can destabilize toric lenses of this design.

b. **Scissor action of lid closure:** *Scissoring action* of lids during closure, destabilizes a contact lens by subjecting it to torque. This torque or induced lens rotation has minimal visual significance for a spherical lens, but causes visual blur for a toric lens by altering its meridional orientation.

As evident from above discussion it cannot be reemphasized that lid factors like-lid tension (tight/flaccid), position (ptosis/ lid retraction) and palpebral aperture play very important roles in adequate functioning of a toric lens.

c. **Watermelon seed principle:** Visualize squeezing a fresh wet watermelon seed with its tapered edges between your thumb and forefinger. The pressing fingers generate force vectors, which aided by 'slippery' wet surface of the seed, expel it from your hand. Extrapolating a similar analogy to toric contact lens with its tapered lens edge (accentuated by prism ballast/double slab-off design), force vector or squeeze contributed by lid and moistness by tears, it is evident that CL faces same expulsion fate of the watermelon seed.[2]

d. **Tear flow:** Tear film, surface tension grips a contact lens tight onto the cornea by capillary action and aids centration. Poor tear volume and/or increased tear viscosity increases hydrostatic force on lens, increases rotational resistance and ultimately reduces lens movement.

e. **Gravity:** Since most stabilizing designs utilize gravity for alignment of a toric lens, where heavier part of lens lies on inferior cornea in erect position, any viewing activity involving reclining, supine or lateral positions results in visual blur.

f. **Lens profile facts:** Lens thickness profile is dictated by lens design, power and magnitude of astigmatic correction. Thinnest meridian of lens moves towards vertical axis during blinking, with the thin zone coming to rest under the upper eyelid. Thus lens movement around vertical axis is rotationally more stable due to direction of blink and thickness differential of lens design.

g. **Type of astigmatism:** Oblique astigmatism cases, *with the rule* and *against the rule* astigmatism result in unstable toric lens fit in descending order of occurrence due to rotational influences.

Types of Toric Lenses

A. **Based on stabilization designs:** To ensure optimal and stable vision a toric lens design needs to maintain meridional orientation to cylindrical axis of eye at all times, resisting destabilizing effect of blinking, eye excursions and tear flow. This requires an effective stabilization design providing rotational stability. Since a fixed lens without any rotational movement is extremely deleterious to corneal health, therefore *all stabilization designs must stop short of being too effective and permit a minimal lens movement.* The different types of designs for stabilizing a toric lens are: Prism ballasting, circular design, truncation, thin zone, peri-ballasting, reverse prism design.

  i. **Prism ballast:** This design creates an increased lens thickness in its inferior portion by incorporating a base down prism of 1 to 1.5 Δ D (prism dioptres). This greater inferior mass utilizes principles of gravity aided weight distribution for lens alignment. The design is based on *watermelon seed* principle and utilizes lid action on the differential thickness taper for proper lens orientation[2,3]

  Problems inherent to this design are:

  – The thickness differential causes **lower lid discomfort and lens feel** due to excessive edge thickness. This problem is partly solved by rounding both front and back surface.

  – Inferior lens thickness is proportional to amount of refractive error and is therefore more for high minus lenses. Such thick edges cause **limited lens movements**, inadequate tear exchange, poor lid resurfacing, 3 and 9 o'clock staining and inferior corneal edema.

  – Excessive prism weight causes lens to ride too low, on the other hand, insufficient prism weight is ineffective in preventing blink induced lens rotations.

  – **Prism induced vertical imbalance** in monocular fitting can cause aesthenopia and higher order aberrations.[4]

  ii. **Circular design:** In this design optical zone is centered using a lower diopter, base down prism. Lid dependency for lens stability is minimal and this design is preferred for patients with lax lower lids or large palpebral apertures. The back optic zone placed symmetrically around the geometric center, makes both manufacturing and reproducibility easier.

  iii. **Truncation/lower lid alignment:** In this design part of inferior lens along a chord length of 0.5–1.5 mm at 6 o'clock position is physically removed, to permit alignment with lower lid margin.[5] Amount of peripheral lens material removed in periphery is proportionate to minus power of lens. This material loss in high power minus lenses, leads to excessive lens rotation with altered dynamics which require additional balancing with prism ballasting. For plus powers, amount of peripheral material removed is less and does not require any compensation by prism ballasting.

Since a truncated lens with prism ballast often rides low, the optic zone needs to be offset superiorly by 0.5 mm in order to maximize pupil coverage and minimize flare. To ensure comfort with a truncated lens, edges of the truncated area also require rounding off.

Problems inherent to this design are:

– Since the truncated lens base has to be matched to lower lid contour, any lid margin pathology reduces effectiveness.

– Flat inferior lens edge causes chaffing and irritation of lid margin

– These lenses are difficult to manufacture and this design is used as a last resort.

In double truncation design, a superior truncation is added in order to increase lens stability and is used in case of tight upper lid or small palpebral apertures.

iv. **Thin zones/dynamic stabilization/ double slab off design:** In this lid dependent design, thin zones placed in superior and inferior zones, reduce peripheral lens thickness. Both lids can easily compress these thin zones and minimize rotation.

Variable lid tone in every individual, however, makes fitting of this lid tone dependent lens extremely individualized, with loose lid patients being poor candidates. Lens diameter needs to be larger to ensure adequate grasping of peripheral edge by lids.[6]

v. **Peri-ballast:** This design incorporates a minus carrier design with superior carrier being slabbed-off/chamfered to reduce its thickness. This slabbing creates a prism base down effect and allows lens periphery to be positioned under the lids. Inferiorly placed minus carriers increase inferior thickness, reduce oxygen transmissibility and induce discomfort along lower lid margin.[6]

vi. **Reverse prism designs:** This design incorporates a base down prism with inferior base up chamfer, thereby ensuring thinness and comfort. The base-to-base line is located *below* geometric center of lens, and prism is not present in optical zone.

Regardless of lens design, all toric soft lenses become bitoric *in situ* when fitted on a toric cornea. This occurs due to the fact that a soft lens conforms to corneal contour and its back surface in apposition to toric cornea, transmits the corneal toricity.

Remember for manufacturing convenience, most toric lenses are manufactured in plus cylinder form.

B. **Based on material**

i. **Soft toric lens:** They are manufactured by crimping or lathe techniques with lathes being used to grind powers of the principal meridians. Variable lens thickness in these lenses affects lens orientation and oxygen transmission.

Indications of soft torics:

• Lenticular or partly non-corneal astigmatism.

• Patients unable to adapt to RGP lenses.

• For astigmatism of >1.0 D, with sphere-cylinder ratio of < 4:1.

ii. **RGP toric lenses:** These lenses are relatively thick lenses with inherent issues like increased lens awareness, reduced oxygen permeability along with 3 and 9 o'clock staining. Lens edge profile has to be meticulously finished to circumvent these problems. The different types are: Front toric, back toric, bitoric or peripheral toric.

a. *Front toric RGP lenses:* These lenses incorporate an astigmatic correction on anterior surface with the posterior lens surface being spherical. They are used to correct *high corneal* astigmatism and residual asigmatism.

b. *Back toric RGP lens:* A spherical RGP lens with a spherical back surface corrects most of corneal astigmatism by virtue of tear lens beneath it (which neutralizes the corneal astigmatism). For a more toric cornea, a back surface toric design is used. The steeper meridian is fit 1/3–1/4th *flatter* than K and flatter meridian is fit on K. Fitting one meridian flatter allows for better tear exchange and fitting of flat meridian on cornea ensures stability. The slightly flat fitting generates a powered tear lens which contributes to total power, ensuring BVP required for steeper meridian to be less and lens to be both thinner and lighter.

c. *Bitoric RGP lens*: A bitoric lens incorporates an anterior toric surface which compensates for residual astigmatism induced by toric posterior surface. These lenses are used when back surface toric lens cause significant induced residual astigmatism

d. *Peripheral toric*: In conditions with excessive peripheral toricity like resolved pellucid marginal degeneration, simple toric lenses fit would result in excessive edge clearance in steep meridian, bubble formation, lens rocking and decentration. A lens with 0.4 – 0.6 mm wide toric peripheral curves distributes this edge clearance uniformly, over entire circumference and allows a smoother fit.

Most toric trial sets have diameter range from 8.80 to 9.20 mm, with small diameter lenses being preferred for fitting steep corneas and larger 9.20 mm diameter for flatter cornea.

Fitting Methodology

Basic principle to be adhered to in fitting a toric lens is to achieve stability of lens in primary gaze, post-blinking and during eye excursions so as to attain meridional orientation of cylindrical component. This is best done by a toric trial lens method.

In this method a trial lens which incorporates a cylinder close to axis and amount of patients' cylinder is fitted on the eye. The trial lens chosen incorporates cylinder with a particular stabilization feature representative of a series. It must be remembered that the final lens prescribed would also needs to be from same series as trial lens to ensure similar stabilization design and behavior.

Determination of cylinder is done with the help of a tracking mechanism. This tracking uses visible reference marks (line/ dot) on the lens surface which serves as *on eye ruler* for evaluating lens rotation and position. These markings made by laser/ mechanical etchings are present just inside lens edge either at vertical meridian (6 o'clock) or horizontally at 3 and 9 o'clock positions. These markings DO **NOT denote lens axis**. In grouped markings, the standard difference between two marks is usually 30°. Deviation of mark/s from its designated vertical or horizontal location quantifies lens mislocation/rotation. Most toric lenses rotate nasally by 5 to 10° (by convention, nasal rotation is rotation of **inferior base of lens**). Lens rotation is assessed from lens base and has to be checked in different positions of gaze especially near gaze.

The technique of fitting is detailed below:

Step 1: After allowing for **minimum stabilization of 10–15 minutes,** lens is checked for centration, stability and movement. An optimal fit covers the cornea, depicts adequate blink induced movement of <0.5 mm and shows a quick recovery on being displaced.

A tight fit centers well but depicts minimal movement and is slow to return to original axis if mislocated. A flat fit shows excessive movement, centers poorly and causes vision fluctuation.

Step 2: An optimal fit is the first step since inadequate fit (steep or flat), reduces effectivity of stabilization designs in orienting lens to cylindrical axis.

Step 3: For meridional stability the direction of rotation is noted from **practitioner's perspective (clockwise rotation is recorded as left and counterclockwise as right)**. Amount of rotation is assessed by clock hours of torsion, with one clock hour equaling 30°.

Step 4: Direction of rotation is evaluated by LARS **acronym** (Left Add, Right Subtract). This formula is used to compensate for rotation of trial lens as determined again from observer's point of view. If the practitioner looks at 6 **o' clock position** of lens, any rotation to the left /clockwise, is added to cylinder axis of spectacle/trial lens, i.e. **LA (left add)**. A rotation is to right, counterclockwise, looking at 6 **o' clock position of lens, is** subtracted from cylinder axis of spectacles, i.e. **RA (right subtract)**. An **axis mislocation greater than 25° requires refitting with a new trial lens.**

Step 5: A well-fitting lens is allowed a settling period of 10–15 minutes, after which a spherocylindrical over refraction is done. The spherical power determined by over refraction is added to spherical power of trial lens after compensating for vertex distance and final prescription is ordered. Theoretically cylinder and axis of over-refraction should coincide with initial ocular refraction. *In the event of this not happening, initial ocular refraction should determine final lens prescription.*

Flowchart 8.1 illustrates the fitting process.

Some Useful Facts

- Uncorrected astigmatism is more acceptable in nondominant eye.

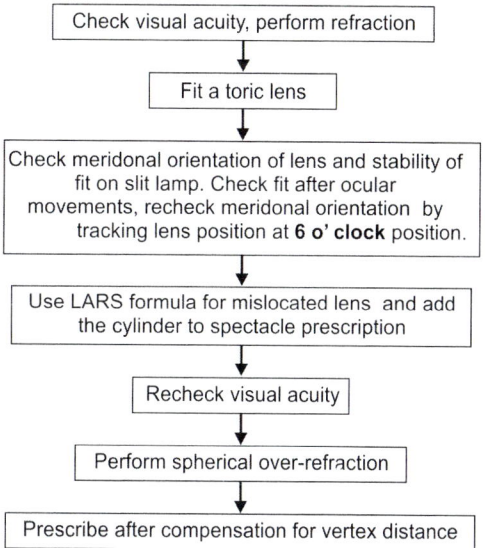

Flowchart 8.1: Fitting process

- **Oxygen transmissibility:** The incorporation of a cylinder along with means to stabilize axis by prism ballast or truncation, usually ensures that a toric lens is thicker than a spherical lens of similar power. This can cause central corneal oedema in hyperopic spherical components or corneal vascularization (inferior and superior) for myopic spherical components by adversely affecting oxygen transmissibility. Therefore, use of high oxygen permeability materials preferred.

- Soft torics are available up to 3.75 to 5 Dc. Customized torics can be made up to 10 Dc.

- Full corneal coverage with minimal movement of 0.2–0.5 mm is aimed at so as to ensure minimal effect of rotation on vision stability.

- Larger diameter (>13.5 mm) and lower water content also aids stabilization.

- **Large inventory of lenses is needed.** A trial set should contain common axis of 180° and 90° in powers ranging from +3 Ds to –3 Ds with BC from 8.5 to 8.7 mm. Maintenance of toric lenses is difficult and adequate hydration, cleaning needs to be done more frequently than for spherical lenses.

- **Dimensional stability:** Shape of toric lens must remain constant over time to ensure compatibility with anterior corneal surface and optical stability. This stability usually deteriorates with time affecting visual performance adversely.

REFERENCES

1. Abraham D. Astigmatism. In Abraham D Eds. Duke-Elder's practice of refraction. 8th ed. New Delhi, BL Churchill Livingstone, 1985, 52.

2. Hanks AJ. The watermelon seed principal CL Forum 1983, 8(9):31–35 IACLE module 3 Unit, 3.5, 233 pg.

3. Tomlinson A, Bibby MM. Movement and rotation of soft contact lenses. Effect of fit and lens design. Am J Optom Physiol Opt. 1980 May;57(5):275–9.

4. Berntsen DA, Merchea MM, Richdale K, Mack CJ, Barr JT. Higher-order aberrations when wearing sphere and toric soft contact lenses. Optom Vis Sci. 2009 Feb;86(2):115–22.

5. Tomlinson A, Bibby MM. Lid interaction and toric soft lens axis location. Am J Optom Physiol Opt. 1982 Mar;59(3):228–33.

6. Tan J, Papas E, Carnt N, Jalbert I, Skotnitsky C, Shiobara M, Lum E, Holden B. Performance standards for toric soft contact lenses. Optom Vis Sci. 2007 May;84(5):422–8.

Reader's Note

Reader's Note

CHAPTER 9

Fit on a Keratoconus Case

Keratoconus is a condition which is characterized by non-inflammatory corneal ectasia accompanied with corneal thinning. The diagnostic parameters of the condition are: Keratometry readings greater than 47 D, inferior corneal steepening greater than 1.20 D compared to superior cornea, and skewing of radial axis of astigmatism by more than 21°.[1,2] Corneal topographic evidence includes: Posterior elevation of >40 µ, irregularity and skewed radial axis in 3 and 5 mm zones and corneal thickness at thinnest point being <500 µ.[3] Primary keratoconus manifests during adolescent years and causes visual impairment due to irregular myopic astigmatism which very often requires visual rehabilitation with contact lenses.[4] The condition manifests as localized usually inferior corneal steepening, increase in myopic astigmatism and decrease in aided visual acuity with standard spectacles. Secondary keratoconus or keratectasia occurs as a sequel to kerato-refractive surgery, trauma or post-keratitis and is usually non-progressive.[5,6]

Contact lenses in this condition provide stable, comfortable vision once spectacles correction fails. Contact lenses succeed in providing better vision than spectacles due to their ability to neutralize irregular astigmatism by modifying the altered anterior optical surface. This neutralization is done more effectively with non-compliant rigid lens. Soft hydrogels by moulding onto anterior corneal surface transmit the corneal properties of irregular surface and are unable to mask the irregular astigmatism. This is corroborated by multicentric studies, including landmark Collaborative Longitudinal Evaluation of Keratoconus (CLEK) Study which report RGP lens usage in 65% of its patients.[4,7] In advanced conus, contact lens usage often averts the need for keratoplasty.[8] In those cases requiring keratoplasty, contact lenses again form the mainstay for correcting induced post-surgical astigmatism.[9] Thus lenses are very useful in visual rehabilitation of this disease.

Since this disease affects adolescents at high school or college levels, during period of intense study and when crucial decisions are being made regarding professional careers, a well-fitted lens goes a long way in shaping these young individuals life and personality.[10,11]

Clinical Aspects of Keratoconus Relevant to CL Fit

The incidence of the disease has increased from prior reported figures of 0.0003% per year to 2.3% in recent studies.[12–14] This increase can be attributed to advent of elegant imaging devices as first line diagnostic investigative modalities in managing irregular astigmatism and if so it is purely a 'tip of iceberg' phenomenon, with subclinical cases being unmasked. However, the phenomenal increase in incidence reported worldwide cannot solely be explained by better pick up rate of forme fruste or subclinical cases. Tear insufficiency subsequent to increased use of video display terminals during plastic stage of corneal growth could be an attributing factor. The associated conditions contributing to the disease are vernal catarrh, floppy eyelid syndrome, sinusitis, hay-fever, atopy and vigorous eye rubbing.[14,15] The latter seems to be definitely indicated as a causative agent since often the most affected eye is invariably the most rubbed eye.[15,16] Ethnicity also plays a role as Asians have a 4 to 8 times increased incidence compared to Caucasian counterparts with the disease manifesting at an earlier age.[17,18] The fact that atopy is less common in Asian population versus Caucasian reinforces role of genetic propensity in Asians.[19] Increased exposure to sunshine, UV light oxidative stress with dry hot climate of India and Middle East could be a possible factor responsible for higher prevalence of disease compared to cooler climes.[20]

Systemic co-morbidities associated with keratoconus are Down syndrome, connective tissue disorders like Ehlers-Danlos, Marfan's, Rieger's, Crouzon's and osteogenesis imper-

fecta. In Down syndrome incidence is often as high as 15% (300 times more than general population) and corneal hydrops occurs more frequently.

Staging of Disease

A. Videotopographic Keratoconus (Preclinical)

This is often the stage at which conus is diagnosed in current times of refractive surgery hopeful. These signs on topography are:

- Inferior steepening of cornea, distortion of photokeratoscope ring images, with narrower ring separations at area of greatest steepening.[21]
- Central or paracentral thinning of cornea, commonly seen in inferior or inferotemporal area with corneal thickness at thinnest point being <500 μ.
- Steeper corneal curvature and irregularity in 3 and 5 mm zones is classical. The topographic picture looks like a *red storm in the calm blue green corneal sea* (Fig. 9.1).
- Asymmetric bowtie (AB) patterns with skewed radial axes (SRAX). This is also known as lazy eight configuration.
- Higher mean posterior elevation of >40 μ.

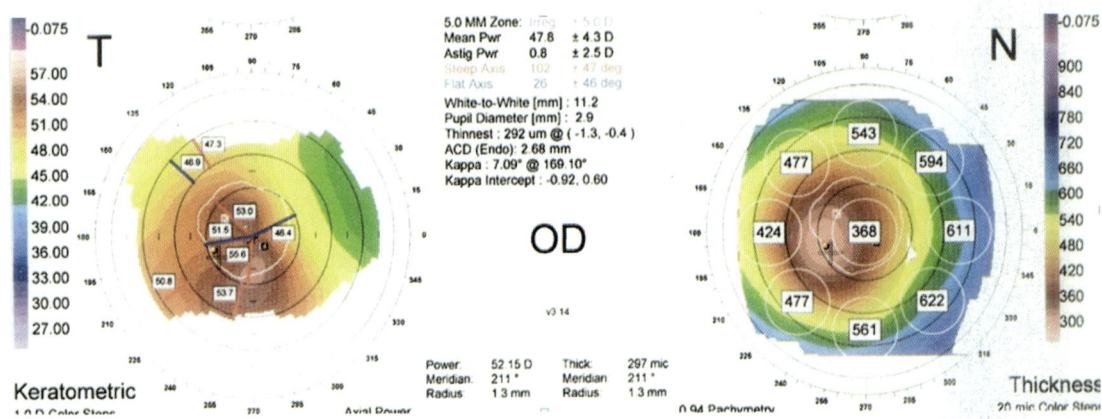

Fig. 9.1: Orbscan of keratoconus patient with steepening depicted by (hot colors) red orange surrounded by yellow and green

B. Clinical Keratoconus

- **Retinoscopy signs**

  The retinoscopy reflex is distorted, non-uniform and manifests as a 'swimming/swirling' effect known as *Charleux sign*. A refractile result of a well-delineated cone retro-illuminated, this sign is best appreciated on a dilated pupil. Shape, size and location of cone can be assessed using this reflex by means of a 4 D lens in Rekoss disc of a direct ophthalmoscope. *Scissoring motion* is another sign, which occurs due to irregular astigmatism. .

- Keratometry signs:

  These include poor focusing, distortion and inability to align mires and/or asymmetric steepening of mires inferiorly or centrally.

- Slit lamp signs (Fig. 9.2):
  - *Vogt striae*: These vertical, rarely horizontal or oblique lines in posterior stroma or Descemet's membrane of cone region represent collagen lamellae under stress. They have a parallel orientation to steepest axis of cone.[22,23]

  - *Fleischer's ring*: This partial or complete ring of iron accumulation surrounding base of cone occurs due to disruption of physiological process of epithelial cell sliding. This ring is best observed using cobalt blue illumination when it assumes a yellow or green color. Ring size is a good clinical tool to assess location and dimensions of the cone (Fig. 9.2).
  - *Prominent corneal nerves*

- Torch light/gross examination (Fig. 9.3):
  a. *Munson's sign:* This is the name given to conical corneal profile manifesting as V-shaped conformation or bulge in lower lid by the ectatic cornea in gaze down position. This sign is only evident in advanced conus.

  b. *Rizzuti's sign:* Formation of an intense, sharp nasal image anterior and parallel to iris plane of a pen light shining from temporal side, it occurs due to internal refraction. This sign can also be seen in high myopic astigmatism.

  c. *Intraocular pressure:* The reduced corneal, possibly scleral, rigidity in advanced keratoconus, causes an

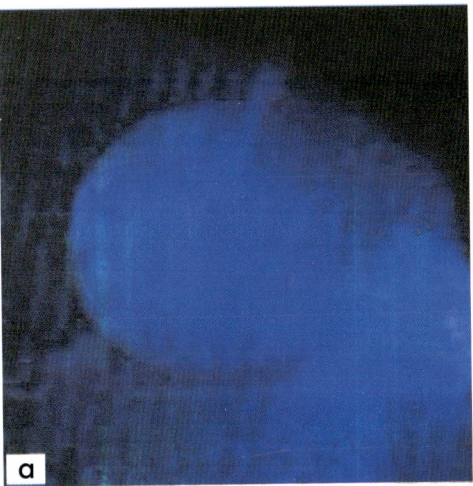

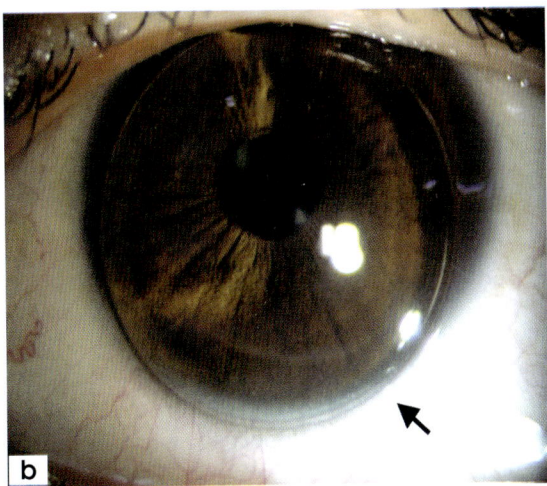

Fig. 9.2: Slit lamp signs: (a) Vogt sign; (b) Fleischer ring

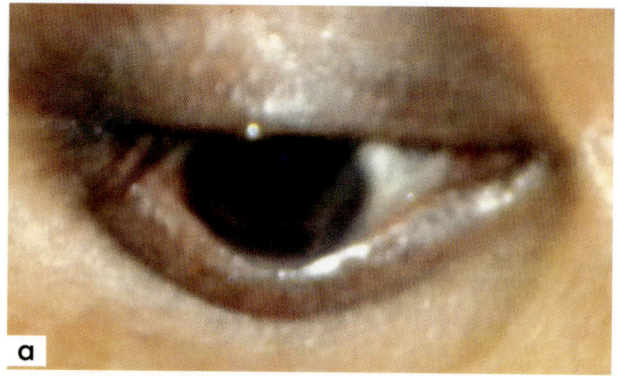 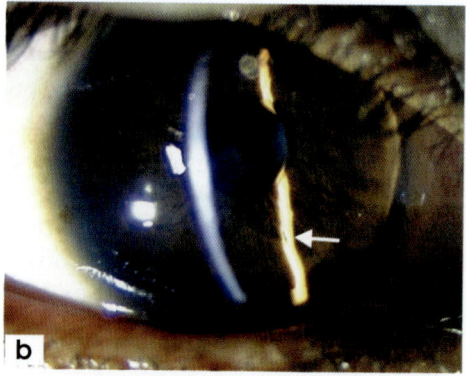

Fig. 9.3: Clinical features: (a) Munson sign; (b) Rizutti sign (note nasal crescentic reflection)

apparent lowering of IOP. In measuring IOP a correction factor for central corneal thickness needs to be applied. A value of 0.8 mmHg needs to be changed for every 10 µ (micron) variation from 520 µ. Corneas thinner than 520 µ need an add of 0.8 to the measured IOP for every 10 µ difference.

Keratoconus can be classified according to disease severity and cone type.

I. Severity

In terms of severity, keratoconus is quantified as mild with steepest keratometrey (K max) reading <45 D, moderate with K max 45–52 D, advanced as K max 52–65 D and severe with keratometry >62 D. Another classification scheme followed is of *Krumeich et al* depicted in Table 9.1.[24]

II. Types of Cones

The three morphological variants of cone are:

- **Nipple cone:** This is the term given to round, small diameter, steep cone with a short radius of curvature located centrally or slightly inferiorly (Fig. 9.4). Although causing significant visual compromise due to their location these cones are easiest to fit with conventional RGP lenses and sometimes even soft lenses.

Table 9.1: Krumeich staging of Keratoconus	
Stage	*Characteristics*
1.	Eccentric corneal steepening, induced myopia and/or astigmatism <5 Dc, corneal radii <48 D, Vogt stria, no central scarring.
2.	Induced myopia and/or astigmatism > 5 but < 8 Dc, corneal radii < 53 D, no central scars, corneal thickness > 400 µ.
3.	Induced myopia and/or astigmatism > 8 but < 10 Dc, corneal radii > 53 D, no central scars, corneal thickness > 200–400 µ.
4.	Refraction not measurable, corneal radii > 55 D, central scars, perforation, corneal thickness < 200 µ.

- **Oval/sagging cone:** These large diameter cones are usually located just inferior and temporal to corneal center (Fig. 9.5). Prone to corneal hydrops and subsequent scarring, they present a challenge to lens practitioner with problem of lens drop out and decentrations. Such cones often require fitting with large diameter lenses or posterior aspheric lenses.
- **Globus cone:** These very large base diameter cones involve more than 75% of corneal area (Fig. 9.6). Fortunately rare, globus cone induced overall steepening of the cornea is difficult to fit with corneal lenses and requires specialized lenses like Rose K or even minisclerals.

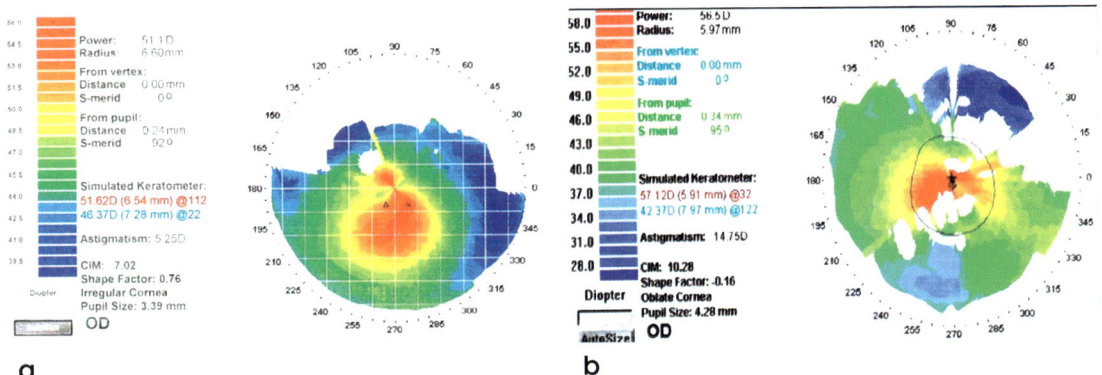

Fig. 9.4: Corneal topography of a keratoconus patient depicting Nipple cone: (a) Inferior location; (b) Central location

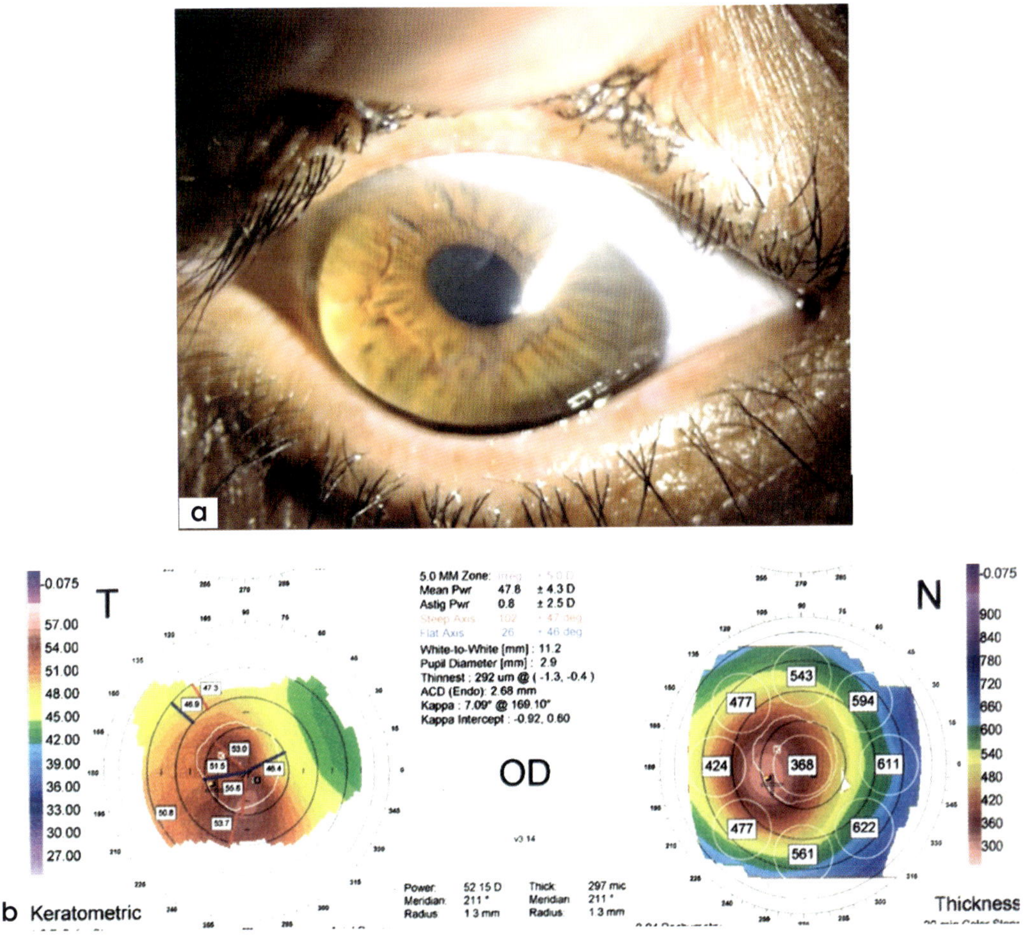

(a) — OD

Power:	51.1 D
Radius:	6.60 mm
From vertex:	
Distance	0.00 mm
S-merid	0 º
From pupil:	
Distance	0.24 mm
S-merid	92 º
Simulated Keratometer:	
51.62D (6.54 mm) @112	
46.37D (7.28 mm) @22	
Astigmatism: 5.25D	
CIM: 7.02	
Shape Factor: 0.76	
Irregular Cornea	
Pupil Size: 3.39 mm	

(b) — OD

Power:	56.5 D
Radius:	5.97 mm
From vertex:	
Distance	0.00 mm
S-merid	0 º
From pupil:	
Distance	0.34 mm
S-merid	95 º
Simulated Keratometer:	
57.12D (5.91 mm) @32	
42.37D (7.97 mm) @122	
Astigmatism: 14.75D	
CIM: 10.28	
Shape Factor: -0.16	
Oblate Cornea	
Pupil Size: 4.28 mm	

Fig. 9.5: (a) Oval sagging cone; (b) Orbscan of the same

5.0 MM Zone:
Mean Pwr 47.8 ± 4.3 D
Astig Pwr 0.8 ± 2.5 D

White-to-White [mm]: 11.2
Pupil Diameter [mm]: 2.9
Thinnest: 292 um @ (-1.3, -0.4)
ACD (Endo): 2.68 mm
Kappa: 7.09° @ 169.10°
Kappa Intercept: -0.92, 0.60

OD

v3.14

	Power	52.15 D	Thick	297 mic
	Meridian	211°	Meridian	211°
	Radius	1.3 mm	Radius	1.3 mm

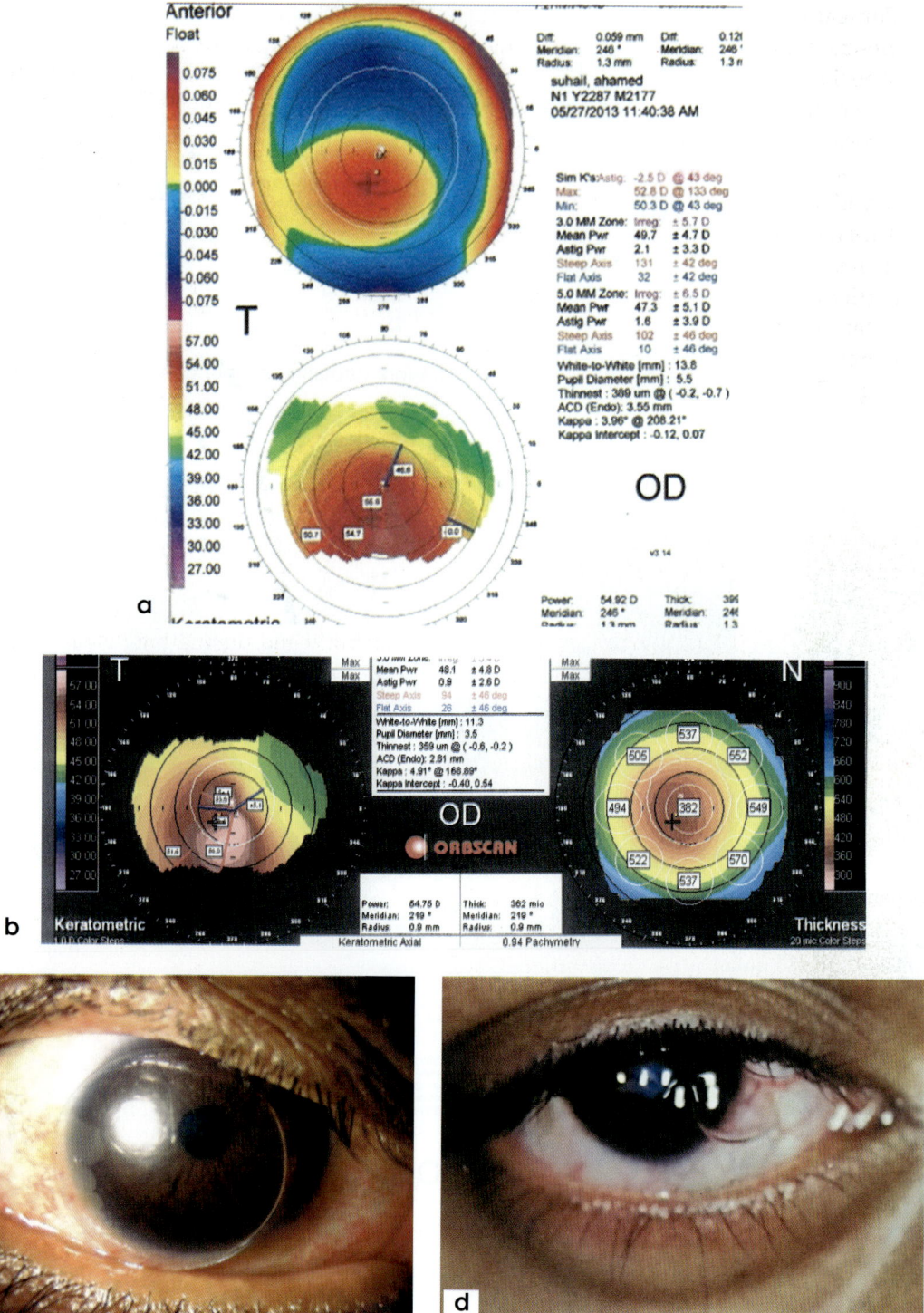

Fig. 9.6: Globus cone: (a and b) Corneal topography; (c and d) Poor centration of conventional RGP lens

– **Corneal hydrops:** This condition patient presents with sudden painful deterioration of vision due to a break in Descemet's membrane causing aqueous inflow into corneal stroma leading to corneal oedema. Visual deterioration persists for a considerable period of time ranging from 3 to 4 months, during which time posterior corneal integrity is re-established and barrier function is restored after scarring. After healing the apex of cone is often flattened resulting in improved lens fitting (Fig. 9.7).

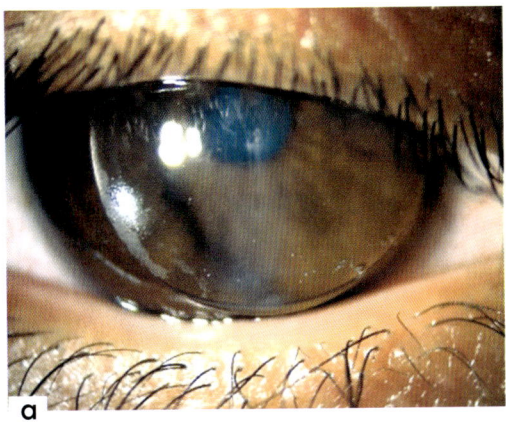

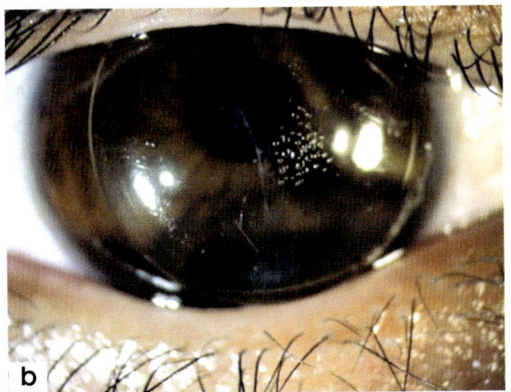

Fig. 9.7: Lens fit on patient after hydrops: (a) Note vertical break in Descemet's membrane; (b) Associated dimple veiling

Lens Fitting Tips

- Posterior surface of conventional contact lens are designed for standard prolate corneas. Since keratoconic corneal surface deviates from this default prolate shape, conventional lenses are not suitable for this condition. Specialized lenses designed with altered posterior spheres incorporating 3 to 4 back curves to accommodate rapid teeing off from steep apex to flatter mid-periphery and periphery are preferred for fitting.[25]

- Contact lenses *gravitate to steeper part of cornea*, which is central cornea for normal corneal contours. This fact aids proper centring of lens on optical axis by allowing rigid lenses to sit on central cornea. In keratoconic corneas, however, the steepest part is usually shifted inferiorly, and lenses gravitate to this inferior steep zone leading to inferior lid touch, discomfort, lens instability and fluctuating vision (Fig. 9.8).

- RGP material with high oxygen transmissibility of 60–100 plus with proven shape stability should be utilized for Kconus. Such lenses are: Flouroperm 90 (CLASSIC Bangalore, India), Silkens, Purecon (Mc Asfeer).

- Mild to moderate cones are fitted with traditional RGP or Rose K contact lens. In advanced cones small diameter (8.7 mm) lenses with base curve 0.2 mm steeper than mean K, can be tried.

- Many patients have associated atopy with lid thickening, blepharitis and floppy eyelids as a sequel of associated allergic diathesis or eye rubbing. Such lax lids require large diameter lenses, whereas tight lids mandate small diameter lenses so as to minimize lid awareness.

- In all fits, excessive bearing on apex of cone is to be avoided so as to prevent apical scaring. To prevent seal-off and lens adherence subsequent to steep peripheral curves, outer peripheral curves need to be

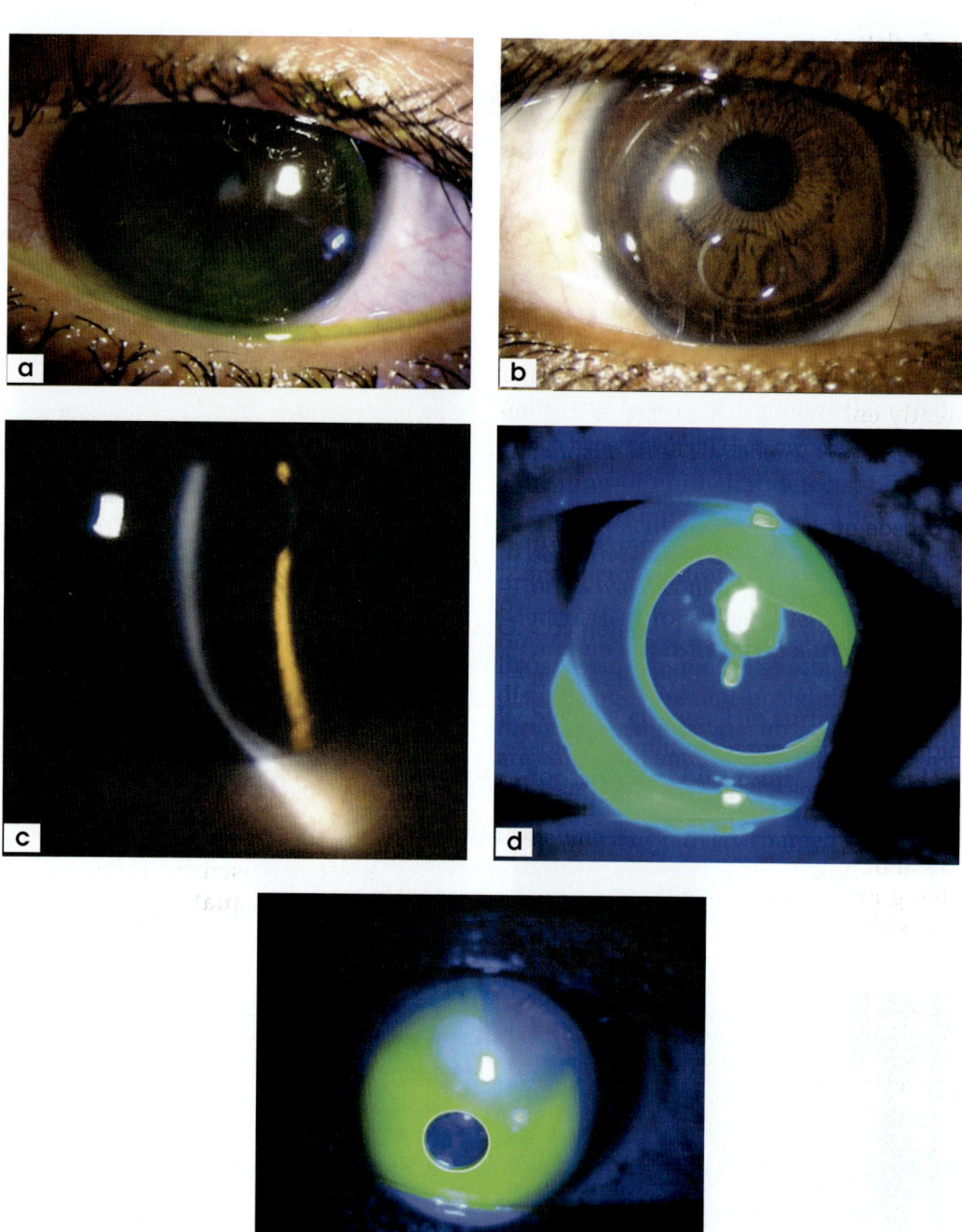

Fig. 9.8: (a and b) Lenses fitted on patients with inferior cone, depicting inferior gravitation of lens; (c) Slit lamp section shows inferior apex with corneal thinning; (d and e) Fluorescein patterns in an inferior positioned lens depicting excessive central cone bearing (an unacceptable fit)

made flatter and wider than conventional designs. Such modified lenses align with flatter superior cornea, redistribute pressure over peripheral cornea by incorporating a rapidly flattening periphery and minimize cone compression.

- Too flat, peripheral curves cause excessive lens movement and repeated lens dislodgement. Too flat a periphery can result in edge lift which causes *lens feel*, irritation and lens dislodgement (Fig. 9.9).
- Concomitant use of tear supplements greatly enhances comfort with a contact lens in keratoconus patients due to peripheral edge issues.[26]

Technique of Fitting

The lens to be selected depends on stage of disease and associated ocular morbidities and patient profile. For mild keratoconus, a soft or soft toric lens suffices but for most cases RGP lens is the lens of choice. Low minus power lens is used for mild keratoconus and high minus trial lenses for advanced cases. Choice of lens diameter is based on location of cone, size, and steepness.[27]

Trial is done from keratoconic set which comes in BC of 5.5 to 7.0 or often till even 7.65 (CLEK guidelines), power in both –3 and –6 Ds with overall diameters from 8.7 to

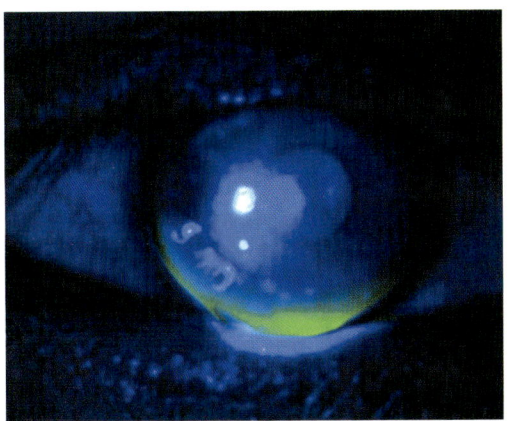

Fig. 9.9: Excess edge lift causing discomfort (in inferior located cone).

9.6 mm. Trial lens BC used has to be as close to midpoint of apical keratometric or videokeratoscopic values (mean K).

The CLEK nomogram dictates using a trial lens 2 dioptres flatter than K reading (K means flattest axis) for 45.0–50.0 dioptres, 3 dioptres flatter than K for 50–55 D, and 4 dioptres flatter than K for values between 55 and 60 dioptres.[28] The initial trial lens diameter should be kept small, a suitable starting point being 8.70 mm. Round nipple cones require diameters of 8.5 to 9.0 mm, whereas oval cones require larger diameter lenses, ranging from 9.2 to 9.7 mm. After lens insertion an adaptation period of 10–15 min is given and both dynamic and static fit are assessed.

Dynamic and static fit: While checking for dynamic fit, a lens movement of 1 mm with each blink needs to be ensured with good stability in different gazes, patient comfort and centration with optic zone covering mesopic pupil at all times. Fluorescein pattern should demonstrate feather apical touch, midperipheral bearing with sufficient edge lift and clearance of 0.5 to 0.7 mm.[29] Assessment of edge lift is equally if not more important as determining the central fit. Steep peripheral curves are diagnosed by restricted lens movement, inadequate peripheral tear reservoir, lens adherence and discomfort.[30] On the other hand, flat peripheral curves cause excessive edge lift with resultant excessive lens movement, repeated lens dislodgement along with lid irritation (Fig. 9.10).

The three different types of static fits (fluorescein pattern) are as follows.

  i. **Apical bearing/touch:** In this fitting pattern posterior surface of optic zone touches apex of cone (steepest part of cornea) and uses that as a fulcrum for its movement (Fig. 9.11). This leads to initial comfort and good, stable vision but causes scarring at apex due to inadequate tear exchange and friction.[31] Rarely heavy bearing can also cause corneal abrasion, epithelial breakdown and lens into-

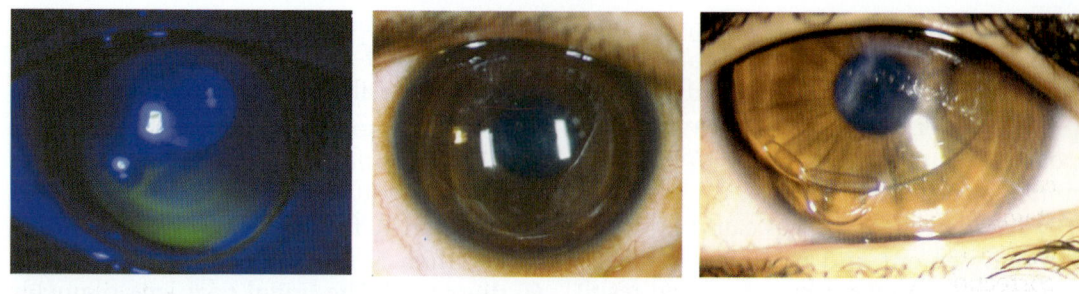

Fig. 9.10: Axial edge lift from 2 to 6 o'clock position causes excessive lens excursion and displacement

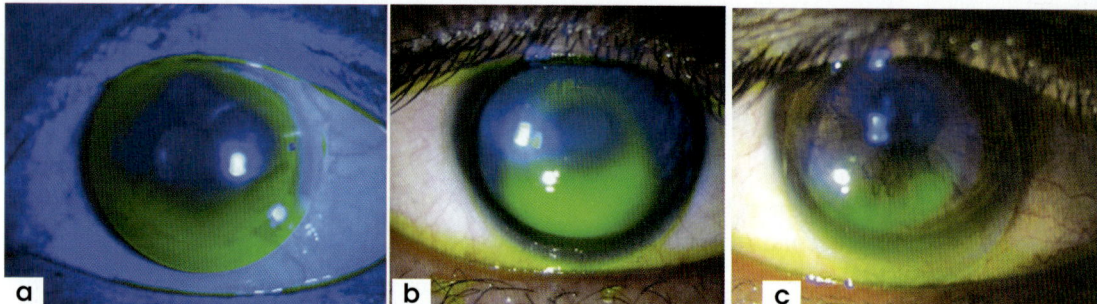

Fig. 9.11: Fluorescein fit demonstrating apical touch in central, superior and inferior area

lerance. This type of fit is thus to be avoided.

ii. **Apical clearance:** In this fitting pattern posterior surface of lens vaults or clears the cone apex and lens support is redirected to paracentral cornea (Fig. 9.12).[28] This technique minimizes apex scarring, whorl keratopathy and corneal staining but is often unacceptable due to uncorrected corneal astigmatism and suboptimal vision. Hard squeeze blinks, pathologic levels of intraocular pressure with vigorous eye rubbing, increase distending forces on apex of cone in apical clearance fits which can accelerate risk of progression.[32,33] Lenses exhibiting apical clearance also have a steep back optic zone radius which is often associated with a smaller back optic zone and smaller overall diameter. Since apex of cone is invariably eccentric from visual axis, lens edge or transition of optic zone often

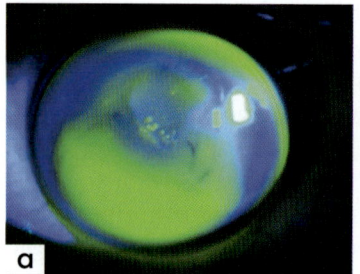
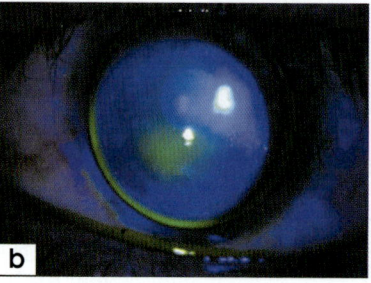
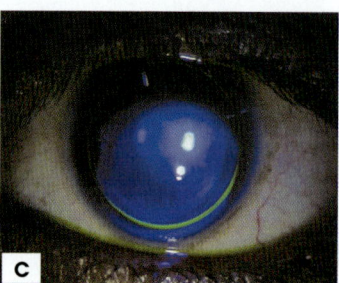

Fig. 9.12: (a) Fluorescein pattern depicting apical clearance over inferior nipple cone; (b and c) The small diameter lens with apical clearance centers well on the eye, but has a reduced peripheral clearance

traverses part of scotopic pupil resulting in flare, monocular diplopia and poor vision in dim light.

In such fits tightening at periphery can cause peripheral 'seal-off' giving rise to a stagnant post-lens tear film which creates a *plus tear lens*.[34] Such a fit requires correction with a more minus powered contact lens to achieve similar dioptric effect.

iii. **Three-point touch/divided support:** This is the *golden mean* fit, between apical bearing and apical touch. It utilizes *divided support* principle by distributing weight of lens over a large area where lens rests lightly on cone apex (feather touch), nasal mid-periphery and temporal mid-periphery. This pattern involves light apical feather touch of 2–3 mm, surrounded by an intermediate clearance zone, a mid-peripheral contact annulus (bearing), a 0.5–0.7 mm edge lift and clearance at lens periphery (*bull's eye pattern*) (Fig. 9.13). As cone advances, lens edge may stand off with pooling and air bubbles under inferior peripheral edge.

This fit minimizes risk of apical scarring, facilitates tear exchange, long-term comfort and stable vision.

After finalizing fit, lens power is finalized by over-refraction through *trial lens which has the same back surface design as final lens to be ordered.*

Specialized Lenses for Keratoconus

A. **Multicurve spherical and aspheric lenses:** Multicurve spherical lenses have a steep spherical central curve in optical center followed by multiple progressively flatter curves in non-optical periphery. Some prototypes are:

– *Soper lens*—a bicurve lens design with steep optical portion and a flatter second curve, with a carrier width of 2.0 mm.

– *McGuire design* incorporates central steep curve with four additional progressively flatter peripheral curves.[35]

These multicurve lens designs fit round nipple cones very well.

B. **Rose K lenses** (Menicon Co. Ltd, Nagoya): These are one of the most commonly used lenses for cases of corneal irregularities. A detailed description of types and techniques of fitting is given below.

Designed by Dr Paul Rose these specialized lenses have a small posterior optic zone with multiple peripheral lens edge options to minimize corneal impingement and aid centration on irregular corneas.[36–38]

The lens has aberration controlled aspheric optics on front surface generated by computerized lathes. The semi-finished lenses require only light polishing at the finishing laboratory. The back surface design is spherical, conical, aspheric or reverse geometry depending on corneal condition.

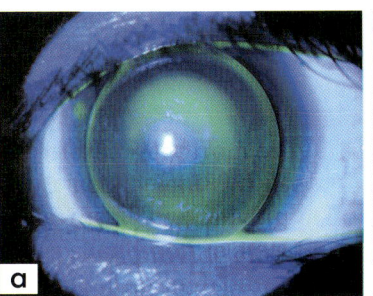 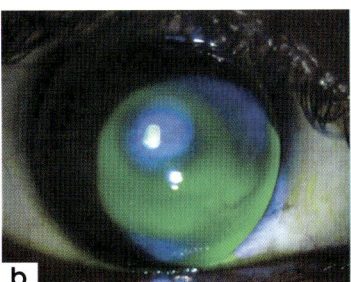 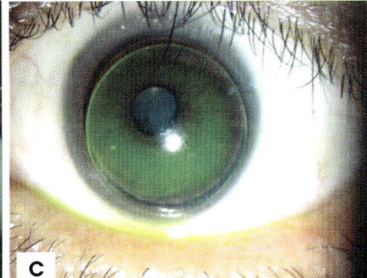

Fig. 9.13: Three-point touch with central feather clearance in a nipple cone. Ideal fit

They are manufactured in six designs: Rose K2 (for fitting oval cones), Rose K2 NC (for nipple cones), Rose K2 IC (for irregular corneas like post-Lasik, PMD, post trauma/keratitis), Rose K2 PG (for post-graft/post-surgical cases), Rose K2 XL Semi Scleral lens and Rose K2 soft lens.

- The prototype *Rose K2* is used to fit oval and early nipple keratoconus and even early pellucid marginal degeneration (PMD). The trial set comes with BC from 4.30 to 8.60 mm, diameters from 7.9 to 10.4 mm and has standard edge lift design which is adequate for most cases.

- *Rose K2 NC* lens is used to fit nipple cones and is available in BC range 4.3 to 7.70 mm with diameter of 7.6 to 9.0 mm. The peripheral edge lift for Rose K2 and K2 NC is available as increased edge lift from 0 (standard) to increased (+) 4.00 in 0.10 steps. Decreased edge lift is available from 0 (standard) to decreased (–) 1.30 in 0.10 steps.

- *Rose K2 IC* is used to fit early/moderate PMD, early keratoglobus, LASIK induced ectasia/irregularity, corneal scars post trauma and keratitis. It may be useful to try this type in oval keratoconus with very inferior cone not being fit with Rose K2. These lenses are available from BC of 5.70 to 9.30 mm, in diameters of 9.4–12.0 mm. Edge lift is available as standard (0), standard flat (+1.00), standard steep (–0.50), double flat (+2.00) and double steep (–2.00).

- *Rose K2 PG (postgraft)* is a reverse geometry back surface design lens used to fit post-keratoplasty cases primarily and also large ablated corneas post-LASIK irregularities. Available in base curves ranging from 5.70 to 9.30 mm, diameters of 9.4 to 12.0 mm, with edge lift of standard (0), standard flat (+1.00), standard steep (–1.00), double flat (+2.00) and double steep (–2.00). Early grafts are usually flatter than donor/host interface,

the latter having raised steep areas of scar tissue. This results in decentration of lens towards steepest cornea and can be rectified by using steeper, larger lenses.

- *K2 XL* is a **Corneo-Scleral design** made of Boston XO (100 Dk M/H), Menicon Z (189 Dk FATT), Optimum Extra (100 Dk M/H) or Optimum Extreme (120 Dk M/H) material and used in fitting irregular corneas intolerant to any lens type. It has an aspheric back optic zone (BOZ) which decreases as BC steepens and reverse geometry design for flatter base curves. Front surface has aberration control with edge lift (EL) from –3.00 to +3.00. Lens diameter ranges from 12.60 to 16.00 mm, back curvature optic radius (BCOR) from 5.60 to 8.6 mm. The manufactures guide recommends choosing first trial lens based on the pathology. For keratoconus a graph which relates to mean K is used, in PMD 0.6 mm steeper than mean K, in post-graft/post-LASIK 0.7 mm steeper and only 0.1 mm steeper in corneal ring/INTACS patients.

- *Rose K2 soft lens* is a daily wear (DW) lens made from Lagado silicone hydrogel (LSH Dk 49) or Menicon 72 hydrogel (MH). High oxygen transmission of these materials allows them to be made thick enough to prevent transmission of optics of irregular corneal shape. It is of reverse geometry design lens with spheric back OZ combined with front surface toricity and surface aberration control. The toricity requires prism ballast technology for stabilization and has options for 5 edge lifts: Standard (0), standard increased (+1.0), double increased (+2.0), standard decreased (–1.0) and double decreased (–2). If asked for, the manufacturers are able to incorporate an ACT option to aid fitting.

The lens is available in BC ranging from 7.4 to 9.0 mm in 0.2 increments with diameters from 14.3 to 15.3 mm in

0.1 increments, standard diameter being 14.80 mm. Power available is –30 D to +30 D and cylinder from–0.25 D to –10.00 D in 0.25 D increments in 0° to 180° axis. The recommended replacement schedule for these DW lenses is 3 months for LSH lenses and 6–12 months for MH.

The manufacturers propagate use of these lenses in patients intolerant to RGP lenses, working in environs or indulging in sporting activities unsuitable for RGP wear, or early keratoconus cases having suboptimal vision with conventional soft lenses or spectacles.

Figure 9.14 gives a thumb sketch of the type of Rose K lenses to be used according to corneal topography/pathology.

The fitting guide recommends these lenses to be fitted in 5 steps in the following order. Evaluation of central fit, evaluation of peripheral fit, checking for overall diameter, lens location and finally lens movement. Selection of first trial lens is based on mean K or mean 3 mm Sim K.

Initial trial lens selection depends on type of lens and extent of disease.

Rose K2: Oval/nipple kconus : For mean K of 7.1 or flatter, first trial lens selected is 0.2 steeper than average K. For a mean K between 6.0 and 7.0, the average K should determine first trial lens. For steeper corneas with average K of 5.9 or more, trial lens should be 0.4 flatter than average K.

The strategy is to fit steeper initially and subsequently modify the BC until a light

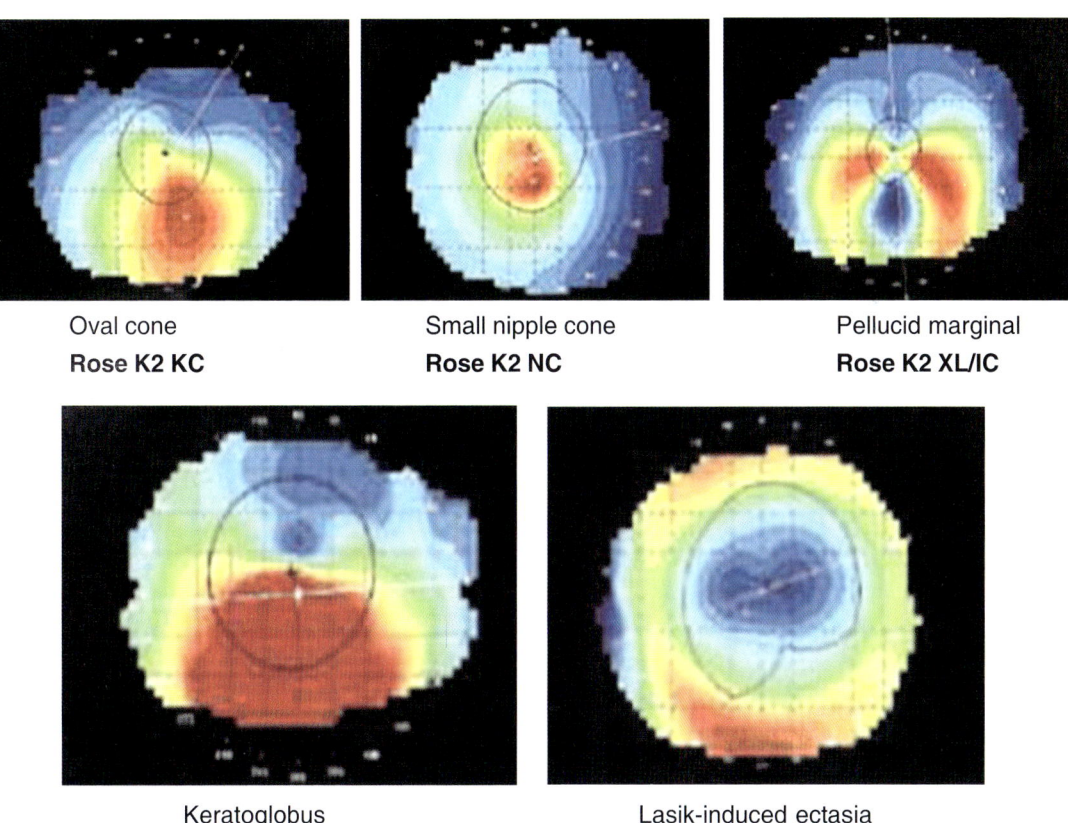

| Oval cone | Small nipple cone | Pellucid marginal |
| **Rose K2 KC** | **Rose K2 NC** | **Rose K2 XL/IC** |

| Keratoglobus | Lasik-induced ectasia |
| **Rose K2XL/IC** | **Rose K2 IC/PG/XL** |

Fig. 9.14: Rose K lens choice as per corneal topography (reprinted with permission from Menicon)

feather touch is first achieved at apex of cone. Poor visibility of cone indicates steep fit. In cases of unexplained poor vision a slight flattening of BC by 0.1–0.2 mm can be tried.

Rose K2 NC (nipple cones only): The first trial lens depends on severity of disease. In mild to moderate disease with mean K flatter than 6.0 mm, first trial lens selected is 0.2 mm steeper than average K. In advanced disease with mean K values of 5.1–6.0 mm, first trial lens equals mean K and for severe disease with mean K steeper than 5.0 mm, it is 0.3 flatter than mean K.

Rose K2 IC (fitting for PMD, keratoglobus, LASIK ectasia/postgraft): The initial trial lens selected is 0.3 mm flatter than steep K meridian.

For Rose K2 postgraft fitting: The initial trial lens is 0.3 mm steeper than mean K.

Table 9.2 gives a guide to initial trial lens BC.

Step 1: Central fit: The central fit should be assessed immediately post-blink with lens centered over pupil. An ideal BC selection aims for *a feather touch at cone apex* except K2 NC design where slightly greater touch is required (Fig. 9.15). In Rose K IC series, for PMD/keratoglobus/post-keratoplasty again a light feather touch is desirable over highest point on the cornea which is often not central.

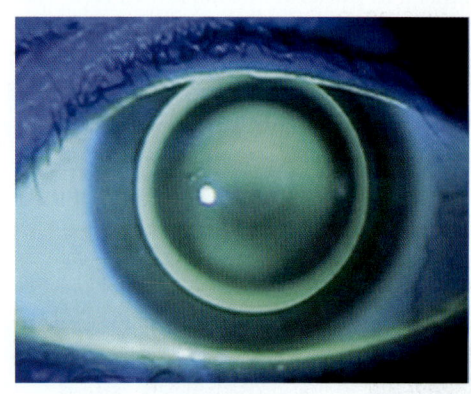

Fig. 9.15: Bull's eye pattern with feather touch at inferior cone

Table 9.2: Guide to initial trial lens BC (reprinted with permission from Menicon)[39]			
Rose K2	*Rose K2 NC*	*Rose K2 IC*	*Rose K2 Postgraft*
Oval keratoconus. Nipple keratoconus	Nipple cone only	Pellucid marginal degeneration, keratoglobus Lasik-induced ectasia and postgraft	For patients who have undergone penetrating keratoplasy
• For K reading 7.1mm and flatter select first trial lens is 0.2 mm steeper than the mean K reading • For K reading from 6.0 to 7.0 mm, select the first trial lens equal to the mean K reading. • For K reading 5.9 mm steeper, select the first trial lens 0.4 mm flatter than the mean K reading (less predictable).	• For mild to moderate cases (where mean K reading is flatter than 6.0 mm), select a first trial lens 0.2 mm steeper than mean K. • For advanced cases (where mean K measures between 5.1 and 6.0 mm), select a first trial lens equivalent to the mean K reading. • If using a corneal topographer, select the first trial lens based on the 3.0 mm Sim K.	**PMD and Globus** Select the first trial lens 0.3 mm flatter than steepest corneal meridian **post-Lasik and graft,** refer to Rose K post-graft section	Select the first trial lens 0.3, steeper than average **K reading.**

In postgraft cases using Rose K2IC or K2 PG series an apical clearing of 0.2–0.3 mm is aimed for in younger oblate or flatter grafts and closer alignment or 0.1 mm flat fit in older grafts.

A common problem is pooling at base of cone which is rectified by reducing OD resulting in reduction of back OZ resulting in a close to cone fitting. Flattening of BC or increasing peripheral lift are other options (Fig. 9.16).

Step 2: Evaluate **peripheral fit/edge lift (EL):** Peripheral fit determines lens movement, tear flow, comfort and ultimate success of lens wear and is assessed in horizontal meridian which is normally where the edge lift is least due to associated *with the rule* astigmatism. It is assessed only once lens has been centralized by manipulating it through eyelid with patient gazing straight ahead.

Edge lift is the term used by Rose K manufacturers to denote optimal peripheral configuration. Fluorescein stained tear film should be able to circulate with a blink under lens edge generating an even band of 0.5 to 0.8 mm.

Approximately 85 % of Rose K lenses fitted use one of the 3 standard edge lifts, 60% standard edge, 20% standard flat (+1.0 flat/increased) and 15% standard steep (–0.5 steep/decreased) for desired peripheral fit. Edge Lift can be specified in 0.1 increments from –1.3 decreased (steep) to +3.0 increased (flat).

Excessive edge lift contributes to lens instability and thus should be avoided. Insufficient edge lift, on the other hand, indents cornea and leads to lens intolerance and 3 and 9 o'clock staining. Early keratoconus cases often require steeper peripheral curves along with larger diameter lenses and advanced cases, flatter peripheral curves (increased edge lift) with smaller diameters. In Rose K2 XL, edge lift can also be altered by changing lens diameter. Narrow band/insufficient fluorescein is corrected by increasing lens diameter or lift and wider band/excess fluorescein by decreasing lens diameter or edge lift.

Irregular band implies presence of peripheral astigmatism and for doubtful situations a flatter or excess lift is preferred over a tight edge.

Rose K2 NC design incorporates a very small posterior back OZ with rapid peripheral flattening. Edge lifts can be ordered in 0.1 steps from –1.3 decreased to +4.00 increased. However, in Rose K2 IC and Rose K2 postgraft series EL options are standard (0), standard steep (decreased –1.00), standard flat (increased +1.00), double steep (–2.00) or double flat (+2.00) (Fig. 9.17).

The final lens is automatically compensated for base curve and power by the manufacturing laboratory so that a change in EL which concomitantly alters sagittal height of lens fit does not affect the final lens central fit.

Unequal corneal flattening around the clock, causes differential edge lift in vertical or horizontal meridians. In such asymmetric corneas, with excessive edge lift in vertical meridian (12 and 6 o'clock) or insufficient in horizontal (3 and 9 o'clock) advance fitting options such as toric (TP design) are used (Figs 9.18–9.21 depict various types of edge life)

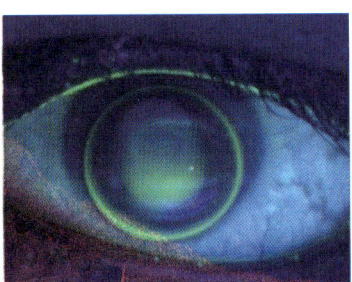 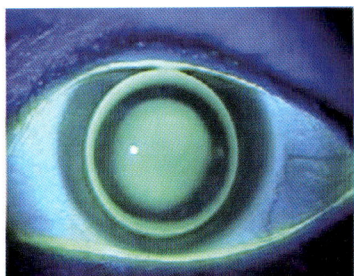 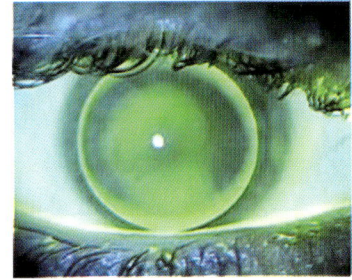

Fig. 9.16: Sequential fitting of starting steep with progressively flattening lens to final optimum fit

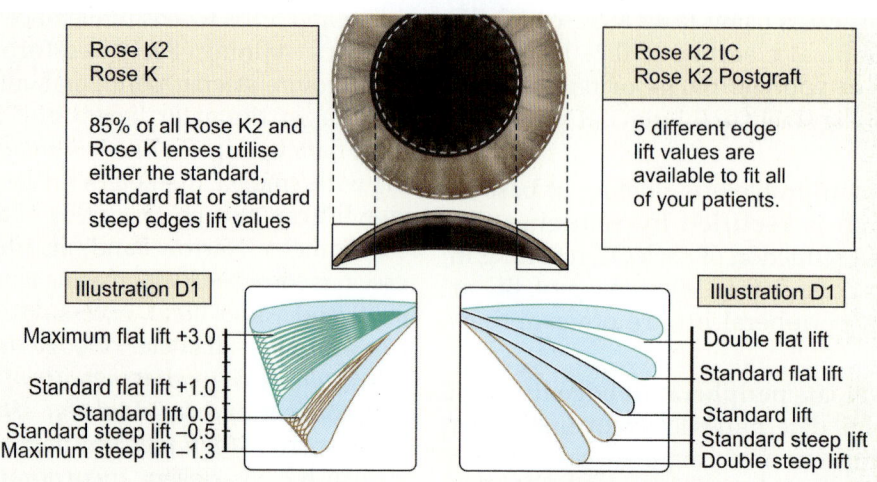

Rose K2 Rose K	Rose K2 IC Rose K2 Postgraft
85% of all Rose K2 and Rose K lenses utilise either the standard, standard flat or standard steep edges lift values	5 different edge lift values are available to fit all of your patients.

Illustration D1

Maximum flat lift +3.0
Standard flat lift +1.0
Standard lift 0.0
Standard steep lift –0.5
Maximum steep lift –1.3

Illustration D1

Double flat lift
Standard flat lift
Standard lift
Standard steep lift
Double steep lift

Fig. 9.17: Edge lifts profile in Rose K lens types (reprinted with permission from Menicon)

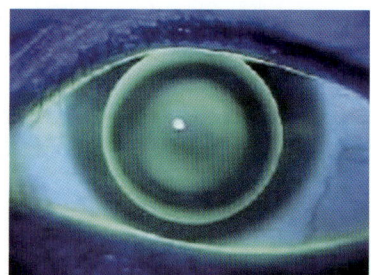

Fig. 9.18: Optimal edge lift

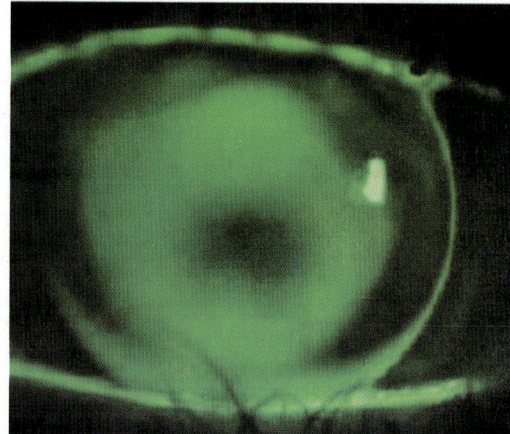

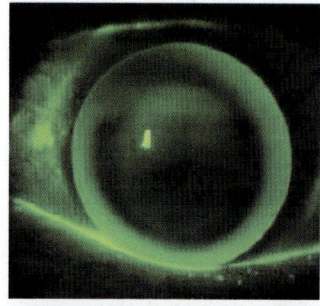

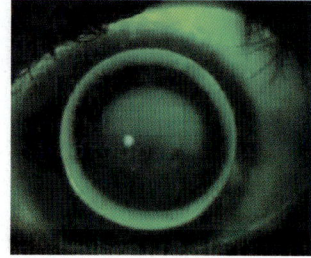

Fig. 9.19: Excessive edge lift

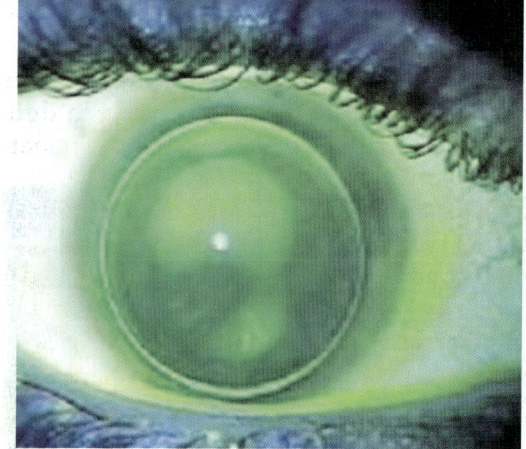

Fig. 9.20: Inadequate edge lift/tight fit

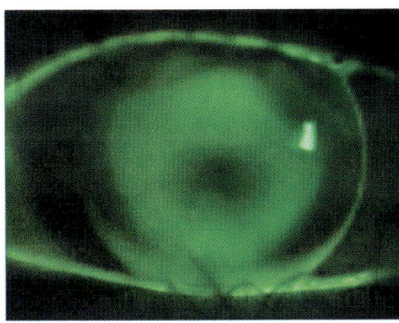

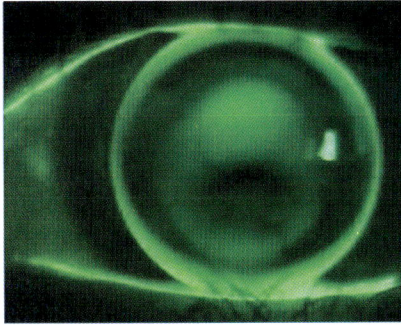

Fig. 9.21: Inadequate edge lift: Tight in the fit on top, which has been modified in fit on bottom by incorporating 1.3 increased lift

For cases with significant edge standoff/ lift off at or around 6 o'clock, asymmetric corneal tuck (ACT) is resorted to whereby lens is tightened in one quadrant. These advanced options are explained on pages 115–116.

Step 3: Assess lens **Overall diameter (OD):** Available lens diameter range from 7.90 to 12.00 mm depending on design. Lens diameter affects lens location, lens movement, lens stability and ultimately lens tolerance. Larger diameters are required for early keratoconus, larger cones, postgraft, irregular scarred corneas and wider palpebral apertures. Smaller diameters lenses are tried in advanced keratoconus, smaller cones and patients with smaller palpebral apertures. The commonest diameter used in Rose K2 is 8.7 mm with a 0.3 mm change being significant. An optimal OD lens aims for lens edge touching upper lid margin also called *hanging off the upper eye lid/lid attachment fit*.

The decision to alter the standard diameter is taken according to the following factors:

a. *Cone severity*: Larger diameters are preferred for early cones, and for patients with PMD to ensure centration and stability. Larger diameter lenses tend to ride higher. For advanced cones smaller diameters need to be considered.

b. *Palpebral aperture*: Larger diameters are preferred for larger palpebral aperture cases. A 9.0 mm diameter is starting lens for larger apertures. *Smaller diameters are required for smaller palpebral apertures.*

c. *Low riding lenses*: The solution is to increase diameter by minimum of 0.3 mm. Another method recommended in manufacturing guide is to measure distance between lower borders of upper lid to upper border of CL. Half of this distance is then added to lens OD for final prescription.

d. *High riding lenses:* The remedy is to reduce OD by at least 0.3 mm.

e. *Corneal staining*: Superior limbal staining necessitates reduction of OD by 0.3 mm. Three and nine o'clock staining imply a lens with larger than required OD, with remedy being reducing diameter by minimal of 0.3 mm. Another option to prevent these staining is to increase edge lift.

f. *Excessive edge lift*: In this situation reduction of diameter and/or steepening of edge lift is the solution.

g. *Vision problems*: Patients who complain of ghosting due to optic zone (OZ) traversing only part of scotopic pupil, increase in diameter with concomitant increase of OZ reduces ghosting and visual blur.

Decisions to alter diameter and/or peripheral systems would change sagittal height and therefore central fit, *e.g. increase diameter would cause base curve flattening*. When these alterations are being incorporated, a fresh calculation needs to be done to generate an appropriate BC ensuring similar sagittal height and central fit (Fig. 9.22). Lens power

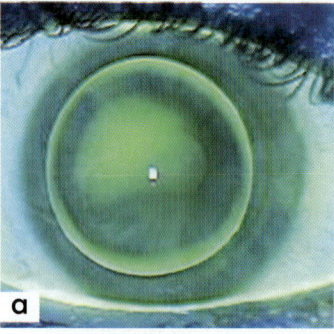 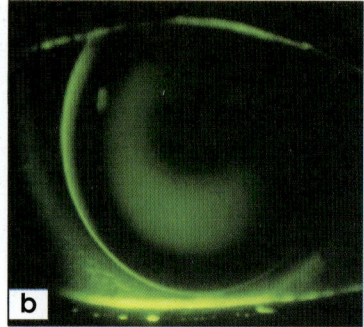 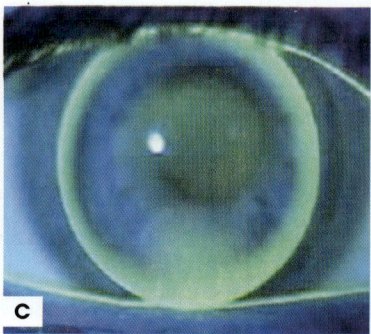

Fig. 9.22: Fluorescein pattern detailing different types of overall diameter lenses; (a) Small insufficient corneal coverage; (b) Large beyond limbus and under top lid (c) Optimal pattern

also alters to compensate for BC change and is calculated by laboratory before finalizing final lens, e.g. altering standard peripheral lift to standard increased lift, BC is compensated by steepening it by 0.05 m and power requires an add of 0.25 D.[39]

Another aspect affecting OD is lens designs with Rose K standard set being available from 7.9 to 10.4 mm, postgraft from 9.4 to 12.0 mm (std 10.4) and IC from 9.4 to 12.0 mm (std 11.4 mm) (Fig. 9.23). For Rose K2 and NC trial set no standard diameter exists as diameter decreases in steeper BC.

Step 4: Evaluate **location of** lens: Location is controlled mostly by overall diameter and less so by edge lift. Low riding lenses settling beyond the limbus are the biggest issue with irregular corneas and cause discomfort, flare/ghost images and lens loss. The modification required is to increase OD, increase edge lift

or flatten BC. A high riding lens, on the other hand, can be optimally positioned by decreasing OD, decreasing edge lift or steepening BC (Fig. 9.24).

The solutions adopted in case of suboptimal location are:

– *High riding lens*: Tighten edge lift, reduce OD, steepen BC
– *Low riding lens*: Increase edge lift, increase OD, flatten BC, address any astigmatism

Step 5: Assess lens **movement:** Movement is primarily controlled by edge lift. A 1–2 mm movement post blink is optimal for tear exchange. Post-blink movement should suffice to carry lens back to its original position of rest. Restricted lens movements cause peripheral corneal drying and staining and indicate a steep fit. Flatter, smaller lenses and those with increased edge lift manifest increased movement.

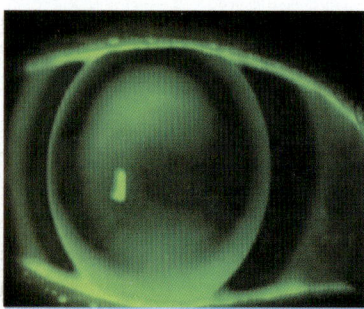 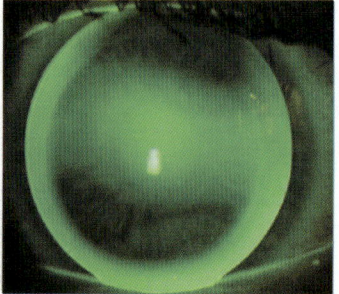 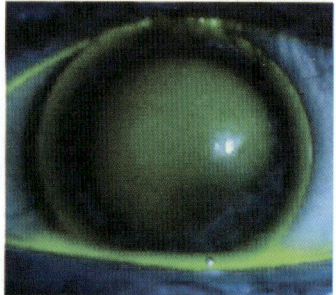

Rose K2   **Postgraft std 10.4 mm**   **IC–std 11.4 mm**

Fig. 9.23: Different diameters used for different corneal conditions

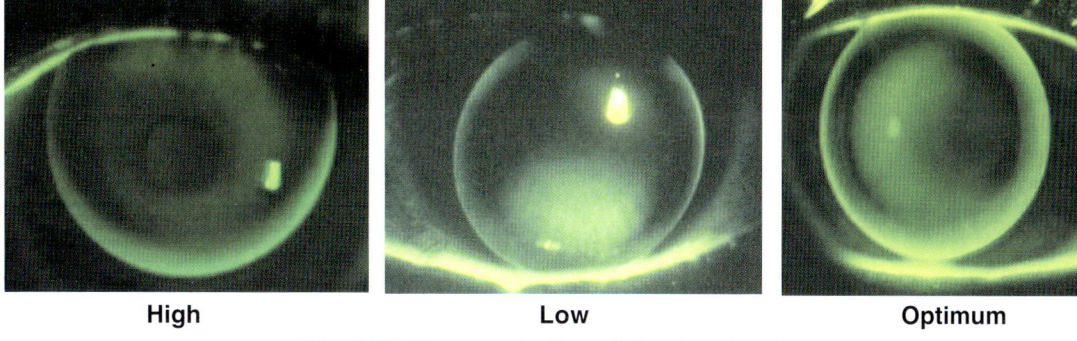

High   **Low**   **Optimum**

Fig. 9.24: Fluorescein fit depicting lens location

Others aspects to be looked for in sequence, in addition to above big 5 of central fit, peripheral fit, edge lift, lens location and movement are:

- **Bubbles/dimple veiling:** Presence of bubbles under lens, indicate poor fit and lead to corneal staining, visual blur and lens intolerance if not corrected. Solutions to rectify dimple veiling are flatten BC, increase edge lift or decrease overall diameter. If despite these the bubbles persist, fenestration of lens at junction of OZ and second curve can be asked for.

- **Advanced fitting options:** These advanced options are: Toric peripheral curves (TP), quadrant specific asymmetric corneal technology (ACT) and toric back/front and bi-toric surface options.

- **Asymmetric corneal technology (ACT):** The usual presentation of keratoconic cornea is asymmetric with inferior quadrant steeper than superior portion, resulting in edge lift at 6 o'clock. In such a situation ACT technology is asked for, to provide alignment at 3, 9 and 12 o'clock and more optimal fit at 6 o'clock (Fig. 9.25). The ACT design is independent of primary BC and EL values and is available for Rose K2, Rose K2 IC, Rose K2 postgraft lens designs. The three grades of ACT available are:
  - *Grade 1 (0.7 mm): Provides slight edge stand off, with pooling at or around 6 o'clock*
  - *Grade 2 (1.0 mm): Provides moderate edge stand off, with pooling and possible bubble at/around 6 o'clock (between 4 and 8 o'clock). The tear meniscus may break up on blinking.*

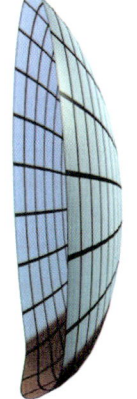
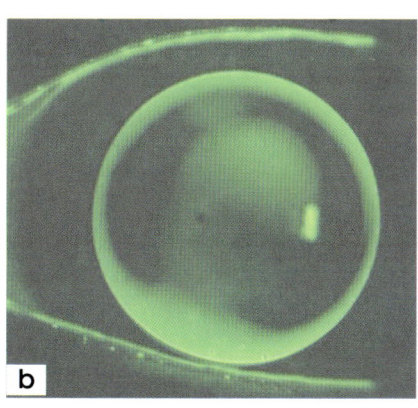
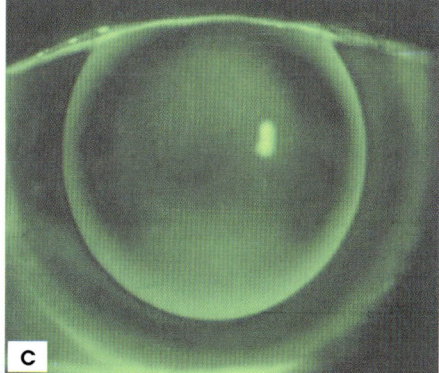

a   b   c

Fig. 9.25: (a) *ACT grade 2:* Lower third of lens periphery steepened at 270°; (b) Lens fit with inferior edge standoff at base of lens; (c) Lens fit after edge standoff corrected by incorporation of ACT

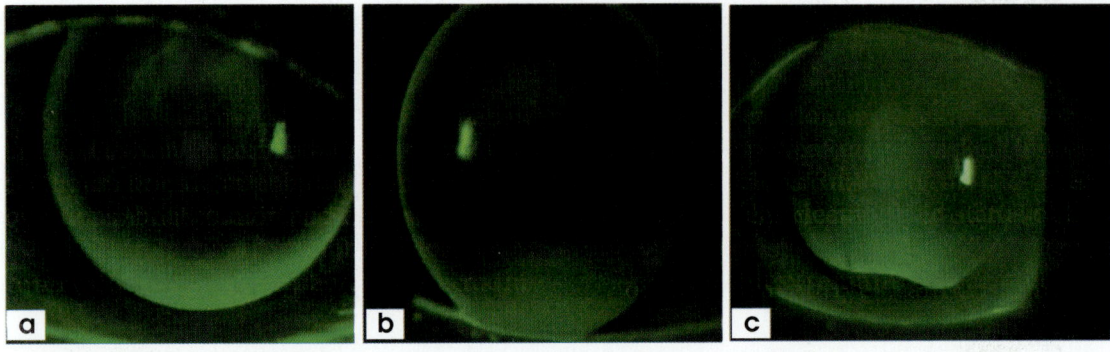

Fig. 9.26: Fluorescein pattern depicting lenses with increasing amounts of tuck; (a) grade 1 (0.7 mm tuck); (b) grade 2 (1.0 mm tuck); (c) grade 3 (1.3 mm tuck)

- *Grade 3 (1.3 mm): Provides significant edge stand off or lift off (tear meniscus break up) at around 6 o'clock.*

Tuck: This technology also serves to improve comfort, lens stability and is specified in degrees in 0.1 steps from 0.4 to 1.5 mm[38] (Fig. 9.26).

Toric periphery (TP): This design incorporates a spherical central optical zone with outermost 1 mm of peripheral curve being made toric. This toric incorporation in periphery is stabilized with truncation or prism ballasting and any degree from 0.4 to 1.3 mm can be ordered. Toric periphery design is often required for larger diameter lenses to combat corneal astigmatism present and when required, toric periphery is preferred option versus a full back surface toric lens. The TP design is available on Rose K2, Rose K2 IC, Rose K2 postgraft lenses.

The following explanation clarifies value of toric periphery design.

Usual presentation of RGP lens fit over a keratoconic cornea depicts tight areas within 20 degrees of horizontal meridian (around 3 and 9 o'clock) and over a PMD cornea with against-the-rule astigmatism, tight fit over vertical meridian (12 and 6 o'clock). This tight pinch at horizontal and vertical meridians respectively can be rectified by TP design (Fig. 9.27).

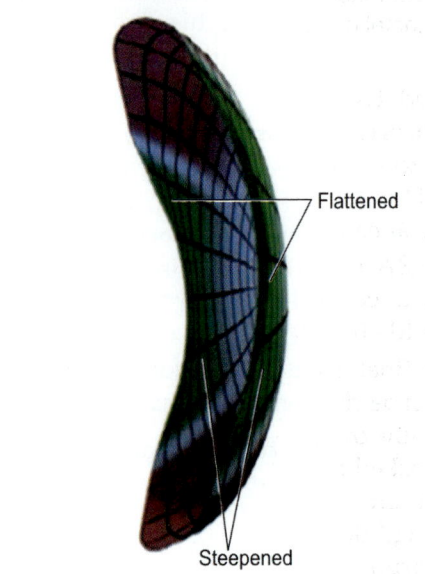

Flattened

Steepened

Fig. 9.27: Toric periphery incorporation

The lens fit depicted in Fig. 9.28 shows fit before and after incorporation of toric periphery.

Step 6: Over-refraction: Finalizing of lens power is done as the last step, only after finalizing fit and 10–15 minutes settling time. Over-refraction should be done in a well lit room with **normal light condition and photopic pupil**. Over minusing of these lenses is common and must be guarded against.

Residual astigmatism (RA): Any residual astigmatism needs to be assessed and a decision taken whether it requires to be

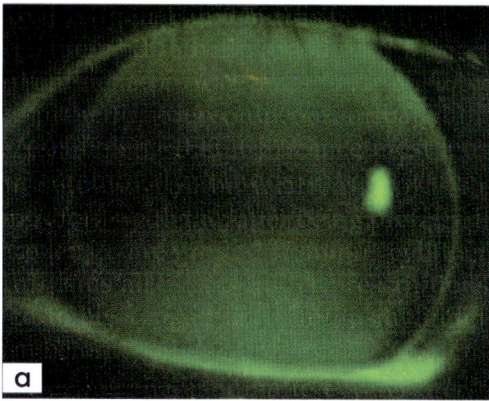 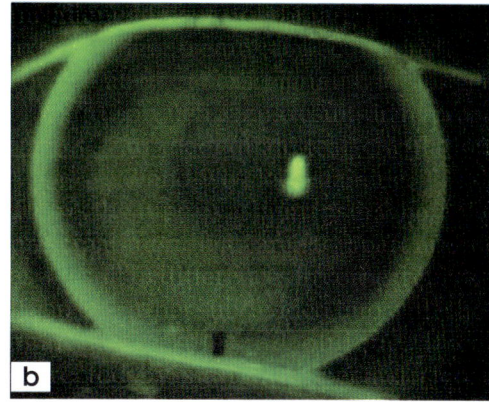

Fig. 9.28: Fluorescein pattern depicting lenses with toric periphery; (a) No toric periphery. Note: Tight fit in horizontal meridian; (b) Toric periphery incorporated

rectified. Usually low quantities of RA can be left uncorrected. For a RA ranging between −1.25 to −1.5 D a spherical equivalent of −0.75 D is added. The usual thumb rule for spherical compensation of RA is:

For RA of −0.25 to −0.50, add −0.25 D of spherical equivalent and for RA of −0.75 to−1.00, add −0.50 D.

The final call is to be taken by the patient and can be checked by placing RA cylinder in trial frame over the CL *in situ*, with the patient being asked for any tangible improvement in vision. In patients who have issues like ghosting/glare during night driving, RA may be incorporated into anti-reflective coating of night glasses worn over lenses.

Step 7 Comfort: This would need to be evaluated after a few days of wear. Use of preservative-free lubricating drops over lens wear is very helpful during initial adaptation period. If persistent discomfort is seen attention should be directed to peripheral system and increasing edge lift often helps.

Use of anti-reflective sunglasses for outdoor activities and meticulous cleaning of lenses with regular de-proteinization regimen and lens edging and polishing at 6–9 months interval are some other measures to enhance lens comfort.

The manufacturing guide recommends use of one drop of local anaesthetic instillation prior to fitting of the first trial lens to reduce tearing, for better evaluation of fluorescein pattern and ultimate reduction of chair time. However, we do not prescribe to this and have been doing optimal fitting without requiring any anaesthetic agent.

Rose K2 Soft Lens

The methodology includes all 5 steps of RGP lens subtypes of Rose K with a few variations. **Central fit**: The BC of first trial lens for keratoconus cases with or without corneal inserts is 0.8–1.0 mm flatter than mean Ks or mean 3 mm Sim Ks (topography) and equal to mean Ks/3 mm Sim K value for post-keratoplasty, PMD, LASIK cases.

After a settling time of 3–5 minutes, fit is evaluated for centration in all gazes with no evidence of tight fit (conjunctival indentation/blanching) or loose fit (evaluated by stability of laser mark at 6 o'clock position). It is better to err on the side of a flat fit, however, a limit should be drawn with 6 o'clock laser mark rotation occurring within 20 degrees in either direction. It is advised that patient squeeze his lids tightly with lens *in situ*. Enhanced visual acuity on opening lids and deteriorating later implies a tight fit. On the other hand, poor vision on opening lids which slowly improves with time implies a flat fit. Thus vision is the main consideration for deciding optimal DC for central fit.

Peripheral fit: This is evaluated independent of central fit and as stated before the options of standard increased, double increased used to loosen fit or standard decreased and double decreased to tighten overall fit are employed. Presence of entrapped air bubbles at limbus, poor lens motility, conjunctival indentation and/or limbal injection after several hours of wear would require ordering a lens with *increased lift.* On the other hand, situations where vision is acceptable but overall fit is loose, are diagnosed by excessive lens motility primarily in up-gaze, fluting in lower quadrants with latter requiring using a lens with **decreased lift.** An extremely loose lenses may cause laser line to locate more than 20 degrees away from 6 o'clock position (Fig. 9.29).

Overall diameter: The dimensions should be such that edge extends 1.5 mm outside limbus. Again it is better to keep OD slightly larger rather than small, stopping short of causing significant conjunctival indentation. In case of the latter situation, OD is either decreased and/or edge lift is increased.

Location: The lens should center equally around limbus and not locate down significantly, the latter being checked on upward gaze. Optimal location is easily verified by presence of laser mark to be within 20 degrees of 6 o'clock. A low location is often seen and is rectified by steepening the BC, increasing OD and/or decreasing edge lift.

Movement: A movement of 1.0–1.5 mm is aimed for post-blink and is most easily observed at bottom of lens, with patient looking straight ahead or slightly superiorly. Push up test can be used to assess adequacy of fit and movement. Poorly moving lens is corrected by increasing edge lift, reducing OD,

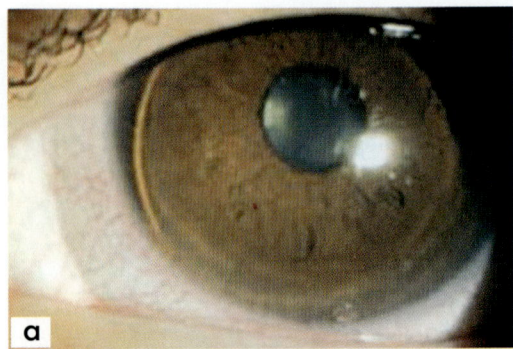

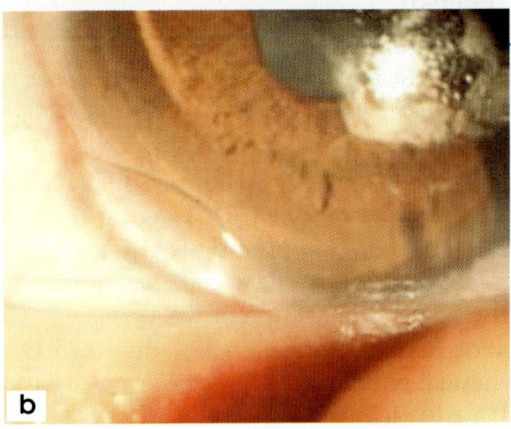

Fig. 9.29: (a) Low riding lens; (b) Fluting of lens in lower quadrant

or flattening the BC. Movement must be evaluated after the lens has settled but within 5 minutes of insertion.

Over-refraction: This is performed after allowing 5–10 minutes settling time and is **performed with lights on, using trial frame,** as pupil size affects final refraction. The cylinder is refined first and if over-refraction throws up a cylinder > 2 Dc, the same is placed in a trial frame and patient is asked to manually rotate lens to choose best vision. This is followed by refining sphere in steps of 1.00 Ds initially and then 0.50 DS.

Any rotation either nasally or temporally of 6 o'clock laser mark beyond 20° of 6 o'clock must be mentioned as "nasal or temporal "in the prescription sent to the laboratory.

Over-refraction is repeated after 20 minutes, confirmed and final prescription written.

ACT: Asymmetric Corneal Technology is usually done in cases of fluting at lower edge of lens and involves tightening/tucking of lens over a single quadrant with axis of steepening to be defined by the fitter. Unless stated by fitter, laboratory would place axis of ACT at 270 degrees (same axis as prism ballast). Two different grades of ACT can be ordered:

– *Standard ACT (1.0)*: This is done when fluting is not apparent in straight ahead gaze, but becomes obvious when patient looks up, down or laterally.

– *Double ACT (2.0)*: It is ordered when fluting is always obvious, even in straight ahead gaze.

Some Pertinent Facts

– Auto-refraction is inaccurate and should not be done. Persisting poor visual acuity is an indication of inadequacy of this design for the case and should be abandoned.

– During over-refraction, push maximum plus since it is easy to over minus the refractive correction.

– Inferior corneal steepening may cause lens to ride low, and fluting may not be apparent until the lens is pushed up via the lid to center over the pupil.

C. KeraSoft IC Lens (UltraVision, UK)

This is lathe cut, front surface aspheric or aspheric, toric, prism ballasted lens whose periphery can be altered independently of base curve. The periphery can be manipulated up to 4 steps flatter or steeper. In addition, the Sector Management Control (SMC) allows independent modification of 1–2 peripheral sectors. These lenses are like soft torics with a single laser mark at 6 o'clock position. In addition to keratoconus, the lens is used in cases of Pellucid Marginal Degeneration (PMD), postgraft, postrefractive surgery and eyes having had INTACs. Table 9.3 gives the parameters available for these lenses.

Lenses are supplied in an 8 lens, 14.50 mm diameter fitting set, including an 8.20:FLT2 (nipple cones) and 8.60:STP2 (for postgraft and other reverse geometry corneal shapes).

Technique of Fitting

A corneal profile chart, that assists in identifying corneal shape and a table suggesting best diagnostic fitting lens for each corneal type is provided by the manufactures. It is advisable to initiate fitting with 8.20 standard (STD) fitting lens and observe fit in straight ahead and upwards gaze within 5 minutes of insertion.

Fit characteristics are remembered by acronym *MoRoCCo VA*, which stands for **Mo**vement, **Ro**tation, **C**entration, **Co**mfort and **V**isual **A**cuity.

Table 9.3: KeraSoft IC lens parameters (reprinted with permission from UltraVision, UK)	
Base curve	7.40 mm to 9.40 mm (0.20 mm steps)
Diameter	14.50 mm standard (diameters of 14.00, 15.00 and 15.50 are available)
Power range	Sphere +30.00 D to –30.00 D
	Cylinder –0.50 to –15.00 (in 0.25 steps)
	Axis 1° to 180° (in 1° steps)
Materials	Flicon II 77% Water content (12 months replacement)[2]
	Etrofilcon A 74% water content (3 months replacement)
DK	[1] 53×10^{11} (cm^2/sec)[mlO$_2$/(ml × mmHg)]
	[2] 60×10^{11} (cm^2/sec)[mlO$_2$/(ml × mmHg)]
Periphery options	Standard, Steep 1, Steep2, Steep3, Steep4, Flat1, Flat2, Flat3, Flat4. Sector Management Control

Movement: Up to 2.0 mm movement is acceptable. *Push-up test should **not be used** to assess movement.*

Rotation is assessed by a vertical laser mark on lens. It is best to aim for as little rotation as possible although rotation up to 10° is acceptable.

Centration is determined by checking front optic zone placement versus pupil.

Comfort is as always a subjective phenomenon and depends on patient characteristics. Immediate, non-resolving discomfort indicates a flat fit and localized discomfort a tight fit at a specific point. It is to be remembered that like any other hydrogel, a tight fit is initially comfortable.

Visual acuity stability is checked after blinking. For a tight lens, VA clears on blink due to pushing down of the lens onto cornea followed by blurring due to lens "springing back" off the surface. A flat lens decenters after blinking, causing blurred vision which clears gradually as lens re-centers.

The fitting characteristics are listed in Table 9.4.

The fitting characteristics as per MoRoC-CoVA are further categorized by the manufactures as optmal fit, reassess fit and change fit as shown in Table 9.5.

Steps of Fitting

1. The **MoRoCCo characteristics** are noted within 5 minutes of lens insertion on slit lamp, in straight ahead and upwards gaze. Rotation is strongest indicator of fit at this point. However, as lens tightens on the eye it is advisable to reassess movement after 30 minutes of lens wear before final prescription. For this lens modification of OD is only resorted to once alterations in BC fail.

Table 9.4: Fitting characteristics of a kerasoft lens (reprinted with permission from UltraVision, UK)

	Optimal	Tight	Flat
↻Ro))	Up to 2.0 mm	Less than 0.50 mm Conjunctival indetation	Greater than 2.0 mm Lens may flute
Ⓒ	No rotation Vertical Laser Mark	Rotation Stable in straight ahead and upward gaze	Rotation Unstable or rotates on upward gaze
Mo⇕	Central	Central	Decentered Front optic zone (FOZ) drops to or below limbus
Co	Comfortable	Comfortable initially gradually becomes uncomfortable in one area	Uncomfortable
VA	Stable	Clearer after blink	Worse after blink

Table 9.5: Optimal fit characteristics in straight ahead gaze. (Reprinted with permission from UltraVision, UK)

	Optimal fit	Reassess fit	Change fit
Movement	**Vertical 1.0– 2.0 mm Movement post-blink:** Till 2.0 mm acceptable if patient comfortable	< 1 mm or > 2 mm <1.0 mm—try one step flatter >2.0 mm—try one step steeper	Mobile = too tight/or too flat. Reassess fit. – Lens too flat : Try 0.40 mm steeper – Lens too tight: Try 0.40 mm flatter
Rotation	Laser mark sits at 6 o'clock, is stable or returns rapidly to position post-blink	Up to 10° stable rotation – Acceptable: If 0.20 mm BC flatter does not rectify problem. – Unstable rotation indicates flat fit : Change to 0.20 mm steeper	>10° rotation – Stable: Lens is tight– remove, try progressively flatter lenses – Unstable: Try 0.04 mm steeper lens
Centration	Centered Minimal decentration acceptable if vision stable. VA clearer after blink indicates tight fit	Significantly decentered – Laterally on straight ahead gaze – Drops to limbus on upward gaze. Indicates flat fit. ...Try 0.20 mm BC steeper	Decentered – Lateral decentration with significant lag BC, OZ drops below limbus on upwards gaze. ...Try 0.40 mm BC steeper
Comfort	Consistently good comfort	Non-settling, discomfort – General edge awareness = Flat – Try 0.20 mm steeper – Increasingly in one position only indicates tight fit. – Try 0.20 mm flatter	Consistent discomfort – Static = Tight – Remove, fit 0.40 mm Flatter mobile may be too tight or too flat .... Reassess fit.
Stable vision	No fluctuation between pre- and post-blink	Unstable vision Worse post-blink = Flat fit Clearer post-blink = Tight fit. Try 0.20 mm BC steeper or flatter accordingly	Very poor vision Caused by tear pooling beneath lens, commonly due to very flat corneal periphery

The same thing is depicted in pictorial format in Fig. 9.30 as optimal, suboptimal and flat fit

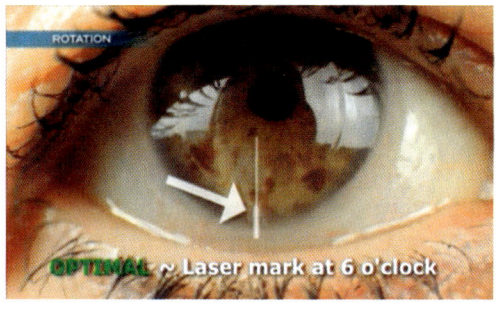

- **Mo**vement 1–2 mm

- **Ro**tation—minimal

- **C**entered

- **C**omfortable

- **VA** stable pre- and post-blink

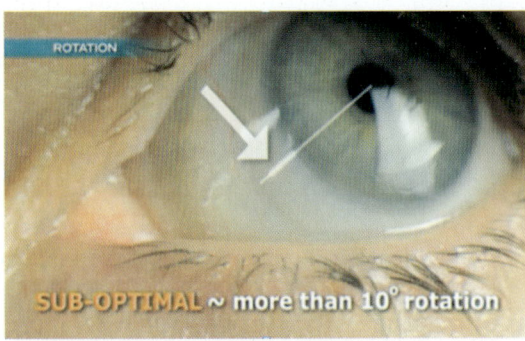

- Stable rotation

- Very little movement

- Centered

- VA clearer after the blink

- Comfortable initially but often progresses to discomfort in one position

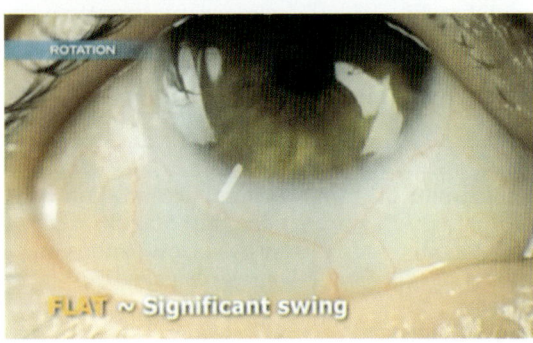

- Significant swing of laser mark between straight ahead and upward gaze

- Excessive movement post-blink

- Drops on upward gaze

- VA worse post-blink—improves with staring

- Uncomfortable

Fig. 9.30: Reprinted with permission from UltraVision, UK.

2. This is followed by **over-refraction**. Subsequently trial lenses are placed in a trial frame and cylindrical followed by spherical powers are refined in 1D steps, like for Rose K2 soft lens.

3. Vision is checked post-blink and fit verified again.

4. **Periphery modifications:** Whenever peripheral change is resorted to, corneal topography needs to be performed to visualize shape. However, in postgraft cases periphery of cornea may not be accurately imaged by topography necessitating use of trial set lenses only.

   a. *Steepening the periphery:* Indication for making the periphery steep are reverse geometry corneas, e.g. postgraft or post refractive surgery and keratoconus cases with steep periphery. Usually a standard lens is tried first. If this lens shows fluting or unstable off axis rotation, steepening the BC can be tried.

   Steepening of entire periphery by one step is equivalent to using periphery of a lens 0.20 steeper in the series, e.g. 8.60:STP2 would mean the periphery is acting like that of an 8.20 BC lens.

   b. *Flattening the periphery:* This is required in cases where all STD diagnostic lenses provide stable off axis rotation, e.g. nipple cones or when STD lenses show mid-peripheral bubbles, poor vision which improves after blink. Flattening the entire periphery allows such a lens to correctly drape over central cornea. Flattening periphery by one step is equivalent to using periphery of a lens 0.20 flatter in the series, e.g. 8.20:FLT2 would mean periphery is acting like that of an 8.60 base curve lens.

5. **Sector management control (SMC):** This is done for more irregular corneas, with 1–2 sectors of periphery being modified independently of base curve. Such corneas

are those with very low/decentered cones, PMD, complex postgraft and significantly toric scleras. Topography in such conditions may be misleading since the lens fits over sclera and not cornea. These are identified by the following fit characteristics.

– All STD lenses persistently drop, imply steep inferior cornea and best fit STD lens usually demonstrates unstable rotation.

– All STD lenses show significant rotation (stable/unstable) implies a lens is either catching or lifting off peripheral cornea at some point.

– STD lenses flute persistently in one position imply reverse geometry cornea.

Angles are recorded counterclockwise around lens circumference as A1, A2, A3 and A4. A1 and A2 define beginning and end of the first sector. A3 and A2 define beginning and end of second sector. Each sector can be ordered as STD, steep 1–4 or flat 1–4 with blend areas being automatically assigned. The classic SMC type is the first one to be tried and is mostly successful. Angles for this design are fixed at: A1=30, A2=150, A3=220, A4= 320 (Fig. 9.31).

Studies evaluating Rose K2 and Kerasoft IC have concluded equivalent visual gain seen in cases of mild and moderate keratoconus with corneal staining occurring more frequently in Rose K fits.[40] However, advanced cones and more irregular cones are better fitted with Rose K.

D. Hybrid Lens

These lenses have a rigid 6.0 mm central optical portion with a hydrogel skirt.[10] The large diameter skirt provides good centration, whereas central RGP portion provides clarity of vision. The prototype being SoftPerm lens (based on historical Saturn hybrid lenses) whose design fuses styrene-based RGP center with low water hydroxyethyl methacrylate (HEMA) soft-lens skirt.[41]

The types are SoftPerm lens, SynergEyes lens (Synerg Eyes, Inc, Carlsbad, CA) with central RGP made of Paragon HDS100 material and peripheral SCL of PolyHEMA hem-iberfilcon A.[27] Overall diameter is 14.5 mm and these lenses can be fitted over any cone severity aiming for apical clearance. Corneal hypoxia and lens adherence are issues and during initial wear and cornea needs to be examined for evidence corneal oedema after 5 hours of lens wear. Complications include hypoxia related changes such as vascularisation, central corneal clouding, endothelial cell loss and neovascularisation over time.[42,43] Other problems include handling difficulties, discomfort, edge pucker, a tendency to tear or split at soft-rigid junction leading to frequent replacements and expense.

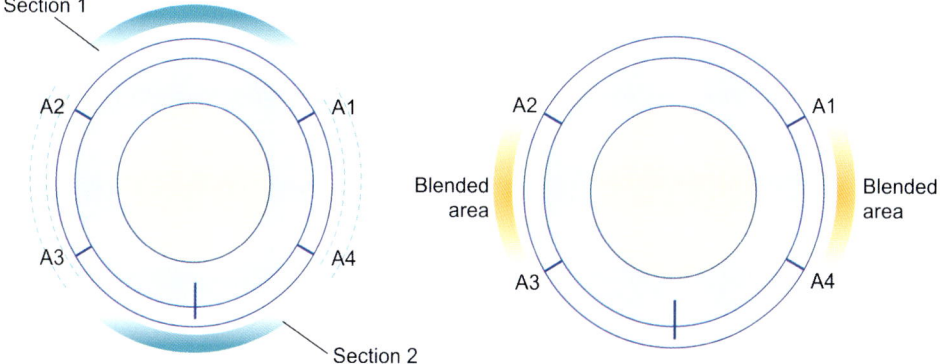

Fig. 9.31: Section management control [reprinted with permission from UltraVision (UK)].

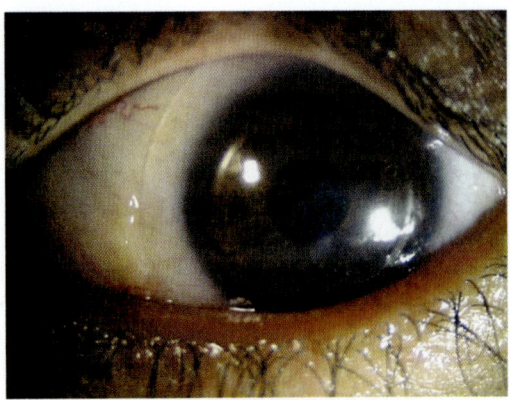

Fig. 9.32: Soft hydrogel in keratoconus patient after collagen cross linkage

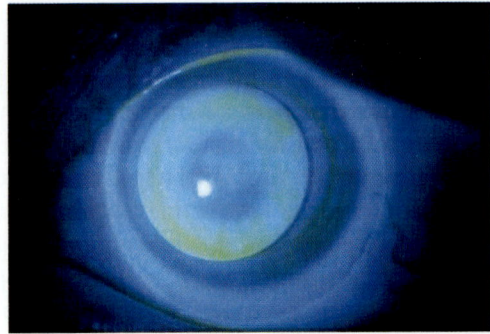

Fig. 9.33: Piggyback lens (*Courtesy:* Abhilekh Aneja)

E. Soft Lenses/Conventional Hydrogels

Indications for soft hydrogels/torics are very few. They are reserved for mild conus, associated high myopia, intolerance or inadequate fit with RGP lenses (Fig. 9.32). Of the hydrogels thicker lenses with low water content should be used to neutralize the irregular astigmatism.[44] The various soft toric lenses, which are available in steeper base curves, are HydroKone (Medlens Innovations), Soft K (Advanced Vision Technologies), Solus Soft K (Strategic Lens Innovations), Special Eyes 59/54 Toric (Special Eyes), and Ocu-Flex Toric (Ocu-Ease).[27] Toric siloxane hydrogel lenses and reverse geometry lenses may be tried in RGP intolerant patients.

F. Piggyback Lens System (PBCL)

This combo lens system uses an ultra-thin lens soft lens which drapes over the cone or a high plus power lens providing bulk with concomitant rigidity, called the **Carrier lens**. This carrier lens serves as base over which a powered RGP lens is fitted (Fig. 9.33). The indications for using this lens fitting are persistent discomfort, dislocation, recurrent abrasions or scarring with RGP lens usage.[45]

A disposable or frequent replacement large diameter soft lens with a low minus power which does not dehydrate easily is fitted first.[46] Siloxane hydrogel material lens is a natural choice due to its superior corneal respiration, however, their hydrophobicity often makes them uncomfortable to wear. This material also has a propensity to cause epithelial erosions and its choice as the most appropriate carrier lens material is not always acceptable.

After ensuring adequate movement of the *carrier lens*, keratometry is performed with hydrogel lens *in situ* to generate a K reading. Subsequently a gas-permeable, thin rigid lens with smallest vault, avoiding edge lift and capturing of central air bubble is fitted over the soft lens base on flat K with diameters ranging between 9 and 9.5 mm.[47] Both lenses should be of high Dk material to minimize the risk of hypoxia. Flatter fit of the RGP lens is preferred and centration, movement of RGP lens has to be titrated to cause minimal lid sensation. High molecular weight fluorescein can be used to evaluate fit in lieu of normal fluorescein which stains the soft lens. The movements of SCL and RGP lenses are independent of each other. Over-refraction is performed and final subjective acceptance is added to RGP power. The final fit of the RGP lens can be modified by altering power of SCL. A plus power SCL is used to flatten the RGP and a minus power to steepen the RGP.[44]

Custom piggyback lenses (Flex lenses piggyback lens, X-Cel Contacts) are lathe cut lenses with a pre-cut groove in the SCL into which a RGP (1 mm smaller than groove diameter) is fitted This enables good centration of RGP, reduces thickness, improves the comfort due to minimal interaction with lids and reduces hypoxia.[27] The sunken well, however, attracts tear debris, solution/environmental contaminants and requires meticulous cleaning.

Problems of this system are:

– **Double lens** care: Unless peroxide lens care system is used, both RGP and soft lens care systems are required which makes it more complex and expensive.
– In addition to patient handling problems, increased thickness of *lens twins* causes giant papillary conjunctivitis (GPC), corneal hypoxia, resulting in corneal neovascularization. Siloxane hydrogel with their high DK values help in overcoming this problem but as mentioned before have their flip side too.
– Lens binding is a frequent problem requiring flattening of BC or increase in edge lift.
– Inter-surface deposits are a common occurrence requiring careful lens cleaning and use of lubricants *in situ*.
– Lost RGP lens.

G. Aspheric Lenses

An aspheric lens has a continuous posterior radius of curvature defined by geometric shape rather than continuation of progressively flatter spherical base curves.[48]

Aspheric lenses are recommended for those patients who develop staining or recurrent erosions with multicurve lenses. They are can be fit slightly steeper than conventional lenses without altering the sagittal depth of lens.

Currently indigenously available post-aspheric lenses, the Mc Asfeer lens, are available in Indian market. Made of Boston XO fluoro silicone acrylate material with DK value of 100, these large diameter 6.0–11.0 mm lens have a large optic zone, reduced edge lift and are designed with customized lathe cutting. These lenses are available in power ranges of – 6.0 Ds to + 6.0 Ds (Fig. 9.34).

Fitting is as for any conventional RGP lens, with conversion of K values in Dioptres to mm by using conversion table. The base curve of initial trial lens is based on Flat K with OD 1.5–2 mm smaller than HVID. Subsequent fitting is as for RGP lens fitting and a static fit of 3-point touch with feather touch in apical zone is aimed at. Peripheral edge clearance aimed at is in the range of 0.5–1.0 mm and can be modified by steepening or flattening edge lift in steps of 1 from 2F–6F (Fig. 9.34).

H. Scleral/Miniscleral Lens

These lenses are reserved for advanced cones or for patients intolerant to conventional RGP lenses. Semi sclerals (diameter 15–18 mm) and sclerals (diameter 18–25 mm) are used when corneal lenses of any reasonable diameter are unable to provide reasonable fit or stable vision. This is often seen in cases with extremely inferior decentered cones or very large globus cone.[49] Recent studies seem to indicate a beneficial role on corneal topography after use of these lenses with a negligible occlusive effect on corneal respiration (Fig. 9.36).[50]

Contact lens fitting in keratoconus is time consuming and challenging. This is the commonest complex situations being handled by the contact lens practitioner and one of most rewarding. Advance cones, younger age and associated atopy make fitting more complex, requiring longer chair time and multiple diagnostic trials. The parameters obtained on corneal topography help in reducing chair time and getting an acceptable fitting.[51]

Recent decades have seen an unprecedented growth in technological advancements and refinements in lenses designed for keratoconus with improvement in visual gains and comfort to the patient. The condition is very well treated by CL fitting with the two requirements being a trained fitter and a motivated patient. The promising advent of collagen cross linkage (CXL) as a modality to

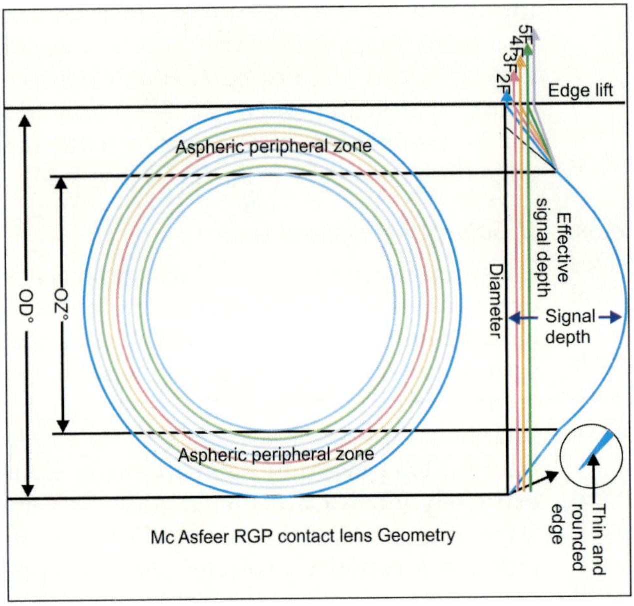

5F
4F
3F
2F
Edge lift
Aspheric peripheral zone
Effective signal depth
Diameter
Signal depth
OD°
OZ°
Aspheric peripheral zone
Thin and rounded edge
Mc Asfeer RGP contact lens Geometry

a

Suggested McAsfeer RGP Trial Set

Diameter (mm)	Base Curvature (mm)	Power (-) (D. Sph.)	Trial Set Categories
9.20	4.50	-16.00	A
	4.60	-16.00	
	4.70	-16.00	
	4.80	-16.00	
	4.90	-16.00	
9.40	5.00	-16.00	B
	5.10	-16.00	
	5.20	-16.00	
	5.30	-16.00	
	5.40	-16.00	
9.60	5.50	-12.00	C
	5.60	-12.00	
	5.70	-12.00	
	5.80	-12.00	
	5.90	-12.00	
	6.00	-12.00	
9.80	6.10	-10.00	D
	6.20	-10.00	
	6.30	-10.00	
	6.40	-10.00	
	6.50	-10.00	
10.00	6.60	-6.00	E
	6.70	-6.00	
	6.80	-6.00	
	6.90	-6.00	
10.50	7.00	-3.00	F
	7.10	-3.00	
	7.20	-3.00	
	7.30	-3.00	
	7.40	-3.00	
	7.50	-3.00	
	7.60	-3.00	
	7.70	-3.00	
	7.80	-3.00	
	7.90	-3.00	
	8.00	-3.00	
	8.10	-3.00	
	8.20	-3.00	
	8.30	-3.00	
	8.40	-3.00	
	8.50	-3.00	
11.00	8.60	-3.00	G
	8.70	-3.00	
	8.80	-3.00	
TOTAL LENSES = 44			

b

Fig. 9.34: (a) McAsfeer lens design; (b) Manufacturers recommendation of lens parameter selection (reprinted with permission from prescription guide)

a
Anterior Float
T
OD
b

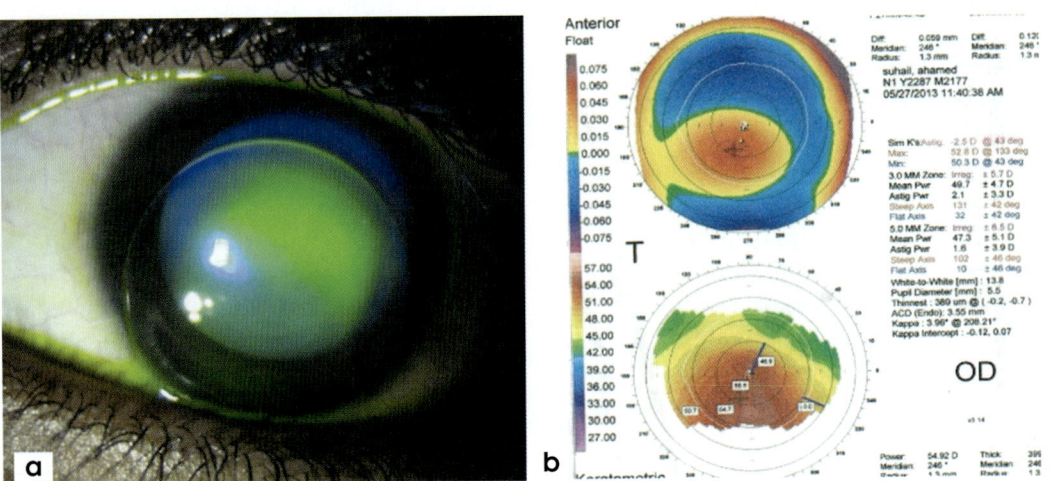

Fig. 9.35: (a) Fit of Mc Asfeer lens over an advanced cone (b) Topography of same patient

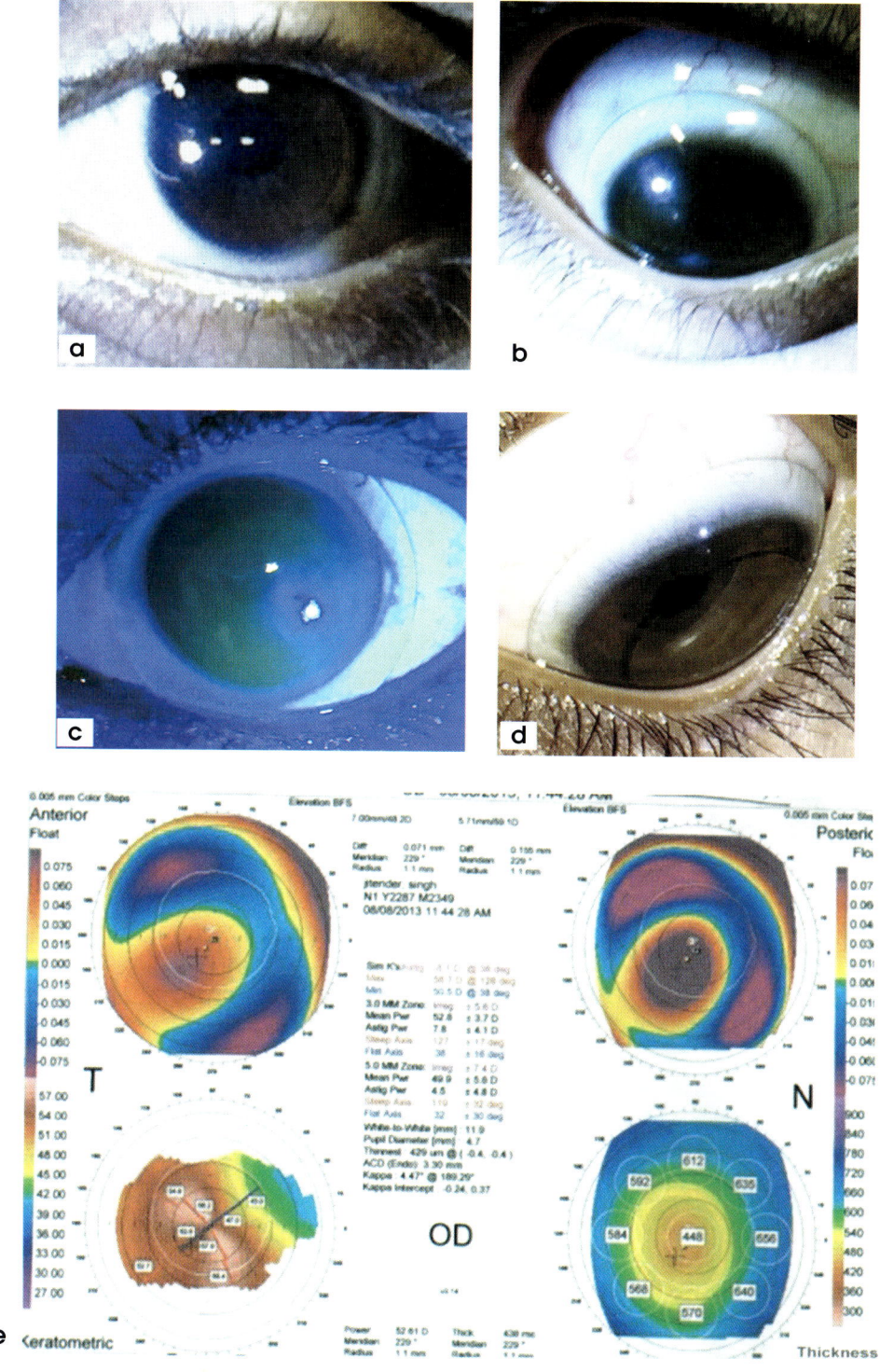

Fig. 9.36: (a, b, c and d) Miniscleral lens; (e) Topography of patient c

arrest the disease had made CL fit more rewarding and effective after this procedure. All short-term and a few long-term studies confirm stabilization of the disease and improvement in vision after collagen cross-linking.[52–54] Personal experience of the author using lenses post-CXL has confirmed enhanced fit, reduced lens drop out, decreased lens intolerance with increase in duration of lens wear from 1.3 ± 1.8 to 9 ± 1.9 hours in moderate to advanced cones (unpublished data).

Use of intracorneal rings improves corneal surface topography and is not a deterrent for RGP lens fit if required.

Complications with lens wear specific to keratoconus

a. Fluctuating vision occurs due to decentration of lens, lens flexure or warpage, progression of the conus and occurrence of presbyopia.

b. Corneal staining—staining at the apex of cone is common. Examination of keratoconus patients should be done by asking the patient to report after 6–8 hours of wear, so that the fitter can assess extent of corneal impingement. Excessive or symptomatic staining requires re-edging with increased peripheral blending or increase frequency of lubricant use.

c. Lens adhesion is commonly seen in inferior cones with low riding lenses which demonstrate limbal compression. Remedy is to refit them with steeper, smaller lenses which are anchored by the upper lid.

d. Ocular surface changes manifesting as decrease in goblet cell densities and tear break up time have been documented after many years of contact lens wear.[55]

e. Accelerated corneal endothelial cell loss has been documented in keratoconus patients wearing contact lenses, more with soft lens wear versus RGP lenses.[42]

REFERENCES

1. Rabinowitz YS, Mc Donnell PJ. Computer assisted corneal topography in keratoconus. Refract Corneal Surg. 1989 Nov-Dec;5(6):400–8
2. Rabinowitz YS. *Keratoconus*. Surv Ophthalmol1998; 42: 297–319.
3. Sonmez B, Doan MD, Hamilton DR. Identification of scanning slit beam topographic parameters important in distinguishing normal from keratoconuic corneal disease. Am J Ophthalmol 2007: 143(3): 401–8
4. Wagner H, Barr JT, Zadnik K. Collaborative Longitudinal Evaluation of Keratoconus (CLEK) Study: methods and findings to date. Cont Lens Anterior Eye. 2007 Sep;30(4):223–32.
5. Wang D, Xie PY, Zhou JL. Clinical study on treatment of secondary keratoconus with special designed rigid gas permeable contact lens. Zhonghua yan ke za Zhi.(Chinese Journal of Ophthalmology) 2013, 49(4):327–33.
6. Hiratsuka Y, Nakayasu K, Kanai A. Secondary keratoconus with corneal epithelial iron ring similar to Fleischer's ring. Jpn J Ophthalmol. 2000 Jul-Aug;44 (4):381–6.

7. Lass JH, Lembach RG, Park SB, Hom DL, Fritz ME, Svilar GM, Nuamah IF, Reinhart WJ, Stocker EG, Keates RH, et al. Clinical management of keratoconus. A multicenter analysis. Ophthalmology. 1990 Apr;97(4):433–45.
8. Bilgin LK, Yilmaz S, Araz B, Yüksel SB, Sezen T. 30 years of contact lens prescribing for keratoconic patients in Turkey. Cont Lens Anterior Eye. 2009 Feb;32(1): 16–21.
9. Prazeres Prazeres S, Malet F, Colin J. Contact lens fitting after keratoplasty for keratoconus. J Fr Ophtalmol. 2008 Nov;31(9):849–54.
10. Erdurmus M, Yildiz EH, Abdalla YF, Hammersmith KM, Rapuano CJ, Cohen EJ. Contact lens related quality of life in patients with keratoconus Eye Contact Lens. 2009 May; 35(3):123–7.
11. Kymes SM, Walline JJ, Zadnik K, Sterling J, Gordon MO; Collaborative Longitudinal Evaluation of Keratoconus Study Group. Changes in the quality-of-life of people with keratoconus. Am J Ophthalmol. 2008 Apr; 145(4):611–7.

12. Kennedy RH, Bourne WM, Dyer JA. A 48-year clinical and epidemiologic study of keratoconus. Am J Ophthalmol. 1986 Mar 15;101 (3): 267–73.

13. Jonas JB, Nangia V, Matin A, Kulkarni M, Bhojwani K. Prevalence and associations of keratoconus in rural Maharashtra in central India: The central India Eye Medical Study. Am J Ophthalmol. 2009 ;148: 760–5.

14. Millodot M, Shneor E, Albou S, Atlani E, Gordon-Shaag A. Prevalence and associated factors of keratoconus in Jerusalem: A cross-sectional study. Ophthalmic Epidemiol. 2011;18:91–7.

15. Bawazeer AM, Hodge WG, Lorimer B. Atopy and keratoconus: a multivariate analysis. Br J Ophthalmol. 2000 Aug;84(8):834–6.

16. Jafri B, Lichter H, Stulting RD. Asymmetric keratoconus attributed to eye rubbing. Cornea. 2004 Aug; 23(6):560–4.

17. Pearson AR, Soneji B, Sarvananthan N, Sandford-Smith JH. Does ethnic origin influence the incidence or severity of keratoconus? Eye (Lond). 2000 Aug;14 (Pt 4):625–8.

18. Saini JS, Saroha V, Singh P, Sukhija JS, Jain AK. Keratoconus in Asian eyes at a tertiary eye care facility Clin Exp Optom. 2004 Mar;87(2):97–101.

19. Georgiou T, Funnell CL, Cassels-Brown A, O'Conor R Influence of ethnic origin on the incidence of keratoconus and associated atopic disease in Asians and white patients. Eye (Lond). 2004 Apr;18(4):379–83

20. Gokhale NS. Epidemiology of keratoconus. Indian J Ophthalmol. 2013 Aug; 61(8): 382–3.

21. Gatinel Damien. Corneal topography and wave front analysis. Pg 921–63 In Albert Jakobiec's Principles and Practice of Ophthalmology, 3rd ed., Eds Albert DM & Miller J W. Saunders Elsevier 2008.

22. Hollingsworth JG, Efron N. Observations of banding patterns (Vogt striae) in keratoconus: a confocal microscopy study. Cornea. 2005 Mar; 24 (2):162–6.

23. Mocan MC, Yilmaz PT, Irkec M, Orhan M. The significance of Vogt's striae in keratoconus as evaluated by in vivo confocal microscopy. Clin Experiment Ophthalmol. 2008 May;36 (4): 329–34.

24. Krumeich JH, Daniel J, Knlle A. Live epikeratophakia for keratoconus. J cat Ref Surg 1998: 24: 456–63.

25. Bhatoa NS, Hau S, Ehrlich DP. A comparison of a topography-based rigid gas permeable contact lens design with a conventionally fitted lens in patients with keratoconus. Cont Lens Anterior Eye. 2010 Jun;33(3):128–35.

26. *Evans* J, Hau S. The therapeutic and optical application of a rigid gas permeable semi-limbal diameter contact lens. Cont Lens Anterior Eye. 2009 Aug;32(4):165–9. Epub 2009 May 12.

27. Rathi VM, Mandathara PS, Dumpati S. Contact lens in keratoconus. Indian J Ophthalmol 2013;61(8):410–5.

28. Edrington TB, Szczotka LB, Barr JT, Achtenberg JF, Burger DS, Janoff AM, Olafsson HE, Chun MW, Boyle JW, Gordon MO, Zadnik K. Rigid contact lens fitting relationships in keratoconus. Collaborative Longitudinal Evaluation of Keratoconus (CLEK) Study Group Optom Vis Sci. 1999 Oct;76(10):692–9.

29. Fink B, Heard C, Schafer J, Cline AR, Mitchell L, Barr JT. Fluorescein pattern interpretation in keratoconus. Optom Vis Sci. 2008 Oct;85(10): E939–46.

30. Edrington TB, Gundel RE, Libassi DP, Wagner H, Pierce GE, Walline JJ, Barr JT, Olafsson HE, Steger-May K, Achtenberg J, Wilson BS, Gordon MO, Zadnik K. CLEK study group. Variables affecting rigid contact lens comfort in the collaborative longitudinal evaluation of keratoconus (CLEK) study. Optom Vis Sci. 2004 Mar;81(3):182–8.

31. Zadnik K, Barr JT, Steger-May K, Edrington TB, McMahon TT, Gordon MO. Collaborative Longitudinal Evaluation of Keratoconus (CLEK) Study Group. Comparison of flat and steep rigid contact lens fitting methods in keratoconus. Optom Vis Sci. 2005 Dec; 82(12):1014–21.

32. McMonnies CW Keratoconus fittings: apical clearance or apical support? Eye Contact Lens. 2004 Jul;30(3):147–55.

33. McMonnies CW. The biomechanics of keratoconus and rigid contact lenses. Eye Contact Lens. 2005 Mar: 31(2):80–92.

34. Leung KK. RGP fitting philosophies for keratoconus. Clin Exp Optom 1999;82:230–5.

35. Coral-Ghanem C, Alves MR. Fitting Monocurve and Bicurve (Soper-McGuire design) rigid gas-permeable contact lenses in keratoconus patients: a prospective randomized comparative clinical trial. Arq Bras Oftalmol. 2008 May-Jun;71(3):328–36.

36. Acharya MC, Mathur U, Barua P. Demographic profile and visual rehabilitation of patients with keratoconus attending contact lens clinic at a tertiary eye care centre. Cont Lens Anterior Eye. 2010 Feb;33(1):19-22.

37. Ozkurt YB, Sengor T, Kurna S, Evciman T, Acikgoz S, Haboðlu M, Aki S. Rose K contact lens fitting for keratoconus. Int Ophthalmol. 2008 Dec; 28(6):395–8.

38. Jain AK, Sukhija J. Rose-K contact lens for keratoconus. Indian J Ophthalmol. 2007 Mar-Apr;55 (2):121–5.

39. Rose K manual Practitioners Fitting guide. Rose K kerotconus set. 2013.

40. Fernandez-Velazquez FJ. Kerasoft IC compared to Rose-K in the management of corneal ectasias. Cont Lens Anterior Eye 2012;35:175–9.

41. Ozkurt Y, Oral Y, Karaman A, Ozgür O, Doðan OK. A retrospective case series: use of SoftPerm contact lenses in patients with keratoconus. Eye Contact Lens. 2007 Mar; 33(2):103–5.

42. Edmonds CR, Wung SF, Husz MJ, Pemberton B. Corneal endothelial cell count in keratoconus patients after contact lens wear. Eye Contact Lens. 2004 Jan;30(1):54–8.

43. Fernandez-Velazquez FJ. Severe epithelial edema in Clearkone SynergEyes contact lens wear for keratoconus. Eye Contact Lens 2011;37:381–5.

44. Barnett M, Mannis MJ. Contact lenses in the management of keratoconus. Cornea 2011; 30:1510–6.

45. Kok JH, van Mil C. Piggyback lenses in keratoconus. Cornea. 1993 Jan;12(1):60–4.

46. Romero-Jimenez M, Santodomingo-Rubido J, Flores-Rodriguez P, Gonzalez-Meijome JM. Which soft contact lens power is better for piggyback fitting in keratoconus? Cont Lens Anterior Eye 2013;36:45–8.

47. Smith KA, Carrell JD. High-Dk piggyback contact lenses over Intacs for keratoconus: a case report. Eye Contact Lens. 2008 Jul; 34(4):238–41.

48. Barnett M, Mannis MJ. Contact lenses in the management of keratoconus. Cornea 2011; 30:1510–6.

49. Kok JH. A European fitting philosophy for **aspheric**, high-Dk RGP contact lenses. CLAO J. 1992 Oct;18(4):232–6.

50. Schornack MM , Patel SV Scleral lenses in the management of keratoconus. Eye Contact Lens. 2010 Jan;36(1):39–44.

51. Soeters N, Visser ES, Imhof SM, Tahzib NG. Scleral lens influence on corneal curvature and pachymetry in keratoconus patients. Cont Lens Anterior Eye. 2015 Aug;38(4):294–7.

52. Mandathara Sudharman P, Rathi V, Dumapati S. Rose K lenses for keratoconus: An Indian experience. Eye Contact Lens 2010;36:220–2.

53. O'Brart DP, Chan E, Samaras K, Patel P, Shah SP. A randomised, prospective study to investigate the efficacy of riboflavin/ ultraviolet A (370 nm) corneal collagen crosslinkage to halt the progression of keratoconus. Br J Ophthalmol. 2011 Nov;95(11):1519–24.

54. Raiskup-Wolf F, Hoyer A, Spoerl E, Pillunat LE. Collagen crosslinking with riboflavin and ultraviolet: A light in keratoconus: long-term results. J Cataract Refract Surg. 2008 May;34(5):796–801.

55. Moon JW, Shin KC, Lee HJ, Wee WR, Lee JH, Kim MK. The effect of contact lens wear on the ocular surface changes in keratoconus. Eye Contact Lens. 2006 Mar;32(2):96–101.

Reader's Note

Reader's Note

CHAPTER 10

Presbyopic Contact Lenses

PRESBYOPIC CONTACT LENSES (PbCL)

Presbyopia is a physiological process afflicting people in their fifth decade onwards as a result of reduced accommodation. The word is derived from Greek *presbys* (old man) + ops (sight), implying *sight like an old man*. In the developed world context, most of the present population spend roughly half their lives as presbyopes.[1]

The people who most often request for a presbyopic contact lens (PbCL) are habitual contact lens wearers, who now require near add to effectively perform near activities. These wearers habituated to lenses are loath to revert to spectacles for near activities and are highly motivated for retaining cosmetic benefits of lens wear. The second category of users comprises emmetropes requiring lenses only for their receding near vision. This subset consists comprises working professionals holding demanding jobs who being at the peak of their careers do not wish a cosmetic or visual compromise. The third category emerging now is the ageing population of myopes, post-refractive surgery, cases developing presbyopia. Thus requirement of PbCL is steadily increasing and this huge market demands effective contact lens technology tailored to their requirements. This demand is, however, largely, unmet by nascent PbCL industry resulting in significant under-prescription of lenses to presbyopes.[2]

Bifocal spectacles have stood the test of time since their invention by Benjamin Franklin in 1784 but the same cannot be said of bifocal CL from their earliest avatar of segmented bifocals, designed by Feinbloom in 1938.[3] Subsequent modifications in design have sought to redress a host of problems both optical and ocular surface related. In 1957, DeCarle attempted to redress the problem of segment rotation in near gaze by developing a simultaneous-vision PbCL.[4] Subsequent modifications brought in nonspherical progressive multifocal lenses and diffraction lenses.[5, 6] However, optical problems preventing mass acceptance of these lenses include reduced stereo-acuity, reduced contrast sensitivity, fluctuating vision/ image jump and altered binocular balance in those with borderline compensated phorias. Ocular issues include age related issues like dry eyes, concurrence of ocular co-morbidities, along with visually demanding environments often involving use of computer terminals.

Fitting Philosophies

Bifocal lenses can be of two types: *alternating vision and simultaneous vision*. In alternating vision type a distant or near object is viewed through the respective lens segment, which comes into play by the wearer by moving his visual axis upward or downward. In the simultaneous vision or segmented type both distant and near images are formed on retina simultaneously. Another method commonly employed is *monovision*, where one eye wears a CL correcting for near vision and other eye a CL correcting for distance vision.

A. Alternating/Translating Vision

This is done by RGP lenses which provide either distance or near vision or alternate two visions by altering positions. Lens moves or 'translates' on the eye with alteration in wearer's gaze, from straight ahead for distance to down for near (Fig. 10.1). Since patient needs to move visual axis downward for near vision, image jump is a common occurrence. Excessive or insufficient lens movement would cause visual blur due to different/ wrong zones occupying pupil in different gazes. For success of this type of fit, lens stability in all gazes is crucial and this is achieved by prism ballasting or truncation.[7] Pupil changes subsequent to altered illumination has a significant impact on quality of vision with this type of lens use.

B. Simultaneous Vision

In normal viewing conditions constant accommodation by natural crystalline lens focuses all images, arising from distant, intermediate and near objects on the retina. To emulate this vision of youth, simultaneous vision lenses (SVL) have been designed. When viewing a distant object with SVL, distance dedicated zone of lens forms one image on retina over which near object image formed by near dedicated zone gets superimposed. The near image is blurred while viewing distance objects and distance image is blurred while viewing distant objects, due to different gaze directions intercepting different portions of the SV lens.

The main disadvantage of this lens is requirement for a "learned behavior" by wearer to ignore blurred image and focus on clearer one.[8] The cumulative effect of multiple *defocused* images, from intermediate and far distances superimposed on *in focus* near image at retinal plane, causes reduction in quality of vision, confusion, ocular fatigue and/or monocular diplopia during initial periods of lens wear. *Best visual acuity is achieved after 1–2 weeks of wear, after brain has adapted to simultaneous vision.* Long-term success of this lens has been reported to be around 40%.[9]

Pupil size and shape is the common denominator for success by either simultaneous or alternating vision.

C. Monovision

In this method, one eye is fitted for distance and other for near vision. Depending on visual needs, dominant eye is fitted for visual task most commonly performed, e.g. for a watchmaker near vision is most important so dominant eye is fitted with lens correcting for near vision. This method is currently the most

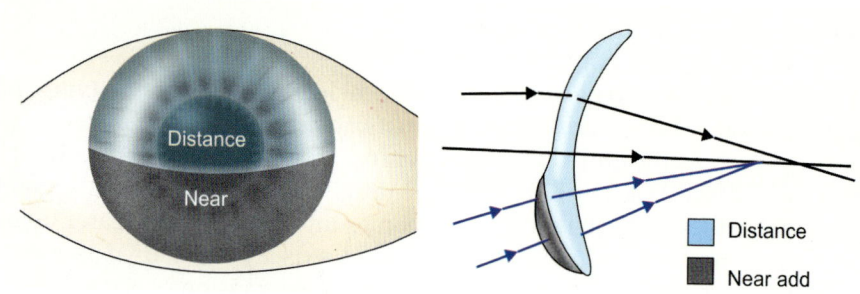

Fig.10.1: Alternating vision: Incorporates plus add for near/down gaze

commonly employed with success ranging from 67 to 88%.[10, 11]

Since only one eye receives focused image of object of interest with other eye perceiving a blurred image of the same object, eye or more specifically brain has to select 'better' image by suppressing or blurring the other image. This sensory inhibitory process has to be acquired and since plasticity of brain is reduced along with elasticity of lens zonules, extreme confusion and fatigue may ensue. The ability to suppress also depends on quality of visual stimuli, e.g. defocused small, bright lights against a dark background (high contrast) are difficult to ignore by most successful monovision wearers.[11] This aspect translates into difficulty in night driving in situations of seeing headlights of oncoming car against inky black darkness. The problem can be rectified by use of distance glasses over monovision CL.[12] Other problems inherent to monovision wear are: Inability to switch on central suppression, decreased contrast sensitivity (20% loss), reduced stereopsis and uniocular blurring.[8] Such visual degradation can cause poor spatial localization, disorientation and imbalance but most patients adapt to it over a period of time.

Interocular suppression is another important phenomenon which must occur for success of monovision lenses. This is determined by pupil size with smaller pupils facilitating interocular suppression by reducing differential blur between two ocular images. The benefit of this method of PbCL is that critical lens fitting is not so essential for success. However, with increasing age and increasing near add, this technique may not suffice once inter-eye difference reaches insurmountable levels for fusion.

In those with no specific requirement for an activity, dominant eye is corrected for distance, but for those with excessive near vision requirement it is corrected for near.[11] This assignment is based on the assumption that patients have a greater need for distance

vision and that suppression is more easily achieved in the non-dominant eye.[13] In myopes the eye with lesser amount of myopia is corrected for distance and more myopic eye for near with lowest plus power add.[11]

The technique is contraindicated for those with high binocular demand, those with prior binocular vision deficits, strong ocular dominance and unequal vision. **Enhanced monovision** is a term used when dominant eye has single vision lens and other eye a bifocal lens for near vision.

Modified monovision term refers to a bifocal contact lens in each eye with one lens providing better distance vision and other eye lens, better near vision.[14] Small additions to power are made as required for dominant eye (distant vision) and extra power for non-dominant eye (near vision).[15]

Technique of selecting the dominant eye

Sighting tests are used like the Dolman Card /hole-in-the-hand. In this technique wearer is asked to hold the special sighting card with *both* hands. He/ she is then asked to look at a nominated letter on a Snellen chart, through central hole of this card keeping both eyes open. After covering one eye of patient, eye which was used for sighting the letter is identified as the dominant eye.[16]

Lens Designs

The commonly available presbyopic lens designs are detailed in the following paragraphs (Flowchart 10.1).

I. Simultaneous vision bifocals/multifocals

   a. Aspheric Design

     This one-piece lens has near segment on front or back surface with the former being preferred. Central zone of lens may be designated for distance (center distance: C-D/DeCarle type) or near (center near: C-N/Alges type).[7] Pupil size as mentioned before, is an important variable in determining

Flowchart 10.1: Types of presbyopic contact lens designs commonly used

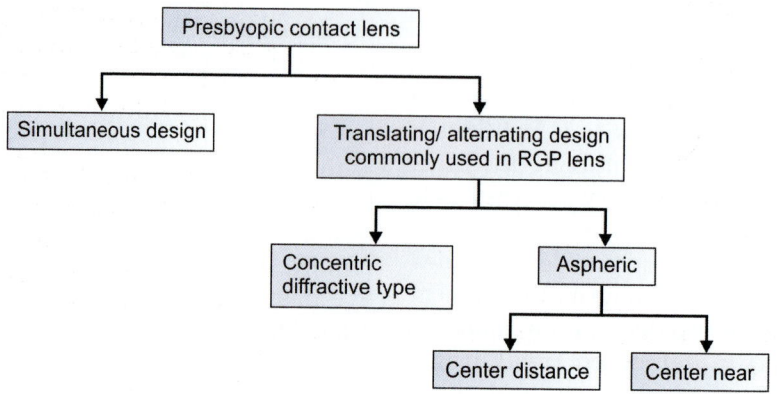

quality of vision and center near configuration lenses design with central zone diameters of <3 mm are able to provide good near vision in both photopic and mesopic conditions. However, physiological alterations in mesopic conditions may adversely affect vision quality. For example, in bright light, a C-N wearer experiences reduction in distance vision quality due to smaller reduced pupil allowing less of distance zone to cover it (Fig. 10.2). Concomitant use of sunglasses during outdoor activities for such patients helps in minimizing this problem. Conversely in dim light near vision may be impaired as the larger scotopic pupil allows light from both distance and near zones, resulting in flare and ghosting.

b. Diffractive Design

There are concentric grooves on posterior surface of these lenses, which cause diffraction of some of the incident light rays (Fig. 10.3). Distance objects are viewed by refraction at center of lens, while near object is viewed as a diffractive image by the circular diffractive zone on inner surface.[7] Conventional concentric bifocal designs encompass two lens powers within pupil, with variable contribution of each component to the final retinal image depending on pupil dimensions. For a diffractive lens entire 'optical' zone directs light to its two focal points and is thus independent of pupil size.

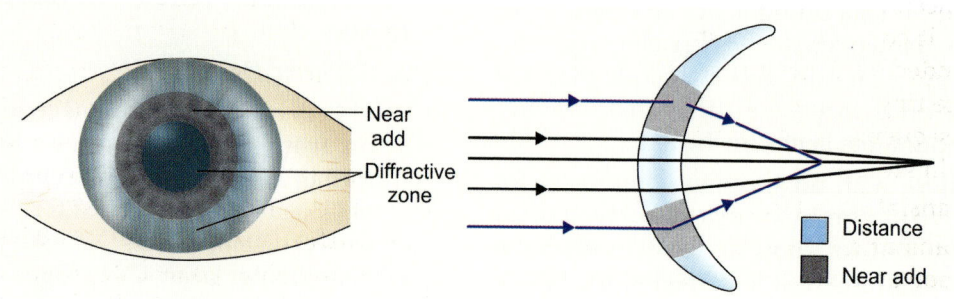

Fig. 10.2: Simultaneous vision: Aspheric center near

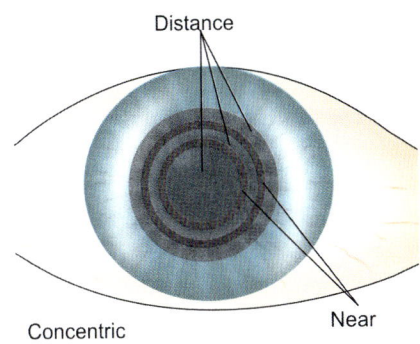

Fig.10.3: Diffractive design:Center distance followed by annular concentric grooves for near and distance.

Such lenses are ideal for patients with moderate adds and for those with small to medium pupil sizes. Incident light is split between both distance and near images, with forty percent light going to each, 20% being lost to higher order diffractive images, scatter, reflection, glare and absorption causing a reduction of contrast.[17] Patients with astigmatism of >0.75 Dc cylinder and prior reduced contrast are not benefited with this design.

Pupil-intelligent lenses utilize diffraction by incorporation of alternate concentric zones for D and N which are relatively independent of pupil size. These lenses are very useful for computer users. The main problem with their use is decreased contrast, due to simultaneous formation of multiple images on retina. A prototype is the Acuvue bifocal, which has five concentric zones to distribute light more evenly. It consists of a central distance zone surrounded by annular first near ring, second distance ring, second near and third distance ring in sequence. This lens minimizes flare and haloes in scotopic illumination.

II. Translating/alternating design

Translating design employs incorporation of two distinct segments or annular concentric design. In *segment design* reading segment is positioned inferiorly and it maintains this position aided by prism ballasting or truncation. Such lens are gaze dependent and are fitted in *low riding position* to enhance reading in conventional downward reading gaze. *Annular concentric* design incorporates reading segment circumferentially and is more suited for near acuity in primary gaze, like computer use. However, these lenses are plagued with problems of flare, ghosting and poor intermediate vision.

III. Nonspherical type

The posterior surface (or both anterior and posterior surface) is nonspherical, with central part being utilized for distant vision with successively increased power to paracentral part, which is utilized for near vision (Fig. 10.4). A RGP lens made from this design moves on the cornea and gives effect of alternating vision with infraversion.[7]

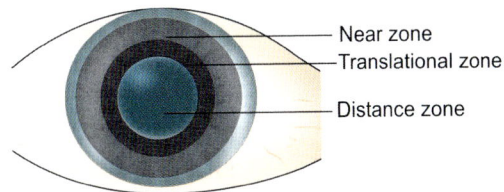

Fig. 10.4: Nonspherical type

Patient Selection and Pre-screening

Information about ocular and systemic co-morbidities, daily activities, occupational needs and patient profile is very important before prescribing presbyopic contact lenses.

1. **Driving activity:** Presbyopic correction can cause reduced distance acuity for safe driving or for renewal of motor driving license. (International standard being corrected vision of 6/12 in at least one eye). This differs in different countries with United Kingdom guidelines being 6/7.5 in better eye with at least 6/60 in other eye,

whereas India and most parts of the USA require 6/12–6/18 vision in the better eye.[18]

2. **Occupational needs/distance at which most work is done:** Precise vision is required in certain professions like navigators, surgeons, fitting of electronic circuits and architects. These people may not be the ideal candidates for use of bifocal lenses due to reduction of stereopsis and contrast. Requirement for crisp night vision, binocular vision and preference of distance *versus* intermediate *versus* near vision would determine design of PbCL if any to be prescribed. Use of computer usage also require correction of near and intermediate vision. Frequency of changes from near to far viewing distances is more relevant for effective vision with translating designs.[11,19] Patients needing fine detailed vision with depth perception, like surgeons, watchmakers, jewelers and commercial night drivers would be very unhappy with monovision quality. Amblyopes also are not good candidates for monovision.[2,10]

3. **Ocular changes with ageing affecting PbCL fit:**

   a. **Anatomical:**
      – Decreased tonus of upper and lower eyelid.
      – Senile miosis
      – Reduced nerve elements in cornea and eyelids which serve to decrease corneal and lid sensitivity.
      – Pinguecula/pterygium at limbal area along with peripheral thinning make fitting of limbal traversing lenses problematic.
      – Increasing ATR astigmatism due to flattening of vertical cornea.
      – Endothelial cell density decrease with concomitant reduction of endothelial pump activity may increase corneal hydration and reduce corneal transparency.

   b. **Physiological:**
      – Decreased contrast sensitivity.
      – Decreased visual acuity for low contrast targets under low illumination[20]
      – Decreased lacrimal secretion.
      – Increased permeability of limbal vasculature permitting leakage of low-density lipoproteins into cornea with alteration of peripheral optics.
      – Increase in refractive index of cornea/crystalline lens due to altered hydration especially in diabetics.

4. **Co-morbidities (ocular/ systemic):** History suggestive of dry eye syndrome, glaucoma, thyroid disorders, diabetes, hand tremors, use of medications like anti-histaminics, decongestants, hormone replacement therapy and diabetes must be taken.[7] Visual quality with bifocals may degrade depending on preexisting ocular aberrations, thus patients with ocular conditions like glaucoma, amblyopia and macular changes are not good candidates for presbyopic lenses. Performing computerized automatic perimetry on patients wearing presbyopic contact lens, which itself induces reduced differential light sensitivity, can causes reduction in global sensitivities (GS) of central visual field.[21]

5. **Pupil size:** Light induced variations in pupil size influence other vision related parameters like contrast sensitivity significantly, thus light levels at work and home must be accounted for and contrast measured at photopic/mesopic light wear before prescribing presbyopic lens.[8, 9, 22]

6. **Personality of wearer:** The reduced quality of vision with use of any bifocal modality makes this option unsuitable for anxious people or perfectionists.[7]

   Lenses must have visible handling tints so as to be easily identified by the presbyopic wearer. For ease of insertion near lens is inserted first and removed last.

REFERENCES

1. Charman WN. Developments in the correction of presbyopia I: spectacle and contact lenses. Ophthalmic Physiol Opt. 2014 Jan; 34(1):8–29.

2. Morgan PB, Efron N, Woods CA; International Contact Lens Prescribing Survey Consortium. An international survey of contact lens prescribing for presbyopia. Clin Exp Optom. 2011 Jan;94(1):87–92.

3. Moss HI. Bifocal contact lens—A review. Am J Ophtom Arch. 1962;39:653–68.

4. DeCarle J. Bifocal and multifocal contact lens. In: Stone J, Anthony PJ, Eds : Contact lenses. 3rd ed. London: Butterworths; 1989. pp. 595–624.

5. Stein HA. The management of presbyopia with contact lens. CLAO J. 1990;16:33–9.

6. Freeman M, Stone J. A new diffractive bifocal contact lens. Transactions BCLA Conference. 1987:15–22.

7. Hiroshi Toshida, Kozo Takahashi, Kazushige Sado, Atsushi Kanai and Akira Murakami Bifocal contact lenses. History, types, characteristics and actual state and problems. Clin Ophthalmol 2008 Dec; 2(4): 869–77.

8. Rajagopalan AS, Bennett ES, Lakshminarayanan V. Visual performance of subjects wearing presbyopic contact lenses. Optom Vis Sci. 2006 Aug;83(8):611–5.

9. Hamano T, Hamano T, Hamano K, et al. 5-year following-up study of 423 wearers of 2-week replacement bifocal contact lenses. J Jpn CL Soc. 2006; 48:2–6.

10. Jain S, Arora I, Azar DT. Success of monovision in presbyopes: review of the literature and potential applications to refractive surgery. Surv Ophthalmol. 1996 May-Jun; 40(6):491–9.

11. Evans BJ. Monovision: A review Ophthalmic Physiol Opt. 2007 Sep;27(5):417–39.

12. Schor C, Landsman L, Erickson P. Ocular dominance and the interocular suppression of blur in monovision. Am J Optom Physiol Opt. 1987 Oct;64(10):723–30.

13. Zheleznyak L, Alarcon A, Dieter KC, Tadin D, Yoon G. The role of sensory ocular dominance on through-focus visual performance in monovision presbyopia corrections. J Vis. 2015;15(6):17.

14. Gohrmlet NR. The hydron ECHELON bifocal contact lens. ICLC. 1989;16:315.

15. Walker JS. Case study: presbyopia and astigmatism. CL Spectrum. 2002;17:6–8.

16. Seijas O, Gómez de Liaño P, Gómez de Liaño R, Roberts C J, Piedrahita E, Diaz E. Ocular dominance diagnosis and its influence in monovision. *American Journal of Ophthalmology* 2007; 144, 209–16.

17. Brenner MB. An objective and subjective comparative analysis of diffractive and front surface aspheric contact lens designs used to correct presbyopia. CLAO J. 1994 Jan;20(1): 19–22.

18. Vision requirement for diving safety with empharic on individual assessment. Report prepared for the international council of ophthalmology of the 30th world opthalmology congress, Sao Paulo, Brazil, Feburary 2016.

19. Cardina G, Lopez S. Pupil diameter working distance and, illumination during habitual talks. Implications for simultaneous vision cancer for presbyopic J optoms 2015:15:5–61.

20. Woods RL. The aging eye and contact lens. A review of ocular characterstics. J Pr contact lens Assoe 1991; 14:115–27.

21. Alongi S, Rolando M, Corallo G, Siniscalchi C, Monaco M, Saccà S, Verrastro G, Menoni S, Ravera GB, Calabria G. Quality of vision with presbyopic contact lens correction: subjective and light sensitivity rating. Graefes Arch Clin Exp Ophthalmol. 2001 Sep;239(9):656–63.

22. Sado K. Bifocal or multifocal contact lenses for presbyopia. J Jpn CL Soc. 2000;42:s3–20.

Reader's Note

CHAPTER 11

Fitting an Aphakic Patient

Aphakia is the term used to denote an eye without its crystalline natural lens. This refractive error was traditionally corrected with aphakic spectacles before the advent of contact lenses and subsequently with intraocular lenses, the last being the most preferred modality. Very perspicacious articles on travails of aphakic glasses written by aphakic physicians, give an insight on the problems created by use of these spectacles.[1,2] As one physician put it, aphakic spectacles created visual invalids despite cataract surgery being the greatest gift to its recipients. The landmark breakthrough of correcting aphakia by intraocular lens, rightly earned Sir Harold Ridley the laurel of ridding the ophthalmological fraternity from *scrounge of aphakia*. Due to the ubiquitous use of intraocular lenses aphakia per se is an uncommon entity, with the maximum cases occurring in paediatric population. Childhood aphakia as a consequence of congenital cataract awaiting an IOL or traumatic cataract where IOL insertion is not feasible, is the commonest condition requiring aphakic contact lenses. Thus this chapter would primarily be referring to childhood aphakia.

Optical Inadequacies of Aphakic Spectacles

Aphakic spectacles suffer from inherent optical inadequacy due to differences in image size and prismatic effects.

a. **Magnification:** Placement of a plus (convex) lens anterior to both crystalline lens position and cornea creates a Galilean telescope, which causes image magnification.[3] This magnification is proportional to distance between zero lens position (of crystalline lens removal) and the plus aphakic correction. The image magnification equals $1/(1-pd)$ where p= lens power, and d = distance in metres between correcting lens and pupil. Thus a contact lens placed on cornea induces a magnification of 5–7%, which is much less compared to 25–30% magnification induced by the more distally placed spectacles (13–15 mm away from cornea) (Fig. 11.1).[4]

b. **Altered spatial perception:** Magnification of objects makes them appear closer than they actually are. This is responsible for

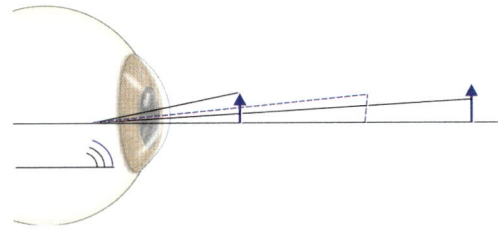

Fig.11.1: Relative spectacle magnification RSM: Similar objects subtend larger visual angle closer they are to eye.1.33 for aphakic glasses, 1.1 for contact lens

spatial element of false orientation and gives rise to "an unpleasant period when tumblers are overturned, when reaching for salt, the unfortunate patient puts his fingers in the gravy-boat, flower vases are upset, ink is spilled, and other similar minor domestic tragedies occur.[1]

c. **Pincushion distortion:** In this optical phenomenon, straight lines appear curved and doorways assume hourglass shape (Figs 11.2 and 11.3). Again this has been comically detailed by an aphakic doctor *"Thus the newly elected aphakic regards a door through which for years he has been accustomed to pass without misadventure and, to his amazement, he finds the jambs in each side curve in toward the middle and leave an aperture only a few inches wide at the centre, through which all reason tells him it will be impossible to wedge his portly person. When mature thought finally persuades him that this is an optical illusion, and he timidly advances to make the test, he finds to his delight that as he approaches the opening, the curves recede gracefully and invitingly to his approach and he finds easy and unimpeded passage"*.[1]

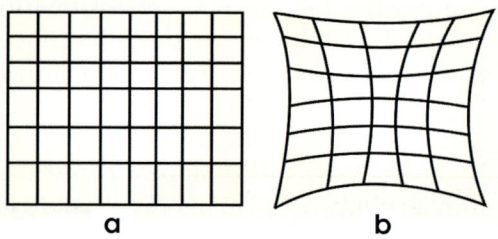

Fig. 11.2: (a) Normal grid or object; (b) Pincushion distortion with a high plus lens

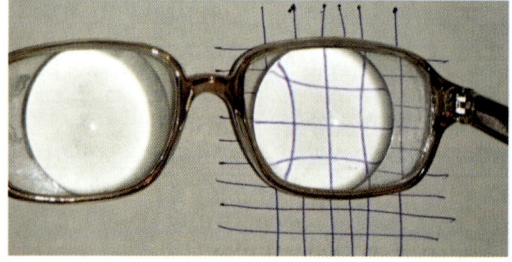

Fig. 11.3: Pincushion distortion as viewed through aphakic spectacle

d. **Prismatic effects:** The base in prism effect of high plus lenses generates a *ring scotoma* between 50° and 65° in the visual field. This obscures objects in mid-peripheral field and makes driving difficult. In addition, it gives rise to *Jack-in-the-box* effect, due to objects suddenly appearing from edge of the scotoma (Fig. 11.4). On the eyes moving laterally behind the aphakic glasses, the scotoma shifts along with eye movements and objects which had been obscured by scotoma are suddenly revealed, emulating a jumping "Jack in box". The patient adapts to this phenomenon by learning to use head movements instead of eye movements while trying to see objects in the lateral field.[3]

e. **Tunnel vision:** Aphakic spectacles cause a 30% restriction of visual fields, due to the ring scotoma and uncorrected visual field outside the spectacles. This creates tunnel vision and restricts navigational mobility.

f. **Diplopia:** This occurs in monocular aphakia, where resultant aniseikonia (difference in image sizes between two eyes) and anisometropia do not permit binocular fusion with spectacle use, leading to intolerable diplopia.[3] Thus aphakic spectacles are not a viable option for unilateral aphakia.

Interrupted binocularity period in case of uniocular aphakia often causes squinting of the aphakic eye. After visual rehabilitation with CL, resultant diplopia becomes an incentive for the squinting eye to resume orthophoric position. Thus it needs to be emphasized that any strabismus in an aphakic eye should be surgically treated only, after an adequate trial of aphakic contact lens has been given for a minimal period of 6 months.

g. **Cosmetic:** The weight of high plus spectacles on the bridge of nose of the young child (despite using lightweight, high index materials) is another hindrance (Fig. 11.5).

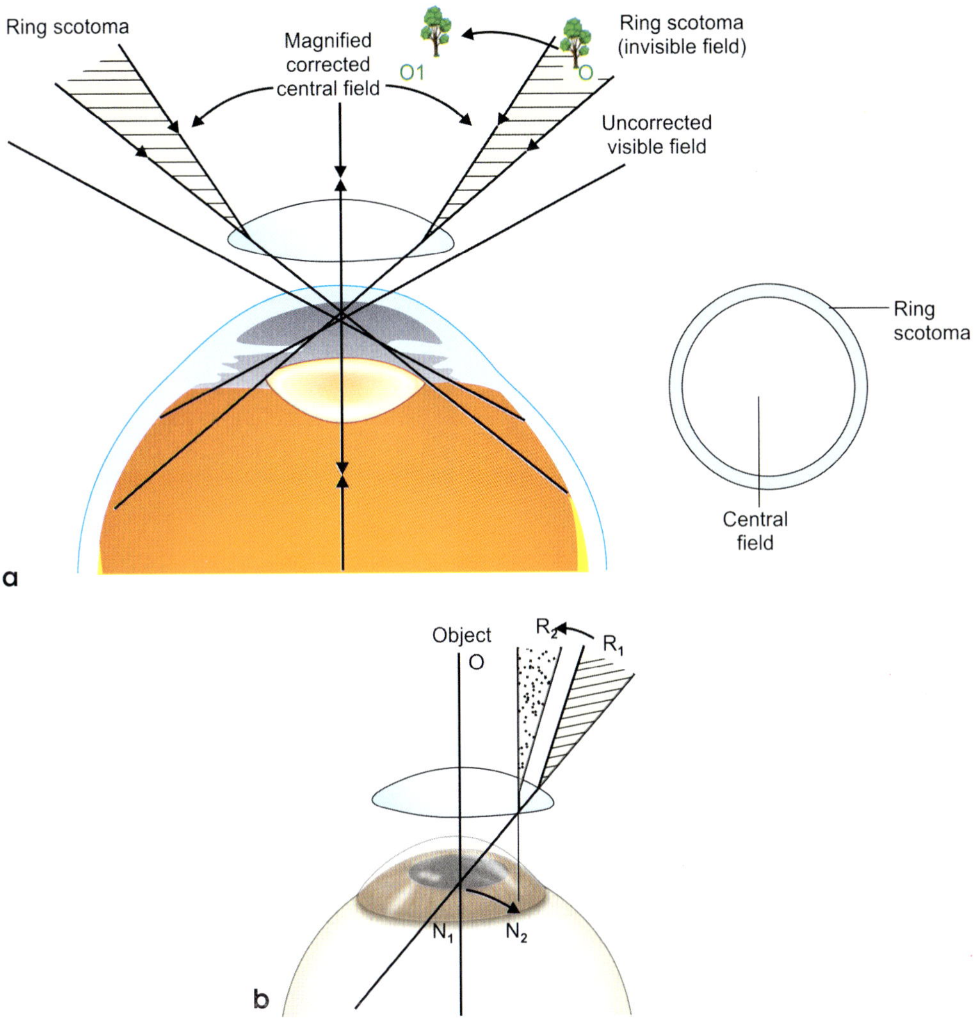

Ring scotoma

Magnified corrected central field

O1

O

Ring scotoma (invisible field)

Uncorrected visible field

Ring scotoma

Central field

a

Object
O

R₂

R₁

N₁

N₂

b

Fig. 11.4: (a) Ring scotoma (b) Giving rise to *Jack in box phenomenon* as object at O is invisible, but suddenly pops into view on moving eye, as it now positions O1 in Fig. a and from R1 to R2 in Fig. b.

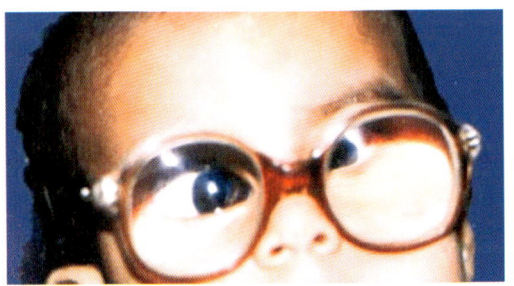

Fig. 11.5: Child wearing heavy aphakic glasses

Contact lenses relieve the aphakic patient of most of these spectacle-related problems and provide better vision for binocular and especially for uniocular aphakes. However, using contact lenses require some amount of manual dexterity and maintenance, which may not be possible or reliable in the very young and very old.

Physiological/anatomical/optical alterations in aphakic eye relevant to contact lens wear

- *Denervation induced reduction in metabolic activity* after cataract surgery results in reduced epithelial oxygen uptake and consumption. This lower basal metabolic rate of cornea coupled with reduced tear production, lax upper lid tone (senile ptosis) makes lens fitting a specialized technique in elderly aphakes. In addition, this age group is behest with corneal degenerative conditions, systemic co-morbidities (diabetes, arthritis) and reduced manual dexterity which makes lens use difficult.

- *Reduced corneal sensitivity*. This is beneficial in ensuring faster adaptation to CL wear, however, warning symptom of pain due to infective keratitis may be delayed.
- *Reduced endothelial cell density* due to operative insult of cataract surgery coupled with age.[6] This makes cornea more vulnerable to lens induced hypoxic insult. This, however, is partly countered by *lower corneal oedema response* to contact lens, since absence of natural lens reduces corneal requirement for available oxygen. Corneal denervation in addition, reduces oxygen consumption of epithelium.[6]
- *Loss of filtering effect of crystalline lens* causes unfiltered excess light to reach retina, thereby causing glare and ultraviolet damage. Removal of natural lens also results in altered color perception like enhanced perception of red colour (erythropsia) or blue color (cyanopsia) during the early postoperative period.
- Poorer quality of *tear film* and blink quality.
- Requirement for *supplementary spectacles* to correct residual astigmatism and a near add.
- Children often develop *strabismus* after advent of monocular aphakia due to interruption of binocularity. This may require squint surgery along with rigorous amblyopia treatment (Fig. 11.6).

Nystagmus may occur in children afflicted with aphakia in early childhood, despite optimal management. This is partly due to stimulus deprivation and partly due to associated motor anomaly. Once it deve-

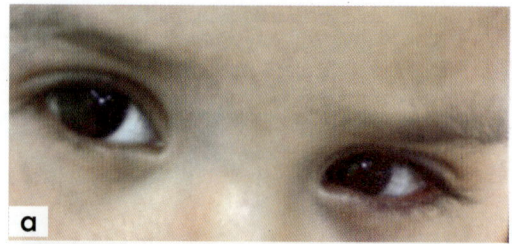
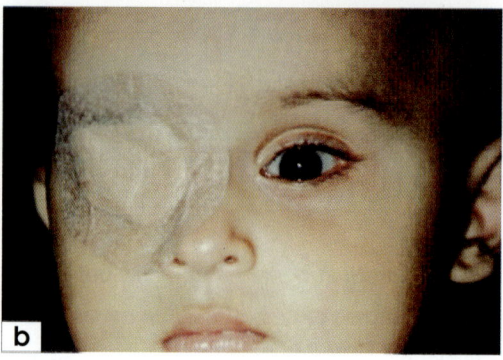

Fig. 11.6: (a) Squinting of left aphakic eye after contact lens correction in a 6-year-old child operated for uniocular cataract; (b) Same child has orthophoria after patching of phakic right eye and contact lens over aphakic left eye

lops, hydrogel, preferably silicone hydrogel lenses only can be used, fitting a RGP lens in such a situation is difficult and unsafe. The vision in aphakic eyes with nystagmus usually is often compatible with navigation and word recognition.

Pediatric Aphakia

Visual rehabilitation with contact lenses in aphakic child permits a more normal development of visual, motor and perceptual skills compared to aphakic spectacles which suffers from multiple optical problems. Contact lenses offer a 15% wider field of view compared to spectacles and are preferred by parents who face a lot of difficulty in convincing the child to wear heavy spectacles. Spectacles are also easily removed, bent or scratched by the active, inquisitive child. In addition, *absence of a prominent nose bridge* in a child makes placement of these inherently heavy spectacles a problem.

Cataract surgery needs to be performed with minimal tissue manipulation to minimize post-operative corneal oedema and conjunctival trauma, so as to ensure a relatively quiet eye for early contact lens fit. In order to prevent amblyopia, contact lens must be fitted within one month of surgery in infants.[7] In the current era, phacoemulsification with anterior and posterior continuous curvilinear capsulorrhexis in infant allows for placement of a secondary intraocular lens a later date. Explaining that lenses are required for a few years before a permanent visual rehabilitation, with an IOL can be performed, is very reassuring to parents who then willingly undertake the daunting task of fitting a lens to their reluctant child.

Despite the fact that contact lens loss is high in the young child (5–6 during initial year) continued formed visual stimuli due to inability of child to remove lenses gives it an edge over the more easily removed aphakic spectacles.[8]

Infant's tears have a higher aqueous component, which is again beneficial when fitting contact lenses. In the interests of continuous visual stimulation, parents should be asked to keep a spare pair of contact lenses in case of lens breakage or loss. For the binocular aphake, a pair of back up spectacles should also be prescribed.

Fitting contact lenses in young children is difficult and requires building up a rapport between parents and practitioner. Parental counselling with requirements and results being explained, has to be done, to avoid lens discontinuation during the initial frustrating period of lens wear. A revealing study by the Infant Aphakia Treatment Study Group which compared visual outcomes of unilateral aphakic children corrected with either IOL or contact lens, revealed parental stress to be similar in the two interventions at 2 years follow up.[9]

Indications and Optical Benefits of Contact Lens in Young Child

- **Aphakia:** This is the commonest indication for use of contact lenses in a child. Contact lenses are preferred method of visual rehabilitation in unilateral aphakia (Fig. 11.7). For bilateral aphakes contacts provide better optics, without image magnification or field reduction of their heavy spectacle counterparts. Results of the recently concluded multicentric Infant Aphakia Treatment Study Group concluded visual outcomes of 114 *unilateral aphakic children* corrected with either primary IOL implantation or contact lens to be similar at 4.5 years.[10] The IOL group had significantly more adverse reactions, more operative procedures including glaucoma and strabismic surgery with fewer adherence to occlusive patching. The group recommended CL rehabilitation to be the preferred alternative in children younger than 7 months.

- **High refractive error** (myopia, hypermetropia): In high myopia contact lens allow larger field of vision and a more normal image size compared to spectacles. In high hyperopes, lenses are better tolerated as they require lesser accommodative demand versus spectacles.

- **Unilateral ametropia:** Stereopsis is better with contact lens correction.

- **Anisometropia:** A combination of part-time occlusion and contact lens wear is done to treat amblyopia. Contact lenses avoid the prismatic effect of spectacles, especially the vertical effects which cause difficulty in reading.

- **Amblyopia:** Special tinted or high plus powered SCLs can be used as an alternative method of occlusion therapy in children, who refuse to wear an occlusive patch.

- **Strabismus with a high refractive error:** By reducing convergence demands in

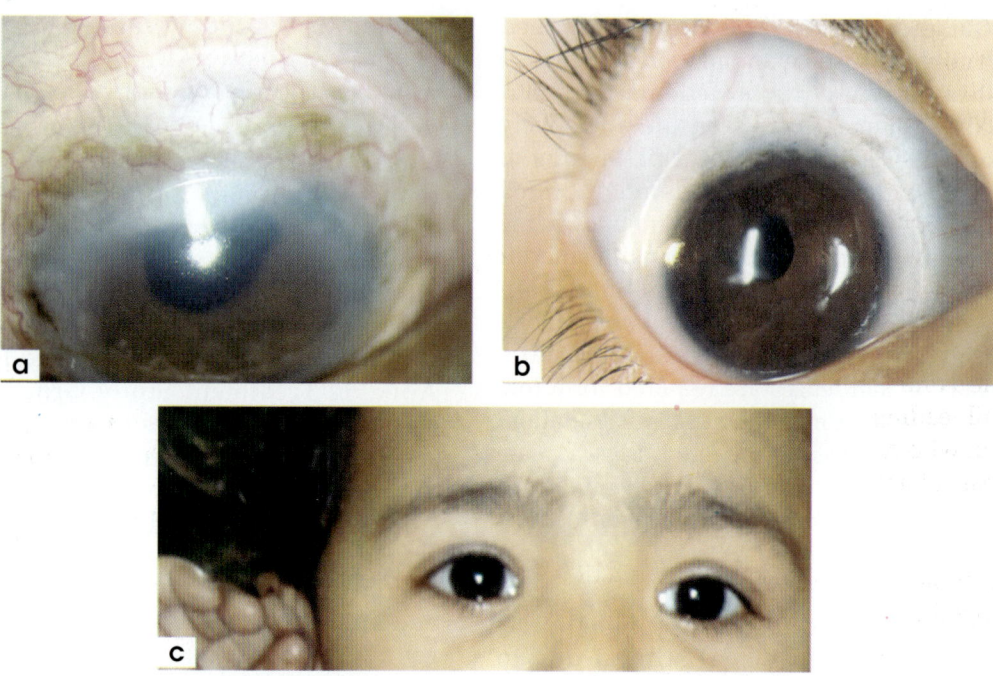

Fig. 11.7: Aphakic contact lens in children: (a) Post-extracapsular cataract surgery; (b) Post-phacoemulsification; (c) Bilateral aphakia in a child

hyperopic patients, lenses help in treating associated accommodative esotropia.

- **Therapeutic lenses** are required for conditions of albinism, aniridia, anisocoria.

Disadvantages with Contact Lens use in Children

- Steep learning curve for parents or care givers in inserting and removing a lens.
- Handling difficulty.
- Cost is high because of frequent lens changes as a consequence of altered refraction and/or lens loss.
- Frequent follow up is mandatory.
- Potential for corneal abrasion and infection.
- Psychological impact on the child and their parents due to daily lens insertion.

Aphakic Contact Lens Design

The shape of a high plus power lens has a thick centre with thin edges. Such lenses tend to position inferiorly due to their weight, gravity

and by inability of lid to pick up and hold the tapered peripheral edge. To aid centration of these lenses, a lenticular design is adopted (for both SCL and RGP) where only the small central zone carries power and the large peripheral skirt has no optics (Fig. 11.8). This

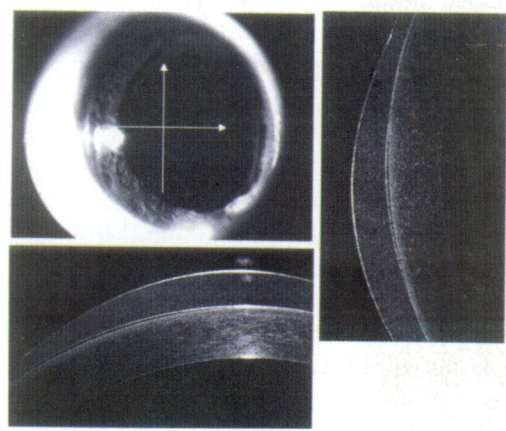

Fig. 11.8: Anterior OCT image of an aphakic contact lens on a child depicting thicker centre and tapering periphery

design serves to decrease lens weight with subsequent increase in Dk/t *value*, alters position of C of G of lens posteriorly and provides upper lid with a plano or minus powered design edge, thereby facilitating upper lid attachment. The back surface may employ spherical or aspheric optics; where the latter reduces spherical aberration inherent in high plus lenses. The flip side of lenticular design is that in case of lens decentration subsequent to child rubbing his eyes, central optic zone may get totally displaced from pupil leading to poor vision and an irritable child, who often has a patch on the sound eye as part of amblyopia treatment (Fig. 11.9).

Aphakic Contact Lens Materials/Options

The choice of lens materials and types has changed over the last few decades reflecting

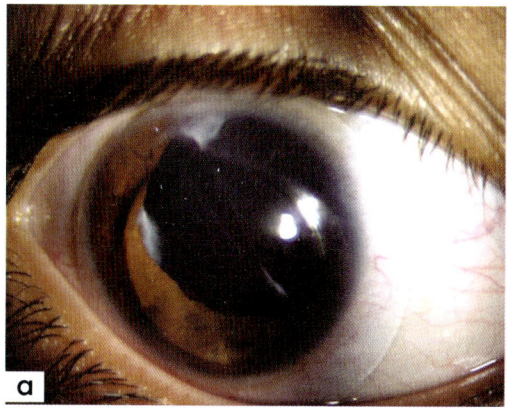

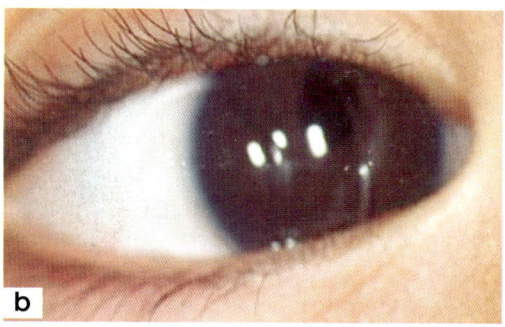

Fig. 11.9: Decentered lenticular aphakic lenses in children with (a) Traumatic aniridia; (b) Updrawn pupil

improvements in lens designs. From hard PMMA lenses to soft lenses to advent of silicone polymer rigid lenses, advances in lens industry has kept the ennui out of fitter's prescriptions.[11, 12]

a. *Soft hydrogels*: These easy to fit lenses are the preferred modality in aphakics with low astigmatism or failed RGP lens wearers. Since aphakic corneal demand for oxygen is reduced, hypoxia under a conventional soft lens is less and the high plus lenses with thicker centre are more effective in masking astigmatism, without the disadvantage of inducing central corneal oedema.

Initial lens to be selected is made smaller and relatively steeper despite its deleterious effect on corneal health, as flat lenses decenter more often and have a high incidence of lens loss. Lens fit in a child is judged more by movement and less by static evaluation. Movement in turn depends on lens thickness. For lenses with smaller central thickness (0.06 mm), movement ranges from 0.25 to 0.5 mm, for a thicker lens (0.12 mm) it ranges from 0.5 to 1.0 mm. In high water content lens, increased volume of water dictates a longer settling (equilibration) time before a valid assessment of lens fit is made. The practical aspect of this is to remember while doing over-refraction for finalizing lens power that a high plus power SCL can lose up to 2.5 D of optical power due to dehydration. These high water content hydrogels are fragile, deposit prone, susceptible to spoilage and require frequent replacement. Meticulous cleaning is essential to decrease risk of infection and frequent dioptric changes are required as power changes rapidly over the first 2 years of life. *Closed eye conditions* are very common due to excessive sleep time of an infant which subjects cornea to hypoxia. Thus for infants *highly oxygen permeable, high water content hydrogel lenses* are preferred. Such lenses have a tendency to dehydrate and be "stuck on" after a nap requiring use of lubricating eye drops prior to attempting lens removal.

During after care visits, corneal health needs to be monitored regularly, using a hand held slit lamp as decompensation can set in due to unregulated lens use coupled with initial surgical insult (phacoemulsification, vitrectomy). Corneal neovascularizartion with soft lens wear can also occur and needs to be monitored especially in presence of corneal sutures (Fig. 11.10).

b. *Silicone elastomer:* These silicone rubber hydrogel lenses are highly oxygen permeable (> 300 Dk value, oxygen transmission of 71), durable lenses.[13] One such lens the SilSoft aphakic lens by Bausch & Lomb, made of elastofilcon, is available in diameters of 11.3, 12.5 mm and powers from +11 to +20 with a Tc of 0.32–0.49 mm. The paediatric variant the *SilSoft* Super Plus comes in powers from +23 D to +32 D, Tc of 0.51 – 0.71 mm and diameter of 11.3 mm.

It is the silicone component which is responsible for oxygen permeability and hydrogel component for flexibility, wettability, fluid transport and lens movement. These lenses are the preferred options for infants and can be safely worn on extended wear basis.[8,14] Initial trial lens is 0.40 to 0.60 mm

flatter than average corneal radius (K readings) and 0.70 mm larger than HVID.[15] To avoid lens adherence, peripheral edge is fitted flat, to the extent of exhibiting a fluted edge which could create an edge lift.[5] Static fit with fluorescein should show minimal apical clearance and some degree of peripheral clearance. Dynamic fit should depict a lens movement of 0.5 mm postblink. The fitting should be checked after 10 and after 60 minutes to observe any changes in fitting pattern and lens movement. An initial lens which fits well tightens with time, so an *assessment of fit must be made after an hour of lens wear*. Drying of lenses and subsequent discomfort are frequent complaints by adults using these lenses due to poor lens wettability (Fig. 11.11). However, in infants, the more watery tears allow better wetting of silicone lenses.

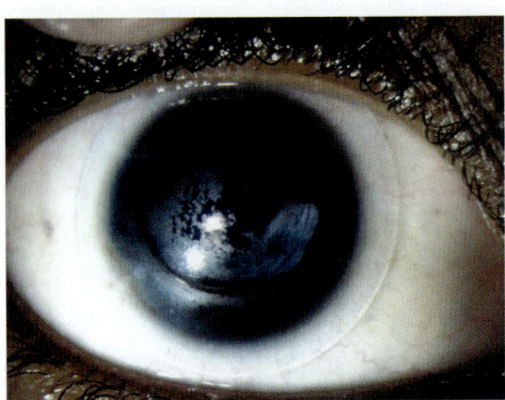

Fig. 11.11: Drying of tear film over the aphakic hydrogel

Hydrophobic silicone material resists tear ingress through its material leading to frequent **lens binding** to ocular surface.[8] This also makes these lenses difficult to remove. The binding needs to be counterbalanced by pressing the lid margin against lens edge to lift lens to allow air to rush in beneath the lens, before attempting lens removal. Parents/caregivers need to be forewarned of this situation; to prevent

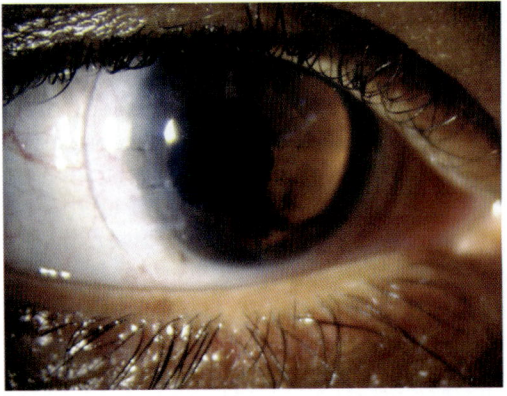

Fig. 11.10: Aphakic SCL with buried corneal sutures

panic at not being able to remove the lens. Long standing adherence causes a painful red eye with chemosed conjunctiva and steamy cornea and requires use of copious lubricating drops before attempting lens removal. The only silver lining to this lens adherence tendency is that it makes it very difficult for the infant to rub out these lenses.

Commercially available materials are Balafilcon (available as Pure Vision By Bausch & Lomb), Lotrafilcon A(available as Focus night and day by CIBA vision), Galyfilcon A (Acuvue by Vistakon). Balafilcon with a 36% water content has a Dk value of 110 barrer. These lenses are surface coated to provide a hydrophilic surface for biocompatibility and good *in situ* wettability. While fitting infants and toddlers it must be remembered that frequent replacements would be required every 3 to 6 months.[8]

c. *RGP lens:* The optics of a RGP lens combined with its property of allowing tear exchange allows clearer and crisper vision. The adequate tear exchange beneath the lens also makes it more salubrious to corneal health. However, the thick plus lens is difficult to fit and more difficult to retain in small eye of the child. The thick, heavy lens is down riding by nature and often falls out of the child's eye, more so after a bout of crying. Due to these reasons, rigid lenses are preferred only for traumatic aphakes with corneal scars, cases of high corneal astigmatism and/or corneal distortion (Fig. 11.12).

Aphakia post-extracapsular cataract surgery, has concomitant *against rule astigmatism,* which again causes lens to decentre down and outwards. Centration of these heavy lenses is difficult with the usual methods employed for its correction being use of large diameters (9.4–9.8 mm) along with a lenticular design. Lenticular design with reduced centre thickness attached to a peripheral minus carrier encourages lid attachment fit and ensures adequate high riding of lens allowing optic zone to cover the pupil. This method is called *blink-induced centration.*

Aphakic RGP ensues are usually fitted a little steep with slight apical clearance to ensure stability, with a slight 1–1.5 mm blink induced movement. Adequate tear exchange needs to be ensured by modifying the peripheral curve clearance if need be. In case of significant peripheral corneal astigmatism (toricity), peripheral curves

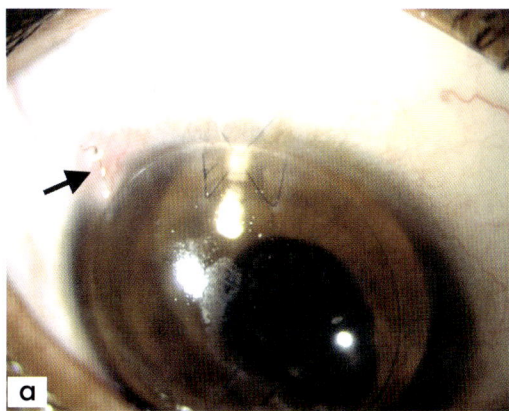 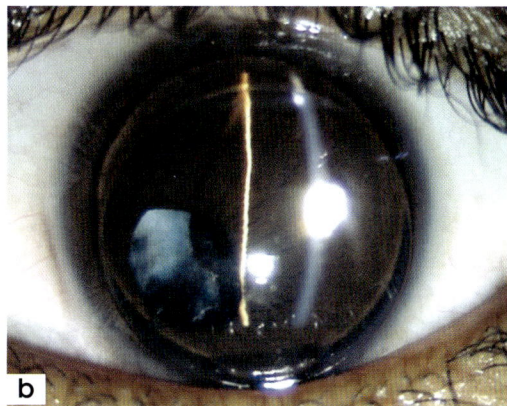

Fig. 11.12: (a) Aphakic RGP contact lens over buried, infinity corneal suture. The supero temporal suture with exposed knots needs to be removed. (b) Aphakic RGP contact lens over inferiorly distorted pupil

can be made toric to aid both lens fit as well as tear exchange.

d. *Scleral/miniscleral lenses:* The large dimensions of this lens make lens loss or decentration a remote possibility. This fact coupled with current, highly oxygen permeable materials, makes sclerals/minisclerals a feasible option for the paediatric aphake. Correction of irregular corneal astigmatism is also better managed with these lenses. Older patients with poor manual dexterity may find these larger lenses easier to handle, after the initial learning period. Despite these benefits these lenses are still reserved as a last resort due to their cost, poor availability and requirement to put tear supplements/saline cushion at regular intervals during lens wear, requiring manual lens removal for the action.

In geriatric aphakes presence of dry eyes, difficulty in lens in insertion due to tremors, arthritis, lax lids which generate ineffective blinking are all factors iniquitous to lens wear. Extended wear lenses with stringent follow up can be resorted to in such scenarios. Despite best intentions to fit lenses, sometimes aphakic spectacles maybe safer options for such patients.

Since many aphakic children have trauma as the preceding event, pupil and corneal co-morbidities like corneal scars, secondary glaucoma are common occurrences (Fig. 11.13). This cases adverse situations like-induced surgical astigmatism and its decay, pupil abnormalities (eccentric, and/or distorted and elongated), presence of corneal sutures and ocular tissue disturbances. All of these determine lens type and dictate lens fit (Fig. 11.14). In addition,

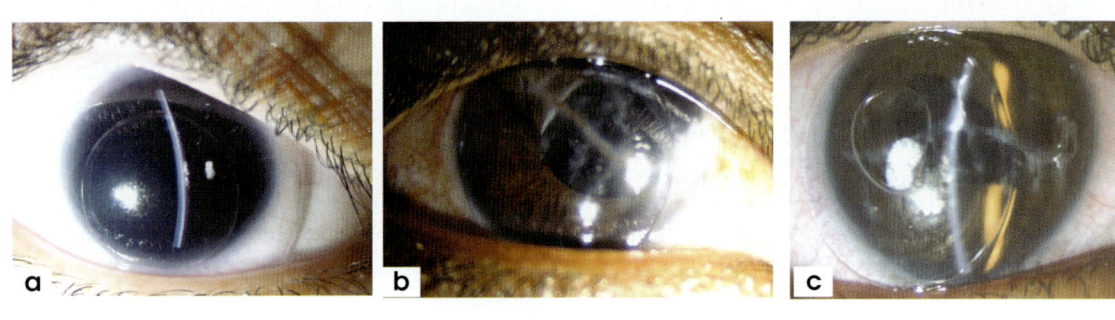

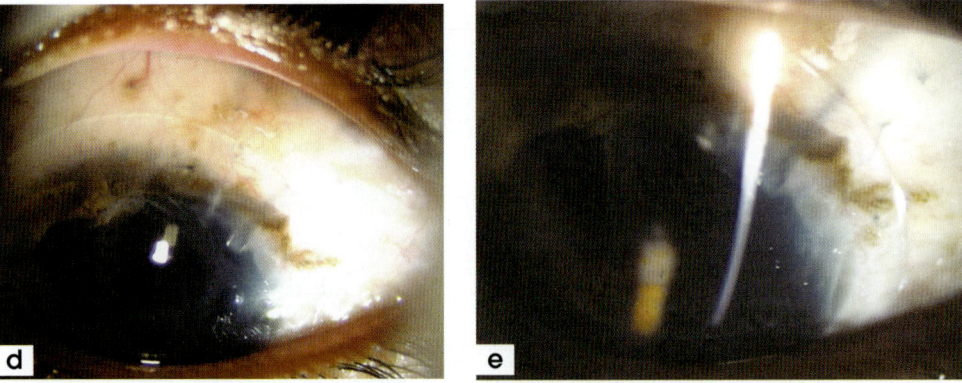

Fig. 11.13: Aphakic contact lens for child with: (a) Traumatic aphakia; (b and c) Coexisting with repaired corneal perforation; (d and e) Over Ahmed glaucoma valve for traumatic glaucoma, (e) Zoom in view of pateint seen in (d)

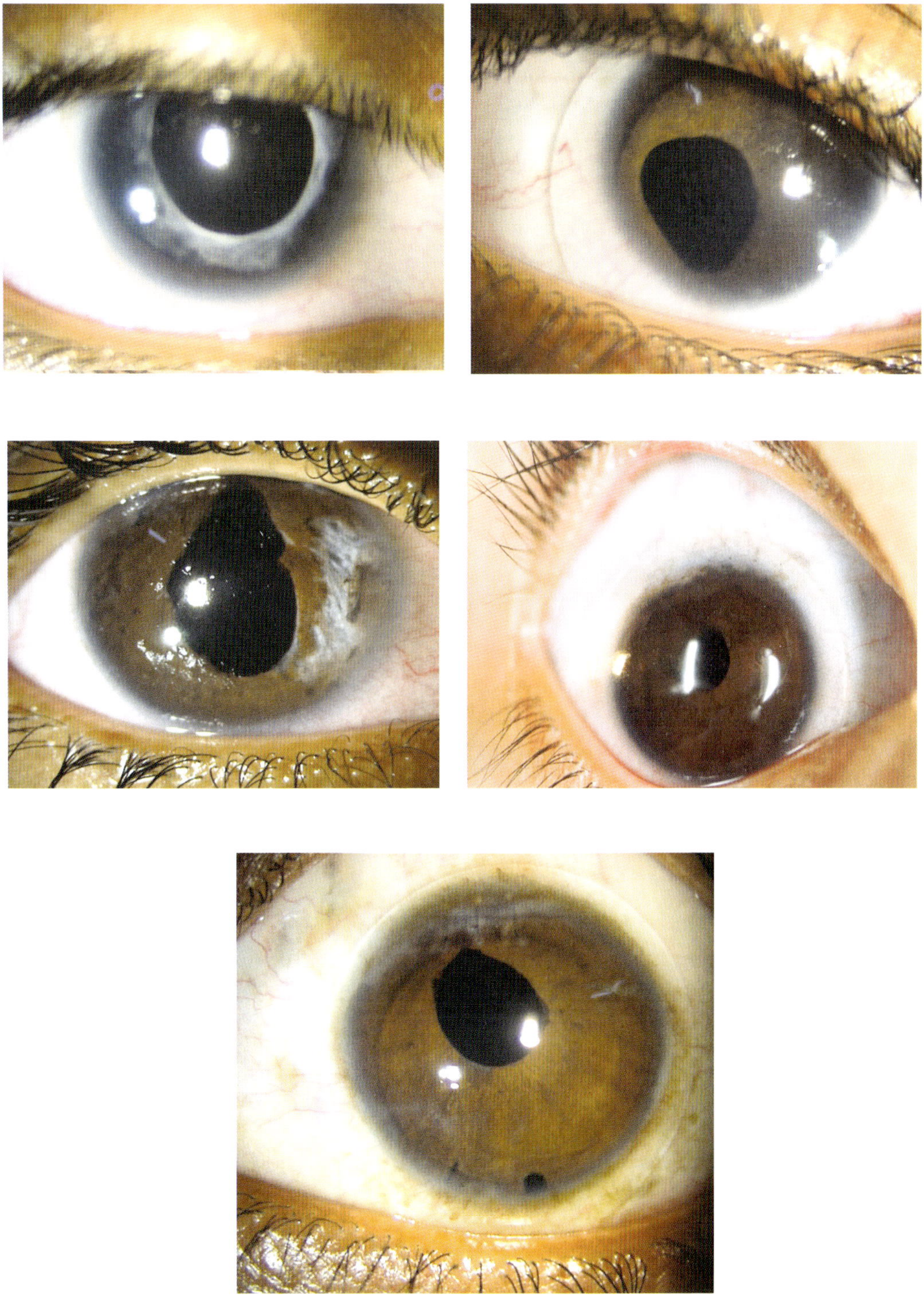

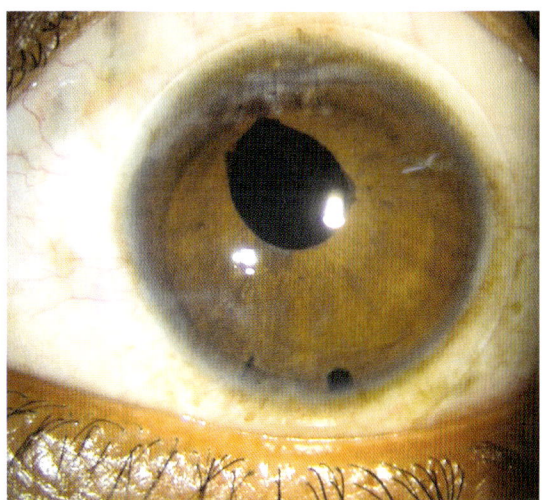

Fig. 11.14: Soft lenses being fitted onto aphakic children with different pupil (eccentric/updrawn) and iris abnormalities

during initial period child is extremely photophobic due to increased ultraviolet and visible light transmission subsequent to removal of absorbing crystalline lens. Additional protective UV filter glasses worn over aphakic contact lens for initial few weeks, may help in adjustments during this phase.

Fitting Methodology of a Soft Lens for an Infant

- **Keratometry:** This is done by using hand held keratometers, alternately conventional keratometer can be used with the child lying on his side, with measurements in vertical and horizontal meridians being interchanged. Standard K value can also be used in cases where keratometry is not possible, as shown in Table 11.1. The same was advocated by de Brabander et al.[8] The values used are: 47.00 D (7.18 mm) to 50.00 D (6.75 mm) for first 2 months and 7.0 to 7.2 mm for first 4 months.[16] Corneal curvature flattens out by preschool age of 3 to 4 years to 43.00 D (7.85 mm)/44.00 D (7.67 mm), except in cases of retinopathy of prematurity, where curvature remains steep.

Table 11.1: Standard K and power according to age of child		
Age (months)	Soft lens BOZR (mm)	BVP(D)
0–6	7.5	+29 to + 32
7–17	7.7/7.9	+26
18–28	7.9	+23
29–34	7.9/8.1	+18

- **Corneal diameter:** The corneal diameter or HVID can be measured with a hand-held rule or similar device. Average corneal diameter at birth is 9.8–10.0 mm, which increases rapidly in first year of life and then tapers over next few years to reach adult diameters of 12 mm by 3–4 years age.

- The common method employed in our clinic is use of trial lens based on standard K reading.
- **Trial lens insertion:** In order to simplify insertion, infant is tightly wrapped in a towel restraining his hands. Fitting a lens in a toddlers is more difficult preposition and often two people are required to hold the child's arms and shoulders, while another inserts trial lens after holding lids apart (Fig. 11.15a). We prefer not to feed the infant before/during lens insertion for fear of aspiration during the accompanying bout of crying. Instead a pacifier or bottle is offered after lens insertion. After a few minutes allowing for tearing to subside, child opens his eyes, at which time a hand held slit lamp is used to evaluate lens fit. A direct ophthalmoscope with the convex lens dialled in (at power of +7 to + 8) also gives a reasonably adequate view of the CL profile *in situ* (Fig. 11.15b).

  Another position used in—Helicopter position of child unable to sit on slit lamp (Fig. 11.15c).

- **Over-refraction:** To confirm final lens power, over-refraction is performed by retinoscopy. Cycloplegic refraction is usually not needed as accommodation is lacking in aphakia. Since poor pupillary dilatation is frequent in aphakic children, powerful mydriasis by atropine ointment application (twice a day for two days) is often necessary. While doing over-refraction, trial lenses must be kept close to eye of infant to minimize risk of prescribing an incorrect contact lens BVP, due to high prescription involved. The arbitrary values to be used if retinoscopy is not possible are: BVP of +34.00 D for a 6-week-old infant, +28.00 D for a 6-month-old baby and by 1 year of age +24.00 D power.[16]

  Distance vision correction would require an aphakic contact lens power ranging from +20 to +35.0 D. As *infant's visual world is usually restricted to near objects*, therefore

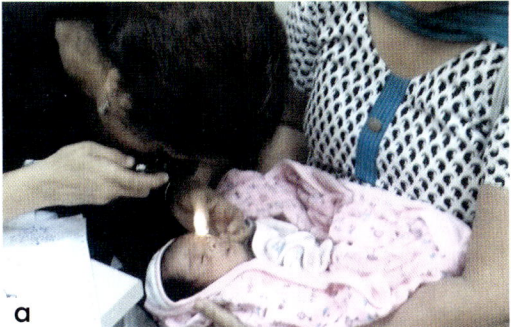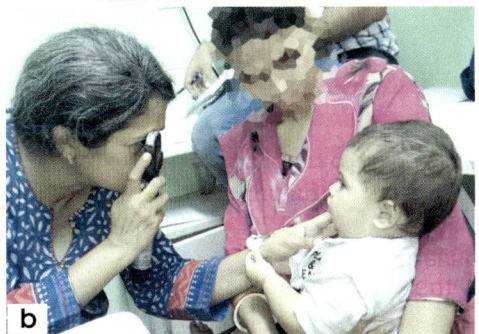

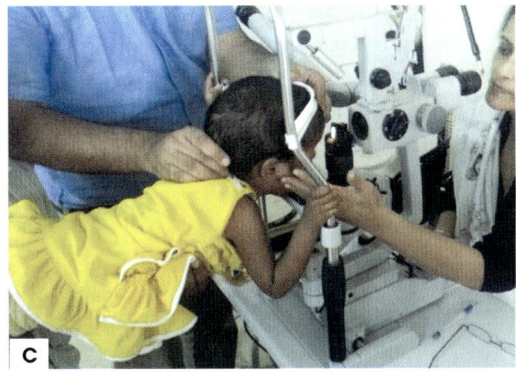

Fig. 11.15: Examination techniques of a young child with CL in eye: (a) Holding lids apart in an infant; (b) Using plus lens dialled into ophthalmoscope for a toddler; (c) Helicopter position to examine young child not able to sit on slit lamp

in order to provide optimum focus, contact lenses need to be over-corrected by +2.00 D to +3.00 D. This near prescription is changed to a distance prescription by the time child goes to school with a bifocal spectacles add given for reading. The spectacles may incorporate any astigmatic correction required.

- **Lens removal:** The child's eye is held wide open, both lower and upper lids are manipulated under lens edge to break suction effect. This procedure may be difficult in deep set eyes and a crying child. Parents are taught the technique of applying and removing the lenses. The initial frustration is quickly replaced by confidence and dexterity in most parents. The first few times parents need to be supervised during contact lens insertion and removal. Older children can be taught to handle and care for their own lenses.

Pediatric Eye

For the pediatric contact lens fitter a basic understanding of ocular dimensions, visual milestones and methods to assess vision is required. These are briefly described.

A. Ocular dimensions

Length of the infant eyeball is approximately 17 mm, as opposed to 24 mm in the adult. Corneal diameter at birth is 10.0 mm, it reaches 11.6–12.0 mm (adult size) by 3–4 years. The radius of curvature of anterior corneal surface is 7.0 mm at birth, which gradually flattens to an adult average of 7.86 mm eye by 10 years. A normal neonate has a moderately hyperopic error with a slight astigmatic component.

B. Vision assessment methods

These depend on age of child with methods differing for preverbal to verbal stage.

i. Preverbal child (infant/toddlers)

Objective tests are required for this age group.

- Fixing and follow light/object (Fig. 11.16a).
- Bruckner test (red reflex test): Difference in intensity of binocular red reflex seen by direct ophthalmoscope, the eye with high error having a paler reflex (Fig. 11.16b)
- Cover test: A child with significant refractive error opposes, resists covering of better eye (Fig. 11.16c).

- Preferential looking tests (Teller and Cardiff acuity charts) (Figs 11.17 and 11.18).
- Otokinetic nystagmus (OKN), pattern VEP (Fig. 11.7b)
- ETDRS charts with LEA symbols consist of four optotypes (circle/square/apple/house) where the child is required to match target with similar shapes available on loose cards.

ii. Verbal child (Schoolgoing)

- Standard ETDRS charts with geometric progression in each line with equal number of letters in each row are used (Fig. 11.19a)

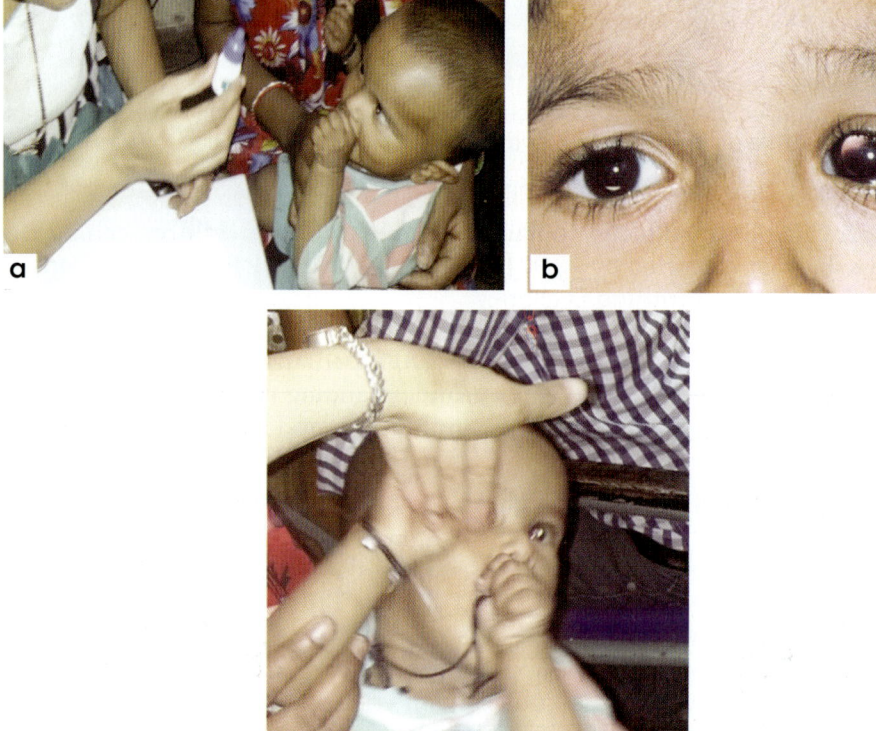

Fig. 11.16: (a) The child is fixing at the colored top of a bottle; (b) Bruckner's red; (c) On covering of right eye the child resists it and tries to force the examiner's hand away.

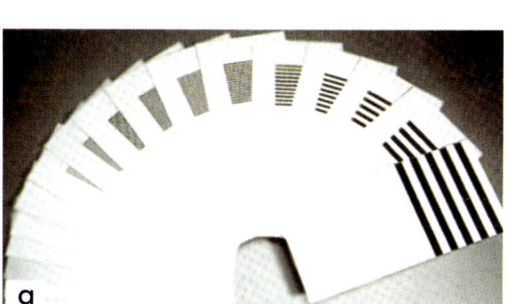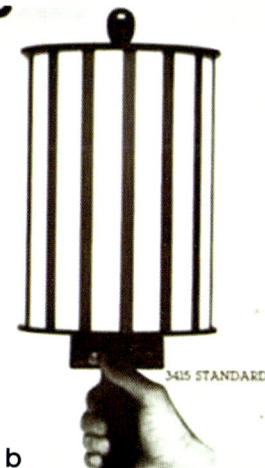

Fig. 11.17: (a) Teller visual acuity chart; (b) Optokinetic nystagmus drum employs OKN reflex where the eyes pursue moving bars in same direction followed by a quick saccade in opposite direction to fixate on next moving bar. Different sized stripes are used to quantify visual acuity

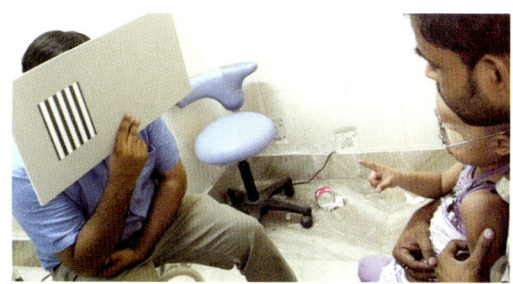

Fig. 11.18: Teller visual acuity chart viewing by a child. Gratings of varying cycles per centimeter against a grey background are presented and finest grating visible is the child's acuity. Concept is based on preferential viewing of patterns. The child will look at sequentially finer pattern till it is visible, in preference to an unpatterned stimulus

– Snellen charts/Allen picture chart/ Tumbling Landolt E chart (Fig. 11.19b to d)

American Academy of Pediatrics recommends that a child aged 3–5 years should be able to read most of letters on 20/40 (6/12 Snellen's equivalent) and children ≥ 6 years should be read beyond 20/30 line.

In addition to vision evaluation, stereopsis should be evaluated to test for binocular function. This is more relevant for uniocular aphakia to confirm if the visual rehabilitation is sufficient to provide stereoscopic vision. Titmus fly test is a good screening test and it is done after ensuring that the aphakic eye is using near add correction over the distance corrected contact lens[7] (Fig. 11.20).

C. Visual milestones

- 6–8 weeks: Eye contact, preferential looking at brightly colored/patterned objects or mother, *social smile*
- 2 months: Protective blink reflex, any crossed eye (eso/exo deviations) straightens out by this time
- 3–4 months: Hand eye coordination, start to reach out for things, non-jerky eye movements, converges on near object, following movement appears.
- 5 months: Gross colour differentiation, stereopsis and binocularity start establishing
- 6 months: Reaches out and grasp toys, objects, recognizes faces, full conjugate eye movements. Watches small rolling balls at 5 ft, macula starts differentiating and fixation becomes stable.

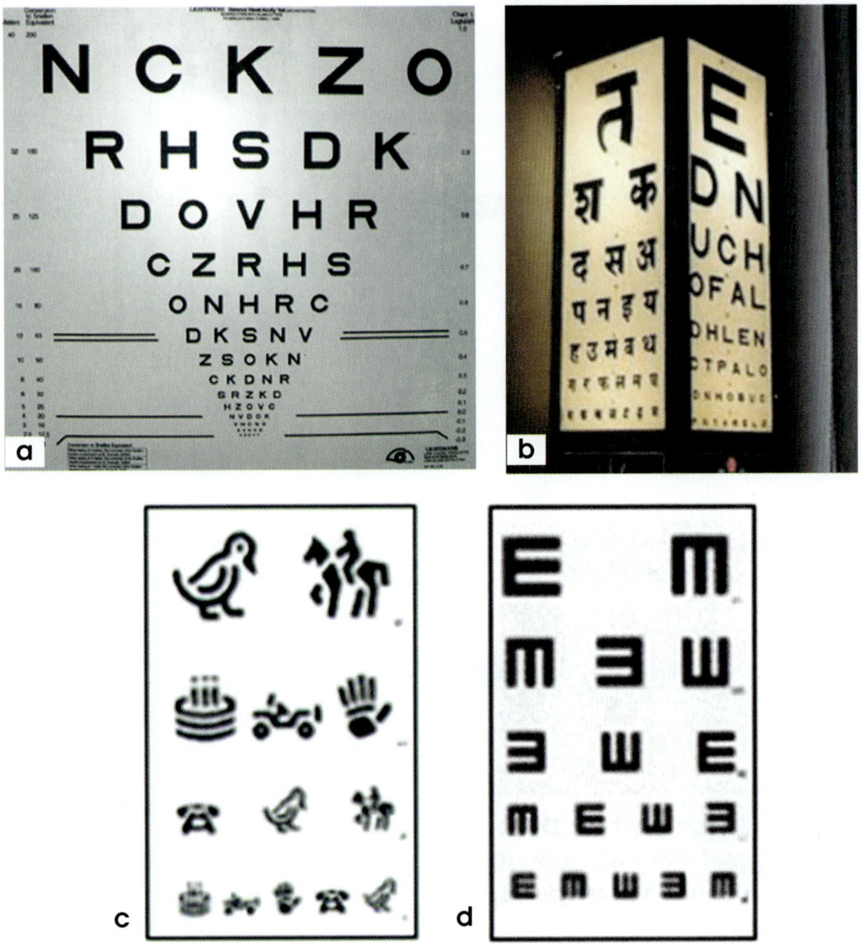

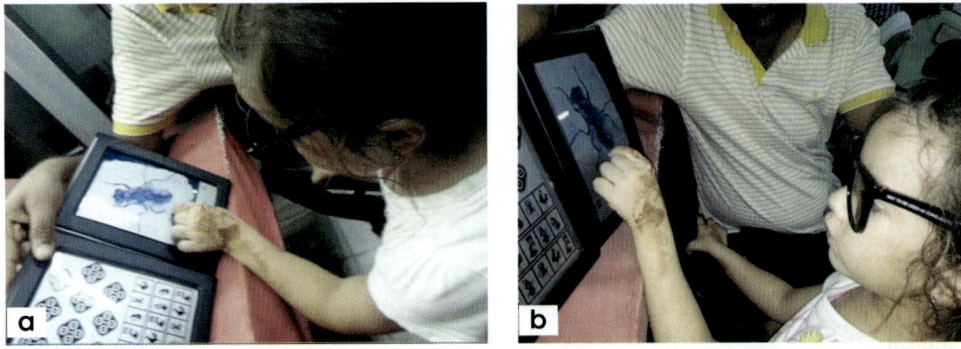

Fig. 11.19: (a) ETDRS chart; (b) Illuminated Snellen chart; (c) Allen picture chart; (d) Landolt's C chart

Fig. 11.20: (a) Titmus fly test: Child wears polarized glasses, test images (housefly, animal, circle) are superimposed stereo pairs presented differently to each eye by the polarized filter; (b) Form is visible as **standing out**/rising out of the page only in child with stereopsis. On monocular viewing or stereo-blind child test images appear in a flat field.

- 9–10 months: Identifies picture books, plays games, imitates, distinguishes strangers, has good hand eye coordination.
- 1 year: Sustained visual interest for both distant and near objects.
- 2 years: Corneal diameter attains adult dimensions. Child points to pictures in books, imitates vertical or horizontal strokes. Letter matching possible, visual acuity can be assessed by picture/Cardiff charts. Steroacuity reaches near adult level.
- 3 years: Draws crude circle, can do colored jigsaw puzzles.
- 4 years: Depth perception, reads and write letters, letter matching tasks possible.
- 5 years: Colors pictures, writes capital letters and in cursive.
- 6 years: Reads texts.

Practical Tips in Fitting a CL in Children

- Small palpebral aperture and tight lids of an infant makes lens insertion very difficult. This is often exacerbated by the crying infant and forceful lid closure. Forcing the lids open leads to lid eversion and inability to introduce the lens. A strong blepharospasm response is concurrent in the crying child, which may either push out the lens and/or cause inside out folding (Fig. 11.21).

- Evaluation of lens fitting in a teary eyed crying child is not possible. Thus persistence in trying to insert a contact lens in a crying child, due to time constraints, benefits no one. In addition, the entire scenario of forcefully inserting a lens into the child's eye creates a distasteful situation and de-motivates other parents. In these cases parents are made partners in the insertion process, remove feelings of guilt or frustration and are called for another sitting. We employ a strategy where mothers who have been comfortably inserting lenses for their children, are asked to help in teaching lens handling technique to new cases/parents.
- High DK value lenses need to be used so that the infant can nap with the lens on without subjecting his cornea to hypoxia.
- Children need to be corrected for near work as infant's world is near world. For schoolgoing children the vision may be corrected for distance with the addition of bifocal spectacles for near work (Fig. 11.22).
- Rarely children with IOL surprise may benefit from contact lens rehabilitation as this uniocular pseudophakic child with a −7D surprise was fitted with a soft contact lens (Fig. 11.23).
- Rapid decrease in refractive correction over first two years of life necessitates a refractive change every 3 months for first

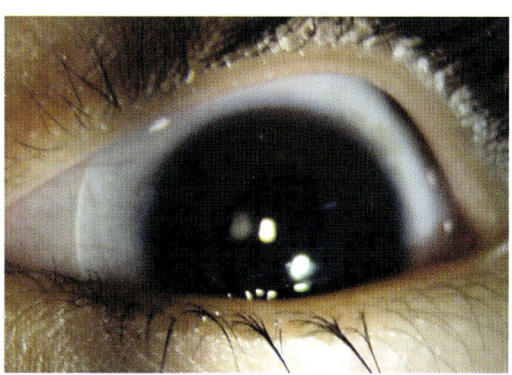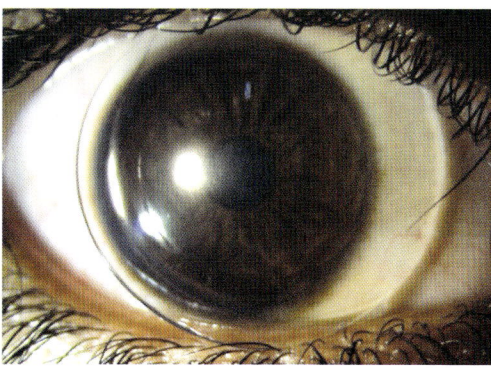

Fig. 11.21: Blepharospasm in a crying child pushes contact lens out

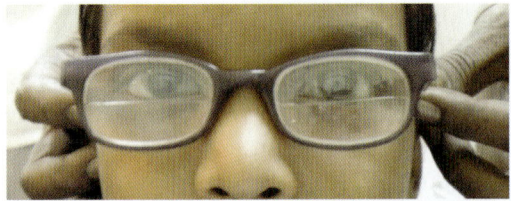

Fig. 11.22: Binocular aphakic child using near add bifocals over distance vision contacts in both eyes

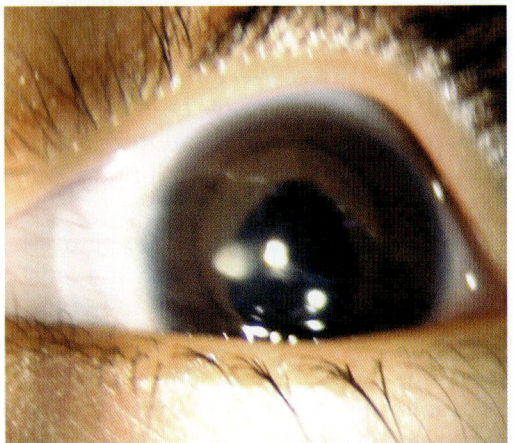

Fig. 11.23: Soft hydrogel over IOL surprise. Note IOL capture in this child.

year and then 6 monthly for next few years. Refraction needs to be performed frequently to pick up this refractive change.

- Minimal astigmatism can be ignored or spherical equivalent incorporated into the spherical lens' power.
- Amblyopia therapy needs to be coupled with use of occlusion and/or penalization (Fig. 11.24).
- A set of spare lenses must be available with the parents at all times.

Follow Up Visits

The first visit is scheduled a week after dispensing the contact lens.

- Lens case is to be checked regularly for signs of poor maintenance.
- Sutures are to be checked for mucous pile up or loosening in which case they need to be removed under anaesthesia (Fig. 11.25).

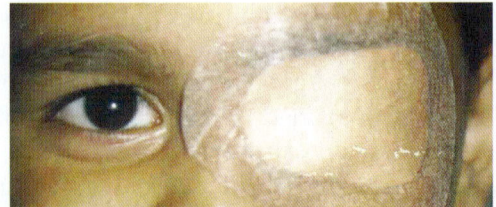

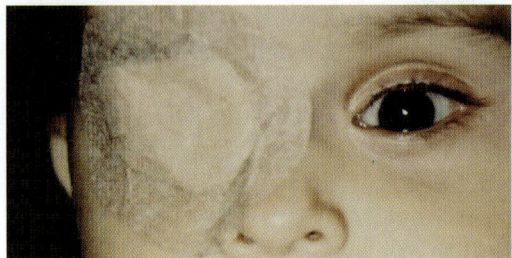

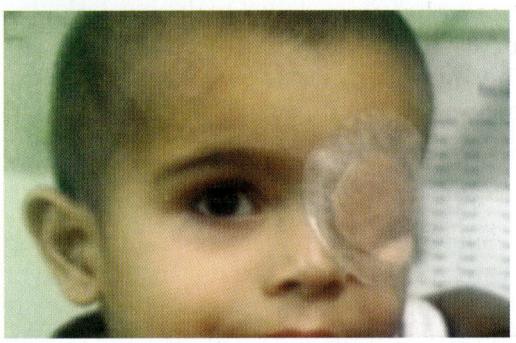

Fig. 11.24: Uniocular aphakic children corrected with contact lens along with opticlude occlusion in phakic eye

- Retinal exam and IOP measure is performed at 3 monthly basis for the initial year and subsequently 6 monthly basis till child starts school. Subsequently it can be scheduled on a yearly basis.

Refraction is done at 3 monthly basis for first year and then at 6 monthly basis till the child is 5–6 years of age. The high hyperopia of a newborn reduces within first weeks of life from 34 D to 18 D by 2 years of age, due to an increasing axial length and flattening corneal curvature. Any deviation from this and a myopic shift could be an early sign of glaucoma. In children with systemic diseases associated with high myopia, e.g. Down's syndrome aphakic power can be as low as +5 D.

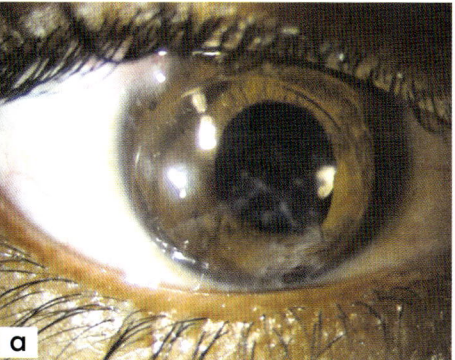 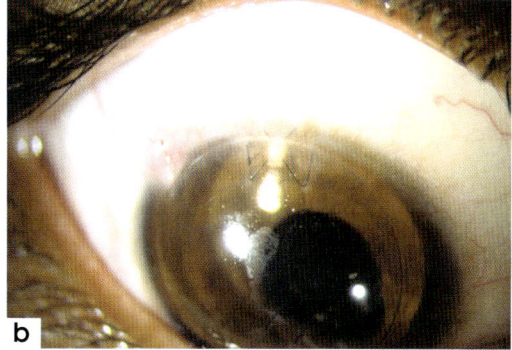

Fig. 11.25: Aphakic lens fitted over. (a) Buried and (b) exposed corneal suture. The suture in patient needs to be removed

Parental Instruction

Parental cooperation is the keystone to a successful paediatric contact lens outcome. The instructions should touch upon the following aspects.

- Normal lens performance characteristics.
- Signs and symptoms of adverse reactions.
- Appropriate emergency responses.
- Proper use of solutions.
- Lens cleaning procedures, wearing schedules.

These must be discussed verbally and supplied in writing.

Successful contact lens wear can improve both vision and quality of life of paediatric patient. This can be very rewarding for child, parents, and contact lens practitioner.

REFERENCES

1. Woods AC. Communications. Patient reactions to disability. The adjustment to aphakia. Br J Ophthal 1964:48, 349.

2. McLemore CS. Aphakic correction from an aphake's point of view. Arch Ophthalmol. 1965;74(3):443.

3. Wong ACM. Optics of Intraocular lens. In Albert Jakobiec's Principles and Practice of Ophthalmology. 3rd ed. Eds Albert DM, Miller JK, Saunders Elsevier 2008: 5295–5315.

4. Boeder P. Spectacle correction of aphakia. Arch Ophthalmol 1962;68:870–4.

5. Rosenthal P. Contact Lenses. In Albert Jakobiec's Principles and Practice of Ophthalmology. 3rd ed. Eds Albert DM, Miller JK, Saunders Elsevier 2008: 5279–94.

6. Dada VK, Mehta MR, Jain AK. Pitfalls in aphakic contact lens fitting. Indian J Ophthalmol 1990;38:27–9.

7. Riise R, Kolstad A, Bruun S, Espeland A. The use of contact lenses in children with unilateral traumatic aphakia. Acta Ophthalmol (Copenh). 1977 Jun; 55(3):386–94.

8. de Brabander J, Kok J, Nuijts R, Wenniger-Prick L (2002). A Practical Approach to and Long-Term Results of Fitting Silicone Contact Lenses in Aphakic Children after Congenital Cataract. CLAO J. 28: 31–35.

9. Celano M, Hartmann EE, Drews-Botsch CD; Infant Aphakia Treatment Study Group. Parenting stress in the infant aphakia treatment study. J Pediatr Psychol. 2013 Jun;38(5):484–93.

10. Infant Aphakia Treatment Study Group. Lambert SR, Lynn MJ, Hartmann EE, DuBois L, Drews-Botsch C, Freedman SF, Plager DA, Buckley EG, Wilson ME. Comparison of contact lens and intraocular lens correction of monocular aphakia during infancy: a

randomized clinical trial of HOTV optotype acuity at age 4.5 years and clinical findings at age 5 years. JAMA Ophthalmol. 2014 Jun; 132(6):676–82.

11. Boyd HH. Hard contact lens corrections in aphakia. Ophthalmology. 1979 Mar; 86(3): 399–402.

12. Aquavella JV. New aspects of contact lenses in ophthalmology. Adv Ophthalmol. 1976; 32:2–34.

13. Ozbeck Z, Durak I, Berk TA. Contact lenses in correction of childhood aphakia. The CLAO Journal 2002, 28(1); 28–30.

14. Aasuri MK, Venkata N, Preetam P, Rao NT. Management of pediatric aphakia with Silsoft contact lenses. CLAO J1999. 25: 209–12.

15. Speedwell L. Contact lens fitting in infants and pre-school children. In: Phillips AJ, Speedwell L (Eds). Contact Lenses. 5th ed., Oxford Butterworth-Heinemann. 2007: 505–18.

16. Morris JA, Taylor D. Contact lenses for children in contact lens practice. Eds MRuben and M Guillon, Chapman 7 Hall. London 1994: 829–38.

Reader's Note

Reader's Note

CHAPTER **12**

Fitting on Post-keratoplasty or Post-corneal Refractive Surgery

PENETRATING KERATOPLASTY

Improved donor storage media, enhancements in surgical procedure, meticulous suturing techniques, modifications like deep lamellar anterior keratoplasty (DALK) and Descemet's stripping automated endothelial keratoplasty (DSAEK), availability of special postoperative care all have led to increased success rate of graft clarity after keratoplasty. However, surgical astigmatism due to suturing, donor-host junction transition and uneven healing still remains as a cause of poor visual recovery despite a clear graft. This aspect often requires contact lens rehabilitation to restore functional visual after a successful keratoplasty with usual indications being: Irregular surgical astigmatism, anisometropia, aphakia or high myopia.[1]

Physiology and Topography in Grafted Eyes Relevant to CL Fit

Grafted cornea is a physiologically vulnerable cornea, where minor inadequacies in CL fitting can give rise to major problems such as dry eyes, graft rejection and graft failure.

- Endothelial density for a grafted eye is lower than age matched normal corneas, which magnifies the *occlusive effect* of a contact lens. Lens material and fit have to carefully chosen to ensure that lens wear does not trigger an edematous response,

which in turn would initiate graft vascularization and subsequently rejection.

- Corneal nerves take 2–3 years or even longer for partial regeneration, with sensations returning to near normal within 12 months of keratoplasty.[2,3] Since donor is desensitized, warning symptoms of pain, photophobia occurring due to epithelial damage or infiltration may be delayed for these patients. The paucity of corneal sensation, however, helps in early adaptation and comfort with lens wear.

- Lid sensitivity, presence of corneal sutures, altered tear film dynamics, use of topical medications may counterbalance lack of corneal sensation and lens wear may not actually be very comfortable during initial period.

- Postgraft astigmatism is determined by graft size, positioning and by uniformity, depth and number of sutures. Eccentric positioning of graft, non-uniform depth of suturing, irregular healing, for example, in herpetic keratitis, loose sutures, interface scarring and episodes of vessel growth also contribute to irregular astigmatism which may range from 5 to 15 Dc.[4,5]

- *Altered corneal topography*: A grafted eye topography differs from the normal and needs imaging by corneal topography. Keratometry in these eyes is insufficient to decide the trial lens dimensions, since

163

central 3 mm² measured by this instrument may suffice in deciding trial lens for a healthy corneas but does not reflect the configuration change occurring in a grafted cornea. Topography, on the other hand, delineates entire donor, host, junction, effect of suturing and in locating high point of graft host junction, with latter being the fulcrum over which an RGP lens would glide.[6] This imaging tool is therefore invaluable in understanding of different topographical variations in a grafted cornea.

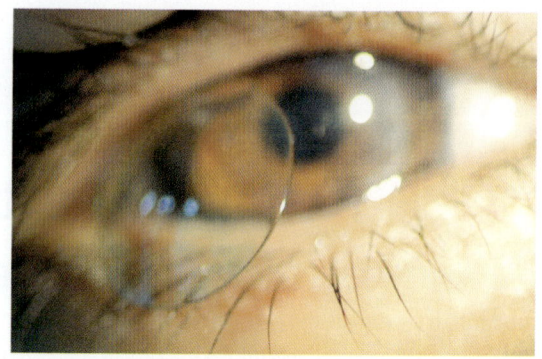

Fig. 12.1: Lens gets ejected out of the eye after blink in a case with proud graft junction

Since this altered topography determines type and pattern of lens fit, a brief understanding of the same is essential.

a. *Proud graft topography:* For a conventional keratoplasty graft size is deliberately kept 0.5 mm larger than host to allow host graft alignment. In situations where graft donor discrepancy is greater than standard 0.5 mm, donor tissue steepens to reduce 'skirt' diameter in order to align with host dimensions, resulting in *proud graft topography.* Such a topography with steep center and flatter periphery is also more likely in case of grafted keratoconus, where host cornea thickness is less than donor button. Resultant raised step at host-graft interface causes an RGP lens to ski off the graft, when displaced by a blinking lid (Fig. 12.1). To circumvent this large diameter, steeper peripheral curve or reverse geometry lenses are used. Other causes for proud graft are tight suturing, irregular healing and occurrence of secondary glaucoma.

b. *Nipple like protrusion:* Scarring at the host donor junction coupled with lower rigidity of graft, causes a central protrusion giving rise to an exaggerated prolate pattern (Fig. 12.2a). *Localized steepness (LS) pattern* occurs when less than 1/4th corneal diameter is steeper

than the residual flatter, and relatively lower power cornea (Fig. 12.2b).[7]

c. *Flat or sunken graft:* This is seen with equal sized donor and recipient, here central cornea is flatter than the peripheral cornea (an exaggerated oblate pattern). An *horseshoe* pattern variant has been identified with a C-shaped area of increased corneal power at the graft host interface.[7]

Lens fit is easier for flat grafts and nipple grafts versus proud graft topography. Lenses with spherical back surface vault over the graft leading to excessive central pooling, and very often bubbles get entrapped in this central pool (Fig. 12.3). Fenestration of the RGP lens can be resorted to, for trapped air to escape from post-lens tear film.

d. *Plateau graft topography:* In this situation reverse geometry lens scores over a spherical lens by minimizing both apical and peripheral edge clearance.

e. *Tilted graft topography:* Discrepancies in thickness of host graft margin, variations in depth of suturing and uneven trephine surface lead to a tilted graft. Lens fitted over such corneas depict excessive *standoff over* recessed area, causing a localized *tear gutter* over this region which may lead to retention of air bubbles. This in turn promotes tear

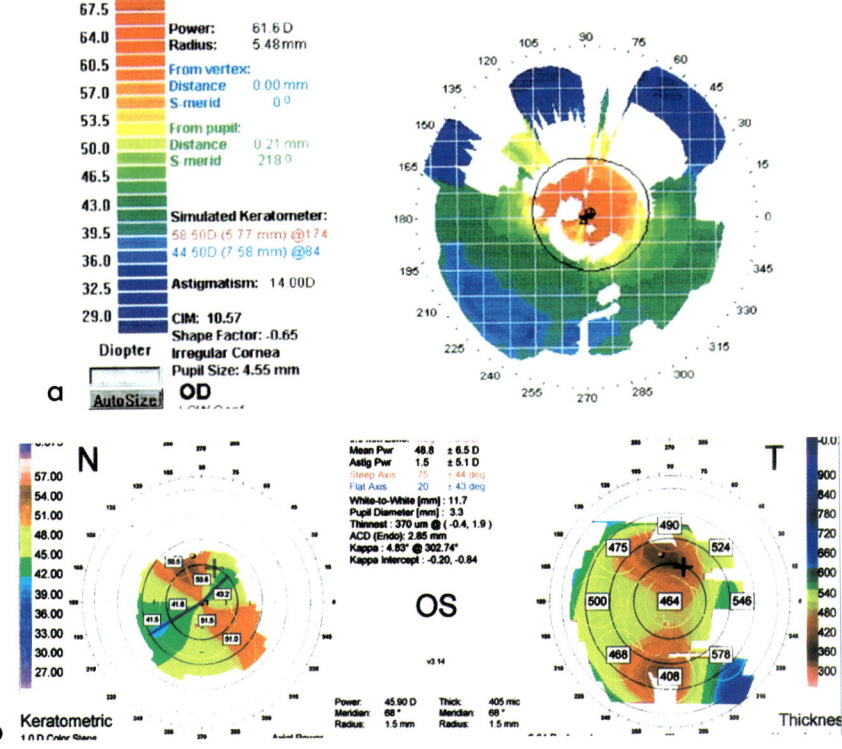

Fig. 12.2: (a) Exaggerated prolate pattern post PK; (b) Localized steep patterns

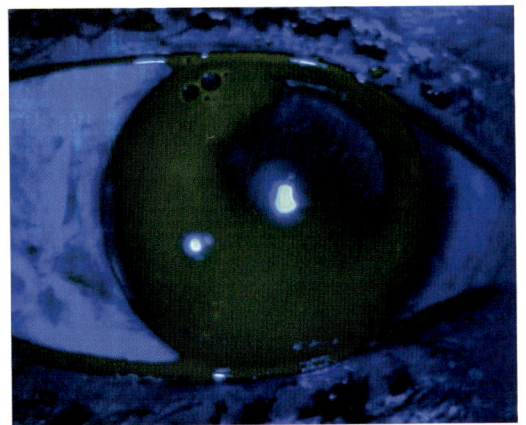

Fig. 12.3: Air bubbles trapped beneath a flat fit RGP lens

desiccation, reduces lens mobility and invites vascularization. Large diameter lenses greater than 10 mm, lens with with tricurve or quadricurve design and

BOZD larger than graft size can be tried for such cases.

f. *Eccentric graft*: In scarred eyes or thinned corneas, the graft centered over the pathological area may not be in the visual axis. Slippage of the trephine while cutting the host is another reason for an eccentric graft (Fig. 12.4).

Timing of Contact Lens Fitting

The usual time elapsed before a contact lens is fitted on a grafted eye ranges from 6 to 18 months, depending on need for functional vision. By this time almost all sutures have been removed and patient is on minimal topical steroids. Corneal integrity and health is also completely restored by 18 to 24 months except nerve regeneration.[1]

Sutures: Fitting over sutures in a grafted eye is very often a necessary evil, and fitters would

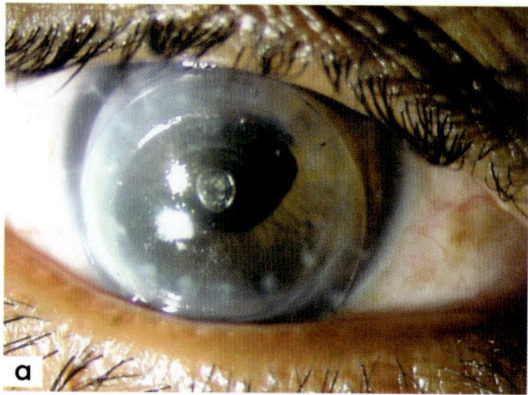 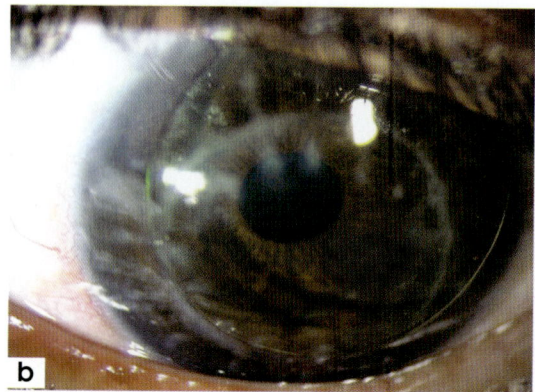

Fig. 12.4: RGP lens over: (a) Tilted; (b) Eccentric graft

be required to fit eyes which have a few *in situ* sutures. The problems while fitting over sutures are the following. Firstly, such fit is technically very demanding and often unfeasible due to irregular host graft topography. Secondly, altered tear film resurfacing causes more hypoxia and can trigger vessel growth near the suture (Fig. 12.5). Thirdly, loose sutures serve as a nidus for mucus build up, cause diminished skiing movement of lens on graft edge, which can lead to either tight fit or a decentered lens. Over time such fits over retained sutures may induce graft vascularization and rejection. Lens decentration and discomfort is also more common. It is thus advisable for all loose sutures to be removed before attempting a CL fit.

In some situations like paediatric aphakia, lens fitting needs to be done prior to suture removal so as to arrest amblyopia, keeping in mind that evolving host graft junction healing, would require frequent lens changes during the initial year. Often a few well-buried sutures are left *in situ* after a year if they do not alter corneal topography. Fitting a contact lens over such sutures can and needs to be done while ensuring frequent, regular follow ups.

Medications: Most PK cases are on long-term medications like topical steroids and less often anti-glaucoma drugs. These drops can be continued safely over RGP lenses but not over a soft lens (another reason for RGP being the lens of choice in PK eyes).

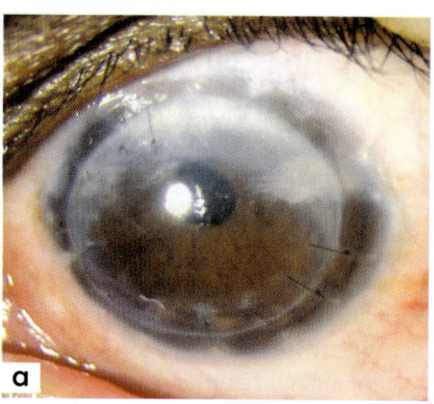 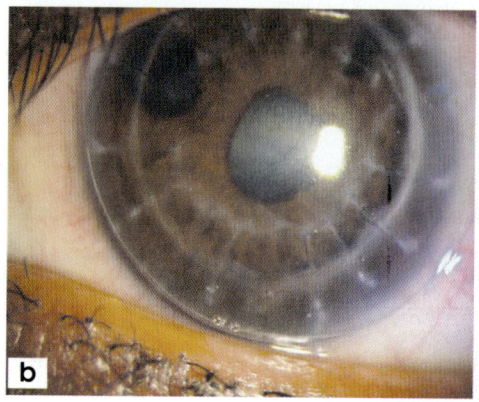

Fig. 12.5: (a) Superior corneal haze after lens wear. Note buried sutures at host graft junction; (b) Rose K lens fitted over a graft, with all sutures removed.

Fitting Technique and Lens Options

In addition to refraction, a detailed slit lamp biomicroscopy examination of the graft size, position, placement, number of sutures, scarring and neovascularization if any is done. A simple diagram should be made documenting these features.

The base curve of the trial lens is chosen based on topographic values on 3 mm Sim K values or on average keratometry values, preferably the former.[6] After a settling in period, fitting is evaluated by both static and dynamic fitting. Fluorescein staining is done to delineate areas of excessive clearance or bearing for RGP lens. The key to a successful fit is optimal use of peripheral host cornea for bearing lens edge. Lens stability is best if horizontal meridian bearing can be achieved.

A steep fit can cause corneal compromise with patient having initial crisp vision followed by edema and blurred vision. A flat lens causes mechanical injury to graft host junction, corneal scarring and lens drop out. Lenses often exhibit a temporal or nasal displacement according to direction of least mechanical resistance. The lens design is chosen to minimize mechanical and physiological stress to the graft. Lens material with high DK values is chosen and lens options are RGP, soft or specialized lenses.

a. RGP lens: They are the lenses of choice, as only they can correct high astigmatism and/or irregular astigmatism exceeding 3–4 D, which is the common scenario in most post-keratoplasty cases (Fig. 12.6).[1,8,9] The masking of astigmatism is very clearly demonstrated in Fig. 12.7.

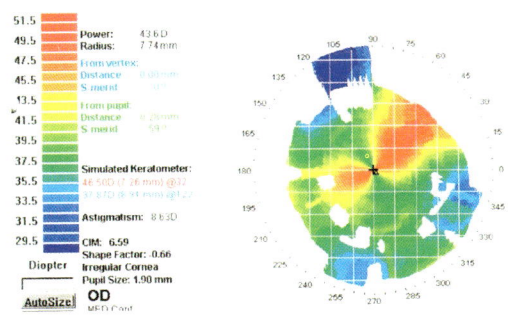

a

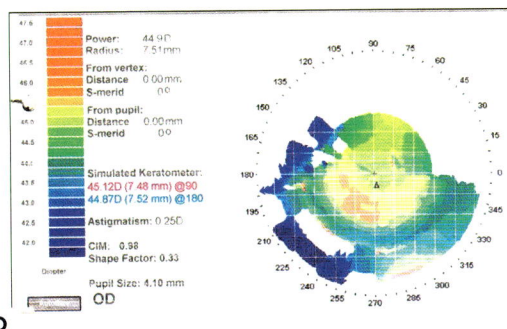

b

Fig. 12.7: (a) Corneal topography showing astigmatism in a grafted case; (b) Topography as imaged after CL *in situ* over same eye. Note regularization of cornea and correction of astigmatism

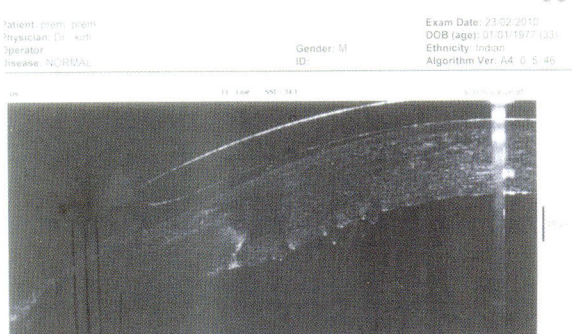

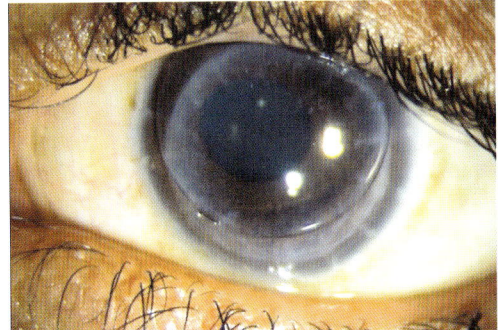

Fig .12.6: Anterior OCT picture of RGP lens fit over a keratoplasty cornea. Note adequate edge clearance and regular posterior tear film beneath the lens.

The trial lens BC is selected on flat K if astigmatism is less than 5 D, and steeper than K for astigmatism greater than 5 D, using a minimum 8.5–9.0 mm diameter. Large diameter lenses >9.5 mm which utilize peripheral host rim for bearing and minimize graft-host bearing, provide improved stability (Fig. 12.8). Large diameter also takes care of inferior edge stand off in such lens fits.[10] Vision in such lenses is more stable and incidence of ghosting is reduced.

Lens decentration is a common phenomenon in grafted eyes. Decentered lenses usually ride high as they are picked up by upper lid.

b. Rose K lenses: These reverse geometry lenses are specially designed keeping in mind the altered topography of a grafted cornea. Centration, movement and comfort is superior to conventional RGP lenses, but cost and availability is the limiting factor (Fig. 12.9). For a more detailed explanation refer to the chapter on keratoconus.

c. Hydrogel or silicone hydrogel lens: Soft lenses are not frequently used in post-keratoplasty eyes because of the following reasons:

- High astigmatism a usual offshoot of keratoplasty, is not amenable to correction by a hydrogel lens
- Irregular corneal surface/host graft junction, irregular healing and corneal scarring in the host is transmitted through soft lens, leading to inadequate visual correction.

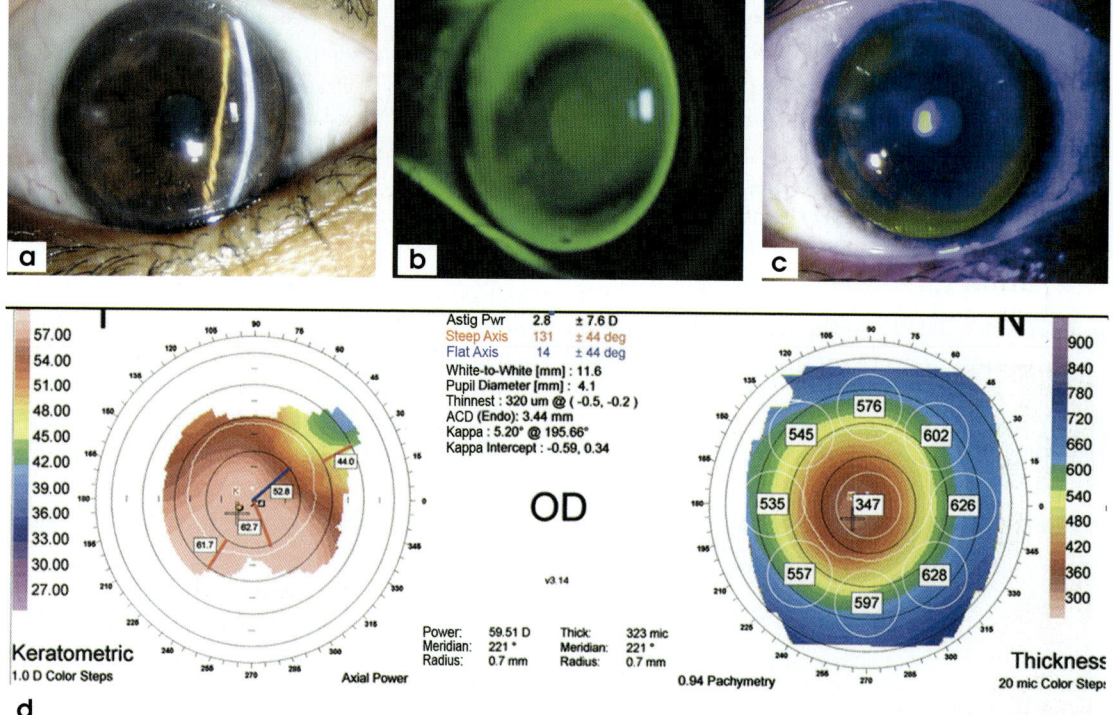

Fig. 12.8: (a, b) Larger diameter 9.6 mm RGP lens over a graft. Note the adequate edge clearance; (b) *Courtesy:* Abhilekh Aneja; (c) Steep fit; (d) Topographic picture of this patient depicts diffuse proud graft

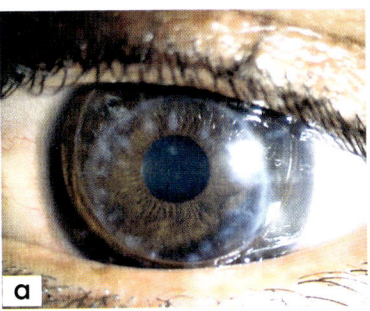 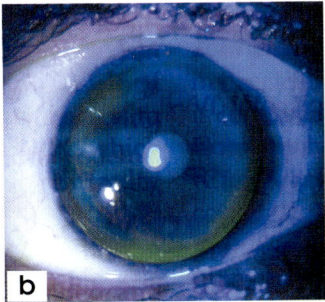 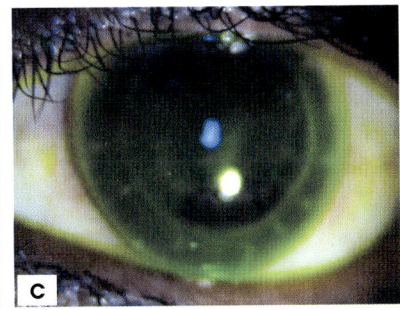

Fig. 12.9: (a) Well-centered Rose K lens over a grafted cornea; (b) Fluorescein pattern shows slightly flat fit with good edge clearance; (c) Optimal fit with diffuse clearance

- A well-fitted soft lens has a greater occlusive effect versus a RGP lens and can induce hypoxia, edema, neovasculrization with subsequent graft rejection (Fig. 12.10).

Indications for use of SCL are: Aphakia, anisometropia, lower degrees of regular astigmatism and patients with intolerance to RGP lenses.[11,12] Materials with high oxygen permeability are required to prevent graft hypoxia. Thicker hydrogels are preferred due to their enhanced stability and optics.

Fitting is commenced by fitting a trial lens of spherical equivalent power. After an adequate settling time of 10–15 minutes of wear, over-refraction is performed. If residual astigmatism is high, soft toric lenses can be used. In

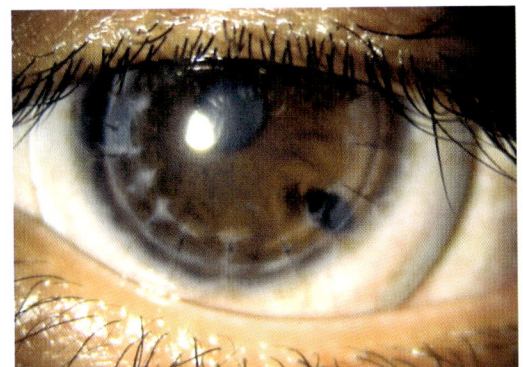

Fig. 12.10: Soft lens over post-keratoplasty cornea. This tight fit presented after a few hours of lens wear

such a situation torics with zonal thinning design are preferred over thick periphery prism ballast designs.

To minimize corneal stress, lens duration has to be regulated with lens holidays being given at weekly off days.

d. *Scleral/semiscleral lenses:* Used when other lens types do not fit, this lens ensures stable on-eye fitting, provides optimum centration with good vision. In addition, the lenses are durable, easy to care and to handle. Cost, availability and long learning curve in inserting the lens are major limiting factors.[13]

e. *Piggyback lenses:* In cases with irregular astigmatism with sensitive lids, a piggy back system which entails a RGP lens fitted over a soft lens may be tried. The soft lens is fitted over graft to smooth over irregular topography at host graft junction. Keratometry readings are then taken over the SCL to decide BC of RGP lens, which is then fitted 0.1 m steeper than this new K reading. The RGP lens neutralizes astigmatism transmitted by soft lens and provides good vision.

The soft lens can be a lenticulated positive power one to aid centration of overlying RGP lens. Alternatively silicone hydrogel with high oxygen permeability can be used.[14] The RGP lens is fitted tight to minimize wobbling or displacement. Follow up regimen is more complicated as two lens care systems have to be followed, one for the RGP lens and one for the soft lens. Lens handling also is more cumbersome; lens loss is more frequent and deposit formation is more common. Thus this method is used as a last resort.

Some Problematic Situations

*   *Vascularisation at graft host interface*:
    Lenses with high oxygen permeability only should be fitted to minimize hypoxia and hypoxic induced graft vascularization. To circumvent this, presence and location of blood vessels near graft interface have to be noted prior to lens fitting (Fig. 12.11). In situations with vascularization encroaching on graft, heavy bearing by contact lens on graft-host interface needs to be avoided or minimized.
*   *Immobile lens*:
    Larger RGP lenses on grafted eyes often exhibit less movement. Old lenses also become tighter and move less with time.[10] An immobile lens impairs corneal health by deranged tear dynamics and oxygen permeability, manifesting with cornea staining, edema and neovascularization. Creating fenestrations in lens, reducing lens diameter and flattening of peripheral curves are some modifications which can

be done to alleviate negative effect of immobility. Use of lubricating drops also helps.
*   *Poor tear resurfacing*:
    This can be diagnosed by presence of bubbles beneath the lens, around graft margins in case of proud grafts and in gutter regions of tilted grafts. Persistent bubbles serve as a nidus for new vessel growth by producing localized xerosis, in addition, they cause fluctuations in vision and discomfort. Modification of peripheral curves (required steepening/flattening) or lens fenestration can solve this problem.
*   *Urrets-Zavalia syndrome*:
    Urrets-Zavalia syndrome term is used for fixed dilated pupil occurring after uncomplicated penetrating keratoplasty for keratoconus in patients who receive mydriatics. The probable cause for the entity being iris ischemia, acute rise in IOP after instillation of strong mydriatics. Lens correcting such eyes would need to have a large optic zone, large overall diameter lens with tinting to reduce glare (Fig. 12.12).

Complications with Lens Wear in Grafted Eyes

Other than the usual complications of lens wear some problems specific to grafted eyes are:

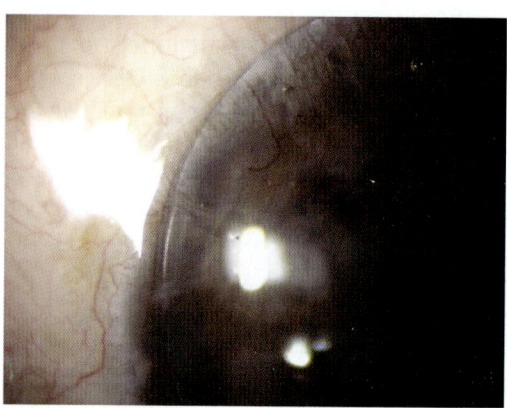

Fig. 12.11: Note the neovascularization at 11 o'clock position, beneath the lens on a postgraft patient

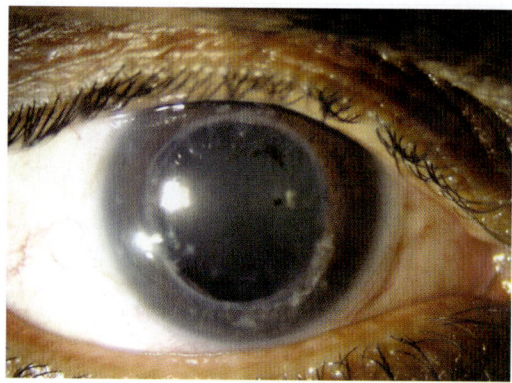

Fig. 12.12: Urrets-Zavalia syndrome post-PK with fixed pupil, corrected with a large OZ soft lens.

- Transitory punctate epithelial keratitis.
- Suture infiltrates and infection. As grafted patients have a depressed corneal sensitivity during the initial few years, warning symptom of pain with infective keratins may be muted.[15] Thus more frequent follow up especially during early post operative years is essential for timely diagnosis of this complication.
- Graft rejection or failure after lens triggered inflammatory episodes. Treatment is by temporary cessation of lens wear, use of steroids and lubricants. Refitting these patients with lenses is not without risk and if attempted only higher Dk materials should be used.[15]
- Monocular diplopia and flare. In decentered grafts, lens tends to position on eccentric and/or steep area. Lens optics may bisect the pupil and give rise to diplopia/flare especially in scotopic viewing. Piggyback lenses may be a solution in this situation.
- Fluctuating vision due to irregular topography graft leading to in wobbly or decentered lens.
- Follow up should be done every 6 months, despite patient having no problems, so as to pick up any early changes like epithelial haze, vascularization and rejection.

Corneal Refractive Surgery/Corneal Refractive Therapy CRT

Historical Aspects

The first forgotten attempt of refractive surgery was in 1885 by Schiötz, the Norwegian ophthalmologist who designed the Schiötz tonometer. Using a 3.5 mm full thickness limbal incision in the steep meridian, he reduced surgical astigmatism induced after cataract surgery from of 19.50 to 7.00 D. Later on Lucciola in 1896, used non-perforating incisions to create astigmatic keratotomies. Bates suggestion in 1894 of corneal incisions at right angles to most convex meridian correcting astigmatism heralded the era of

lmbal relaxing incisions. However, refractive surgery started in earnest in 1939 after pioneering work of Sato of Russia. Sato was the first one to performed radial keratomy (RK) to correct myopia. The incisions made by his team were in both anterior and posterior corneal surfaces, which resulted in corneal decompensation over time and led to the discovery that corneal endothelium lacks regenerating power. The surgery was then abandoned to be later revived by Fydorov, Barraquer and Kaufman. This ingenious trio also devised keratomileusis and epikeratophakia for correction of myopia and apakia by cryo lathing of self/donor corneal tissue or synthetic material (inlay) respectively The surgeries involving freezing and lathing of donor tissue to a pre-calculated power, and storing of freeze created lenticule lost popularity due to occurrence of corneal haze and irregular astigmatism.

Excimer LASERs emerged in 1975 by combining molecules of inert argon gas with fluorine into an unstable association under influence of an external energy (high-voltage discharges). Electrons knocked off from argon molecules electrostatically combined with negative (electron-rich) fluorine molecules, producing argon fluoride. The resultant energy-rich, excited, diatomic, gaseous, transient halide (excited dimer) while seeking a lower energy/ground-state pre-excitement level separates into its component gases with simultaneous release of UV energy of 193 nm wavelength. Controlled repetition of this excitation and dissociation cycle, excimer produced short repeatable pulses. This surgery was replaced by **Laser-Assisted Epithelial Keratectomy (LASEK),** wherein an intact epithelium flap was created using 20% alcohol. The hinged flap is lifted, swept back and LASER ablation performed at stromal bed, after which the flap is reposited. **Epi-LASIK** developed by Pallikaris uses an epikeratome oscillating at high speed as it sweeps across the cornea and separates a hinged flap of epithelium alone from Bowman's layer. As separation occurs beneath the basement membrane, above Bowman's layer both epithelial and stromal integrity are maintained. This epikeratome produces a more precise, reproducible delamination of epithelium and minimizes risk of haze, striae and sub-epithelial debris. Ongoing efforts in improvement have sidelined contact microkeratome with inherent complications of inadvertent slippage and irregular trauma and evolved to use of infrared femtosecond laser (**INTRALASE**). This laser generates a controlled flap by process of photodisruption, with eye being held in position by a negative low-pressure suction ring.

Refinement in refractive surgeries over the ages has made the technique more predictable and safe. However, refractive surprises/regression and complications often require visual rehabilitation with contact lenses, due to inadequate correction, regression or complications.

Altered Corneal Topography Relevant to CL Fit

Refractive surgeries alter corneal topography by inducing central corneal flattening. They alter normal prolate cornea (steeper in center and flatter in periphery) into an oblate cornea (flatter centrally). This induced central flattening creates an elbow at transition of flat center with steeper periphery. Conventional lenses designed for fit on a regular prolate cornea are consequently difficult to fit for post-CRT patients, which have a flatter central cornea (oblate) (Fig. 12.13a and b). Higher refractive errors corrected generate greater amount of iatrogenic corneal flattening which makes lens fitting more difficult. In addition, the hyperopic shift experienced over time in radial keratotomy cases compounds the refractive add to be prescribed.[16]

Fitting contact lenses for patients who had undergone refractive surgeries with a specific desire to discard their spectacles are taxing. These patients are frustrated on being faced

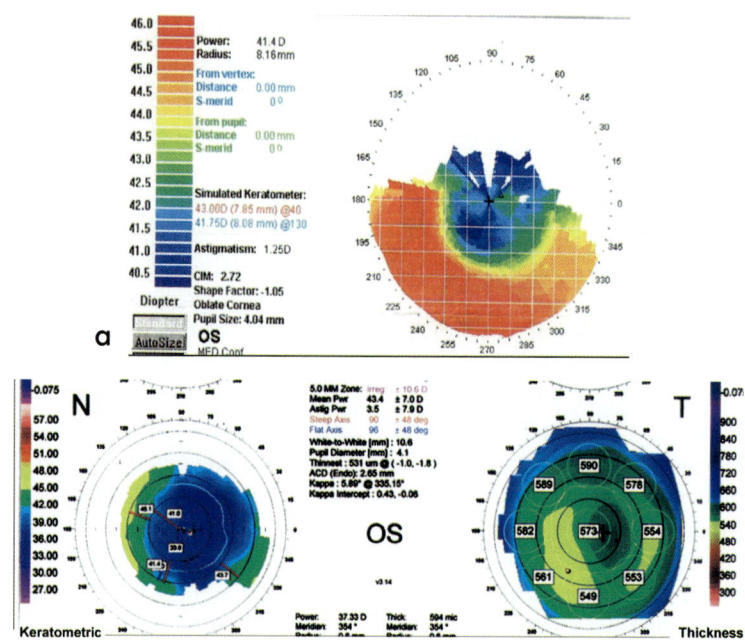

Fig. 12.13: Corneal topography depicting oblate corneas (flatter center, steeper periphery); (a) Post- RK; (b) Post-PRK

with need to re-use a visual aid again and have unrealistic goals with their contact lenses. Fitting lenses on these disillusioned and demanding patients is both challenging and rewarding.

Indications of CL

- As a bandage lens for corneal protection in immediate postoperative period to enhance healing.
- Over and under correction of the refractive error.[17]
- Refractive regression especially in cases of radial keratotomy.
- Eccentric/decentered ablations resulting in large dioptric shifts in central zone. This causes irregular astigmatism resulting in poor vision, glare, halos and even monocular diplopia. An extreme variant of this is occurrence of *paracentral steep island*. This is the name given to a well circumscribed area of greater refractive power, with power variations ranging till 20.00 D in pupil zone.
- Irregular ATR astigmatism with inferior corneal steepening
- Corneal scarring/secondary ectasia.[18]

Lens Options and Fitting Methodology

Corneal sensations and topography stabilize by 6 months post CRT. Thus fitting of a CL must be deferred till at least that much time has elapsed.[19] The different types of lenses which can be fitted are detailed below. The lenses prescribed should be of high diffusion coefficient material as they need to be fitted over corneas subjected to prior surgery.[20]

a. *RGP lenses:* The ability of RGP lenses to vault over altered corneal topography and generate a smooth, regular, artificial anterior surface corrects irregular astigmatism.[18,21] In CRT corneas too the lens vaults over flattened plateau cornea in center and is the lens of choice.

  In cases subjected to older surgery of radial keratomy, diurnal visual fluctuations due to altered fluid tissue interface of these scarred corneas is common. The malleable tear lens present under a RGP lens is able to correct this aspect of RK corneas.[22]

Lenses are fitted using *superior alignment technique* where lens is positioned high and moves in conjunction with upper lid movement. Interpalpebral fit is used for small steep lenses or reverse geometry design (flatter in center and steeper in periphery). In eccentric corneas with corneal apex displaced towards mid-periphery, lens gravitates to this steepest area and is liable to decenter, thus for such topographies large diameter lenses are preferred which would vault over the corneo-scleral junction. At the same time it needs to be ensured that limbal compression does not occur since that would stimulate vascularization.

While calculating the base curve, knowledge of preoperative flat K value is beneficial. The BC of trial lens based on flat original K value usually gives rise to a *steep lens* aligned with mid-periphery vaulting over postsurgical flattened apical zone. This steep lens has to be subsequently modified. But more often than not, these initial K values are not available. In such situations a base curve 1.5–2.5 D steeper to postoperative K value is chosen as initial trial lens.[24]

Static fit pattern: It usually demonstrates *apical clearance* by the lens surface vaulting over the flattened central cornea. This manifests as large central pool of fluorescein stained tears surrounded by a zone of mid-peripheral bearing at the elbow. A common pattern seen in a steep fit as in (Fig. 12.14). Large diameter lenses >9.5 mm along with small optic zones reduce this apical clearance and result in a better fit.

Since peripheral cornea outside zone of ablation is less altered in LASIK/PTK versus RK, it permits better fitting with conventional RGP design. However, modifications are often required to peripheral

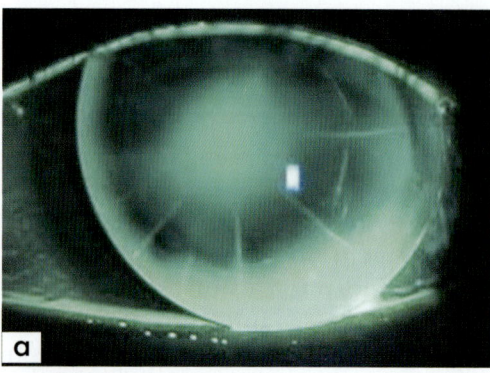
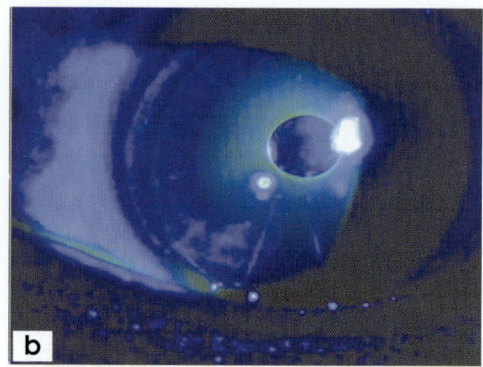

a b

Fig. 12.14: (a) Conventional RGP lens over a RK cornea; (b) Steep fit. A reverse geometry design would be better suited for this case

curve to ensure tear exchange with customized peripheral curves steeper than base curve being often required.[25]

The flattened central topography of the post CRT cornea generates a malleable tear lens between it and posterior lens surface. This tear lens usually attains a plus lens configuration, and needs to be accounted for while finalizing lens power during over-refraction.[26] Another corneal condition requiring large diameter RGP lens fitting is marginal corneal degeneration especially pellucid marginal degeneration (PMD). Corneal topographic picture of "kissing birds' is classical for this condition (Fig. 12.15).

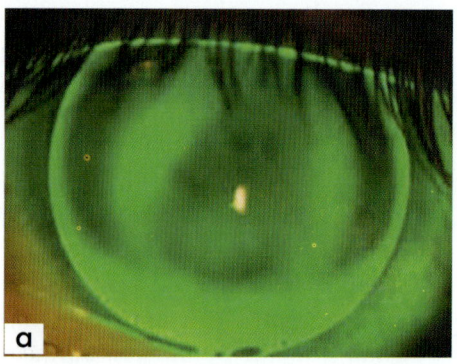
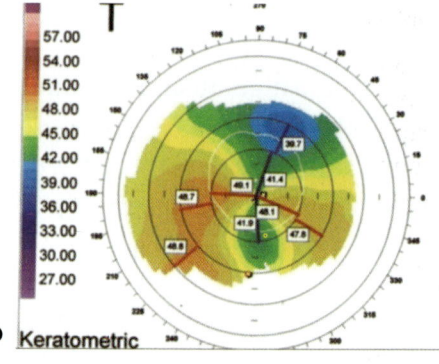

a b Keratometric

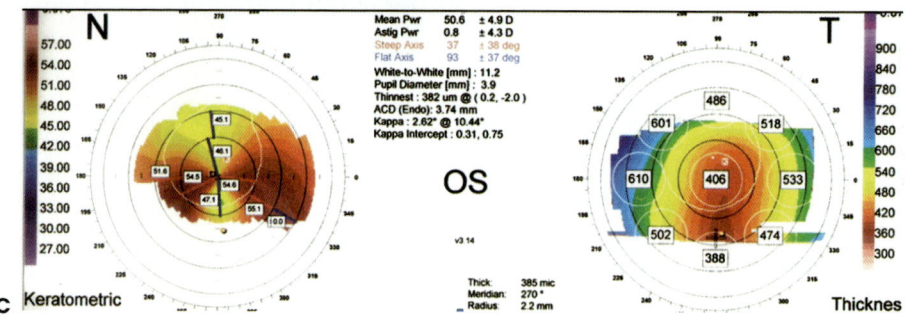

c Keratometric

Mean Pwr	50.6	± 4.9 D
Astig Pwr	0.8	± 4.3 D
Steep Axis	37	± 38 deg
Flat Axis	93	± 37 deg

White-to-White [mm] : 11.2
Pupil Diameter [mm] : 3.9
Thinnest : 382 um @ (0.2, -2.0)
ACD (Endo): 3.74 mm
Kappa : 2.62° @ 10.44°
Kappa Intercept : 0.31, 0.75

OS

v3 14

Thick: 385 mic
Meridian: 270°
Radius: 2.2 mm

Thicknes

Fig. 12.15: (a) RGP lens fit over pellucid marginal degeneration (PMD); (b) Corneal topography of same case; (c) Topography depicting classical "kissing birds" appearance on topography which diagnostic of PMD

b. **Hydrogel lenses/hydrogels:** These lenses drape over contours of a post CRT cornea without the benefit of a tear lens blanket and are therefore unable to mask irregular astigmatism or greater than 1.0 D of regular astigmatism.[21,27] Hydrogels can also induce corneal oedema with resultant corneal vascularization along the RK incisions due to poor oxygen and tear exchange.[28] For these reasons soft lenses are only indicated for short periods of wear and only in cases with simple mild over/under corrections. At all times high Dk value hydrogels only should be used.

c. **Piggyback lenses:** As discussed before two genre of lenses are used: Silicone or thick hydrogel coupled with RGP lens, where optics of the latter is responsible for vision and support of former for stability. Silicone hydrogels are preferred as the base since their high oxygen permeability reduces hypoxic insult arising from twin lenses on the cornea.[26]

d. **Reverse geometry lenses:** These case designed with steeper secondary curves confirming to altered topography of post CRT cornea. The secondary or reverse curve is 2–4 dioptres steeper than central base curve. Interpalpebral fit can be used for such lenses and adequate tear exchange needs to be ensured.[29]

Timing of Lens Wear After PRK

For photorefractive keratectomy case three types of healing responses have been identified, based on which timing and indication of contact lens wear can be determined. Karpecki et al have categorized corneal healing as type I, II or III.[30] In the commonest type I (seen in 95 % case), an initial mild corneal haze occurs along with accompanying slight hyperopia, which converts to emmetropia within a few months. The cornea regains normal epithelial thickness by 6 months post procedure. Contact lens if required should only be prescribed after 9 months. Type II has poor healing, excess flattening, secondary hyperopia, no stromal haze and minimal inflammation. In this type contact lenses are prescribed early on, so as to incite inflammation and reduce the hyperopia. In type III marked corneal haze and significant undercorrection (residual myopia), is seen by 1–3 months of laser, here contact lenses are not prescribed since the inflammation triggered by lens use would promote more regression. Lens wear in this uncommon healing should be reserved after 2 years of the procedure.[31]

Over-refraction should always be done to estimate final lens power. A simple mathematical transposition is never reliable in finalizing lens power over these corneas.[26]

Complications

- Epithelial staining occurs due to friction/rubbing/bearing effect of the lens back surface on proud areas of the cornea.

- Disturbed epithelial basement membrane dynamics post CRT may result in recurrent corneal erosions with use of contact lens.

- Vascularization of post-RK cornea especially at incision lines with conventional hydrogels.

- Dry eyes

- Reduced night vision/ghosting/monocular diplopia due to non-uniform corneal refractive indices, decentration of ablated zone or mismatch between pupil and optical zone of lens (Fig. 12.16).

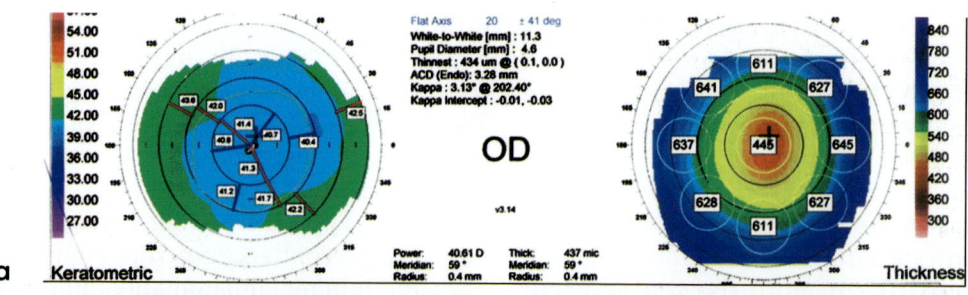

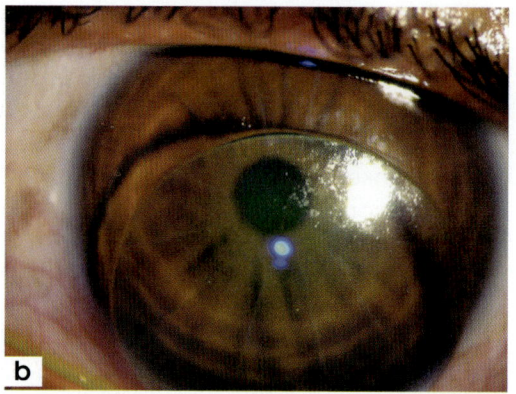

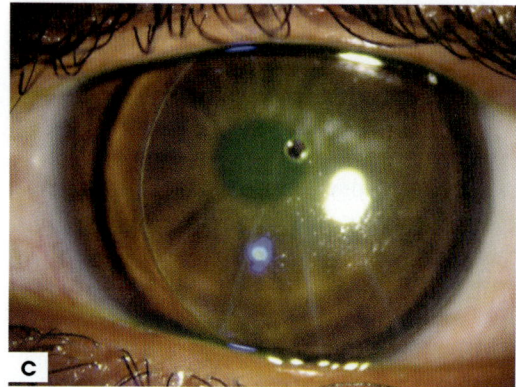

Fig. 12.16: (a) Orbscan of post-LASIK eye showing excessive oblate pattern; (b) CL fitted over same eye is decentered leading to ghosting in scotopic pupil conditions (unacceptable decentration); (c) Over a case of RK: Optic zone of contact lens well centered over pupil, unlikely to cause scotopic viewing visual problems (acceptable decentration)

REFERENCES

1. Wietharn BE, Driebe WT Jr. Fitting contact lenses for visual rehabilitation after penetrating keratoplasty. Eye Contact Lens. 2004 Jan;30(1): 31–3.

2. Darwish T, Brahma A, Efron N, O'Donnell C. Subbasal Nerve Regeneration After Penetrating Keratoplasty. Cornea: 2007; 26(8) : 935–40.

3. Rao GN, John T, Ishida N, Aquavella JV. .Recovery of corneal sensitivity in grafts following penetrating keratoplasty. Ophthalmology. 1985 Oct;92(10):1408–11.

4. Sepehr Feizi and Mohammad Zare. Current Approaches for Management of Postpenetrating Keratoplasty Astigmatism J Ophthalmol. 2011;;2011:708–36.

5. Jorge E. Valdez-Garcia, Juan J. Cueto-Gómez, Juan F. Lozano-Ramírez, and Alejandro E. Tamez-Peña Management of Extreme Ametropia after Penetrating Keratoplasty: A Series of Surgical Procedures for High Myopia and Astigmatism. Case Rep Ophthalmol. 2014; 5(2): 255–61.

6. Lopatynsky M, Cohen EJ, Leavitt KG, Laibson PR. Corneal topography for rigid gas permeable lens fitting after penetrating keratoplasty. CLAO J. 1993 Jan;19(1):41–4.

7. H Karabatsas CH, Cook SD, M Sparrow JM. Proposed classification for topographic patterns seen after penetrating keratoplasty. Br J Ophthalmol 1999;83:403–9.

8. Ozbek Z, Cohen EJ. Use of intralimbal rigid gas-permeable lenses for pellucid marginal degeneration, keratoconus, and after penetrating keratoplasty. Eye Contact Lens. 2006 Jan; 32(1):33–6.

9. Genvert GI, Cohen EJ, Arentsen JJ, Laibson PR. Fitting gas-permeable contact lenses after penetrating keratoplasty. Am J Ophthalmol. 1985; 15; 99(5):511–4.

10. Geerards AJ, Vreugdenhil W, Khazen A. Incidence of rigid gas-permeable contact lens wear after keratoplasty for keratoconus.. Eye Contact Lens. 2006 Jul;32(4):207–10.

11. Chung CW, Santim R, Heng WJ, Cohen EJ. Use of SoftPerm contact lenses when rigid gas permeable lenses fail. CLAO J. 2001 Oct;27(4): 202–8.

12. Katsoulos C, Nick V, Lefteris K, Theodore M. Fitting the post-keratoplasty cornea with hydrogel lenses. Cont Lens Anterior Eye. 2009 Feb;32(1):22–6.

13. Barnett M, Lien V, Li JY, Durbin-Johnson B, Mannis MJ. Use of Scleral Lenses and Mini-scleral Lenses After Penetrating Keratoplasty. Eye Contact Lens. 2015 Jul 24. [Epub ahead of print]

14. López-Alemany A, González-Méijome JM, Almeida JB, Parafita MA, Refojo MF. Oxygen transmissibility of piggyback systems with conventional soft and silicone hydrogel contact lenses. Cornea. 2006 Feb;25(2):214–9.

15. Gomes JA, Rapuano CJ, Cohen EJ. Topographic stability and safety of contact lens use after penetrating keratoplasty. CLAO J. 1996 Jan;22(1):64–9.

16. Waring GO, Lynn MJ, McDonnell PJ. Results of the prospective evaluation of radial keratotomy (PERK) study 10 years after surgery. Arch Ophthalmol. 1994 Oct;112 (10):1298–308.

17. Steele C, Davidson J. Contact lens fitting post-laser-in situ keratomileusis (LASIK). Cont Lens Anterior Eye. 2007 May;30(2):84–93. Epub 2007 Feb 27.

18. Woodward MA, Randleman JB, Russell B, Lynn MJ, Ward MA, Stulting RD. Visual rehabilitation and outcomes for ectasia after corneal refractive surgery. J Cataract Refract Surg. 2008 Mar;34(3):383–8. 597–603.

19. MA Bragheeth and HS Dua. Corneal sensation after myopic and hyperopic LASIK: clinical and confocal microscopic study Br J Ophthalmol. 2005 May; 89(5): 580–85.

20. Lim L, Siow KL, Sakamoto R, Chong JS, Tan DT. Reverse geometry contact lens wear after photorefractive keratectomy, radial kerato-tomy, or penetrating keratoplasty. Cornea. 2000 May;19(3):320–4.

21. Bufidis T, Konstas AG, Pallikaris IG, Siganos DS, Georgiadis N. Contact lens fitting difficulties following refractive surgery for high myopia. CLAO J. 2000 Apr;26(2):106–10.

22. Lee AM, Kastl PR. *Rigid gas permeable contact lens fitting after radial keratotomy.* CLAO J. 1998; 24: 33–35.

23. Villa-Collar C, González-Méijome JM, Gutiérrez-Ortega R. Objective evaluation of the visual benefit in contact lens fitting after complicated LASIK. J Refract Surg. 2009;25(7):591–8.

24. CL Astin, DS Gartry, and AD McG Steele Contact lens fitting after photorefractive keratectomy. Br J Ophthalmol. 1996; 80(7): 597–603.

25. Choi HJ, Kim MK, Lee JL. Optimization of contact lens fitting in keratectasia patients after laser in situ keratomileusis J Cataract Refract Surg. 2004:30 (5):1057–66.

26. Ward MA. Contact lens management following corneal refractive surgery. Ophthalmol Clin North Am. 2003 Sep: 16 (3):395–403.

27. Toda I, Yoshida A, Sakai C, Hori-Komai Y, Tsubota K. Visual performance after reduced blinking in eyes with soft contact lenses or after LASIK. J Refract Surg. 2009 Jan;25(1):69–73.

28. Waring GO 3rd, Lynn MJ, ulbertson W et al.Three-year results of the prospective evaluation of radial keratotomy (PERK) study. Ophthalmology 1987, 94(10); 1339–54.

29. Martin R, Rodriguez G. Reverse geometry contact lens fitting after corneal refractive surgery. J Refract Surg. 2005 Nov–Dec;21(6): 753–6.

30. Karpecki CM, Smith JM, Durrie DS. What you can do to improve PRK outcomes? Rev Optomety 1996, 133(3): 127–133.

31. Mc Mohan T, Szczotka Flynn L. Fitting the abnormal cornea. In Eds Krachmer JH, Mannis MJ, Holland EJ. Cornea. Fundamentals, diagnosis and management Vol 1. 2nd ed., Elsevier Mosby, Philadelphia. 1313–24.

Reader's Note

CHAPTER 13

Fitting on Scarred Corneas

CORNEAL SCARS/ OPACITIES

Ocular trauma or healed keratitis constitutes a large chunk of patients presenting with diminished vision. The reasons for poor vision in these patients are visual axis obscuration, irregular astigmatism, diffraction of light rays by the corneal opacity.[1] Many of these cases have associated post-traumatic aphakia which introduces its own unique optical problems. Spectacles are not an optimal method of visual rehabilitation in these cases, due to their inability to correct irregular astigmatism and/ or uniocular aphakia. Contact lenses remain the only viable option with the preferred lenses being rigid gas permeable contact lenses with their high oxygen permeability, high optical transmission and ability to neutralize corneal astigmatism by generating a tear lens. In addition to optical performance, dynamic tear exchange, ease of cleaning and handling combined with reduced incidence of keratitis make rigid lens preferred modalities for these vulnerable corneas.[2] However, in higher degrees of astigmatism conventional RGP design may not be able to generate an adequate tear lens and provide functional visual gain due to unstable fit.[3] These patients may require specialized lenses like Rose K, post-aspheric and minisclerals. Soft lenses are only indicated in correcting concomitant traumatic aphakia or where suboptimal vision

is tolerated due to comfort and ease of insertion of hydrogels over RGP lenses.[4]

Fitting methodology in patients with corneal scars is same as for conventional lenses with special care being needed to ensure adequate tear exchange. Corneal topography is a better guide than keratometry in fitting these corneas, as it identifies the corneal apex, which invariably does not coincide with geometric axis along with corneal shape, thereby making pairing with appropriate lens more accurate. Common topographic findings are: Flattening in area of penetrating scar, rarely ectasia in scar area, but most often no specific pattern is seen in these damaged corneas (Fig. 13.1).

Factors Determining Visual Gain

The factors determining visual gain with lenses are: Density of scar, size of scar, associated co-morbidities of aphakia, ocular surface disorders, patient expectations and work profile.

a. **Density of opacity** determines success of CL fitting with nebular and nebulo-macular corneal opacities benefiting from corrective RGP lenses (Fig. 13.2).[5–7] Leuco-matous opacities due to total opaqueness and proud elevated surface associated with adherent leucoma makes lens fitting both difficult and often ineffective in these type of opacities.[6]

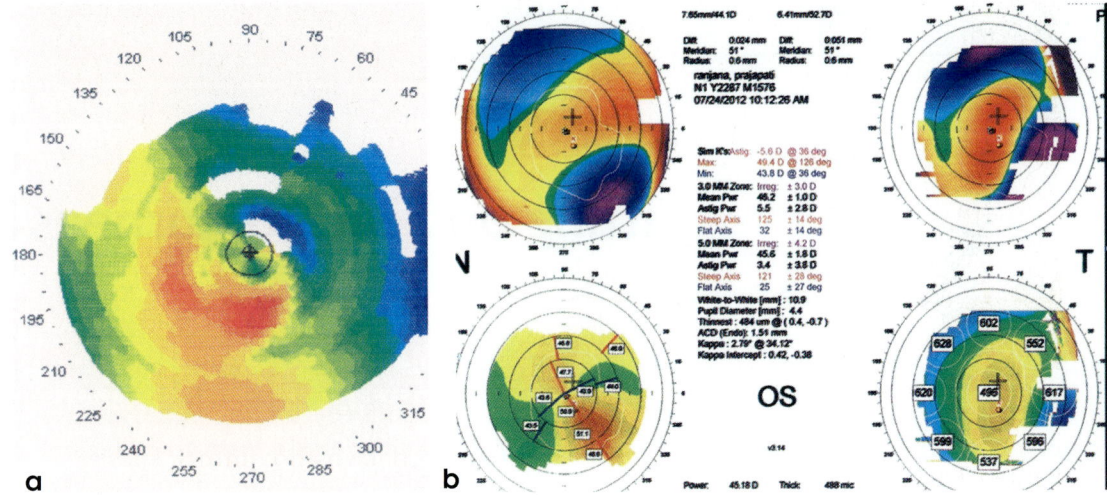

Fig. 13.1: Distorted topography after corneal injury

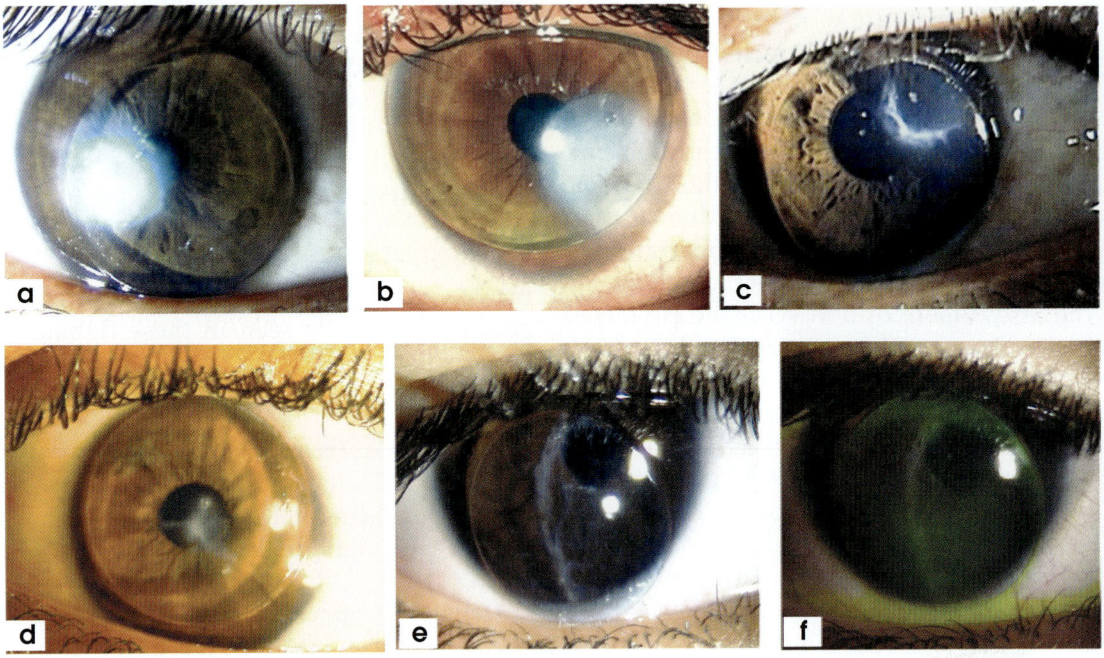

Fig. 13.2: Contact lens rehabilitation in different types and extent of corneal scarring

b. Size and location of scar: Scars causing a central flattening are usually good candidates for successful contact lens fit. Lenses fitted over such depressed scars vault over the opacity, generate a stagnant tear pool and remain well centered (Fig. 13.3). For limbal to limbal scars larger diameter lenses of 9.6–10.0 mm are required. Lenses design with posterior toric surface are best suited and semi-sclerals being often

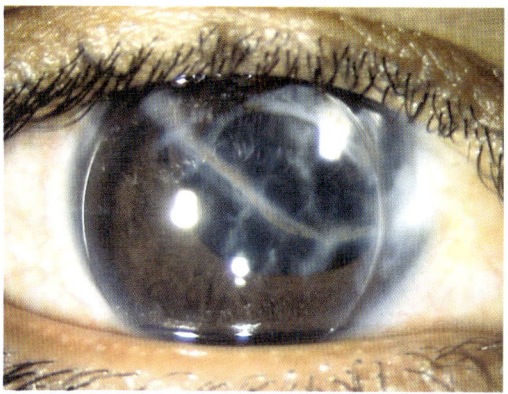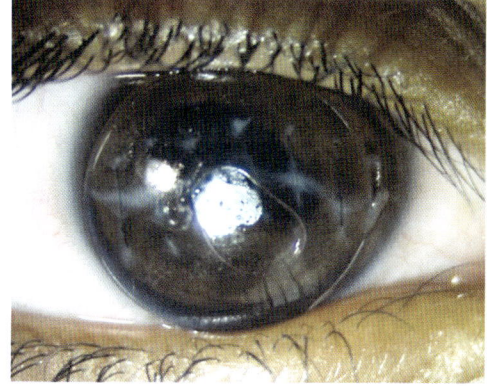

Fig. 13.3: Conventional RGP lens over scarred cornea

required. Larger scars are difficult to fit and lens decentration, epithelial desiccation along with fluctuating vision is common (Fig. 13.2e and f).

Conventional RGP design lenses are tried first and in cases with suboptimal fit, trial of post-aspheric, reverse geometry as required is done (Fig. 13.4). In regular lenses larger overall diameter and optic zone is often required to aid centration and papillary coverage.[8] Attention should always be given to adequate peripheral clearance so as to permit free circulation of tears. Failure to take care of this detail would give rise to lens intolerance after a few hours of wear and corneal hypoxia, which is more detrimental to these already traumatized corneas.

Invariably the fitter is faced with pooling of fluoresecin adjacent to scar (due to depressed topography in areas around scar) (Fig. 13.5). This pattern is acceptable but pooling should stop short of causing dimple veiling.

Another important fact to be kept in mind while fitting scarred corneas is *lens decentration*. Often the lens would decenter and center on steepest part of cornea, which is invariably not the center, for these traumatized cornea (Fig. 13.6a). If decentration is not severe enough to cause limbal bearing, and optic zone is able to adequately cover pupil, such decentered lens fit may be acceptable (Fig. 13.6b). *The use of large diameter lenses, large optic zone lenses and then steep lenses in that order*

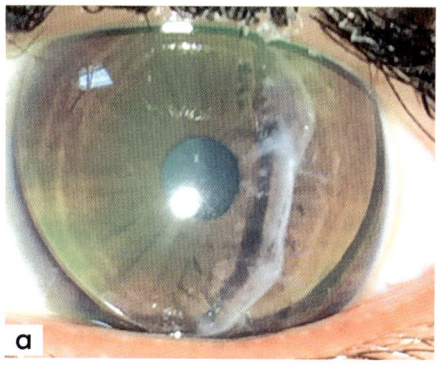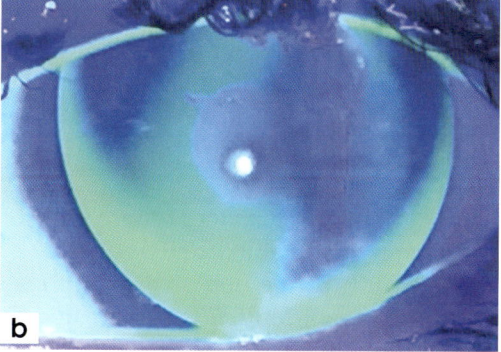

Fig. 13.4: (a) Posterior aspheric RGP (Mc Asfeer) lens fit; (b) Fluorescein staining of same

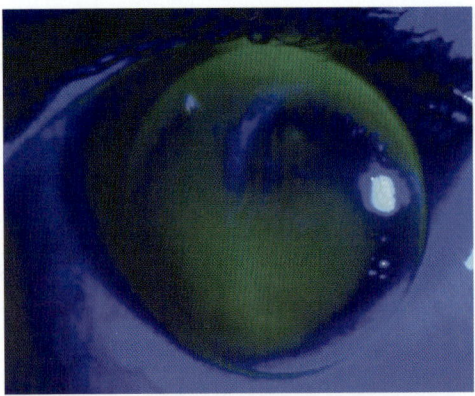
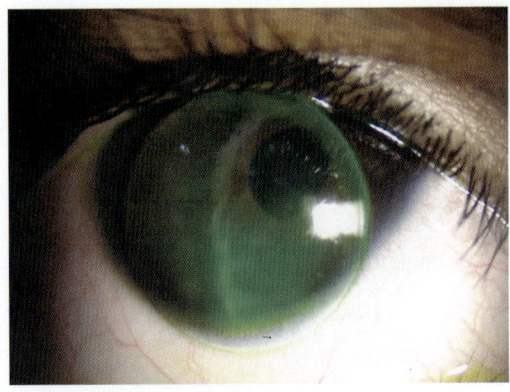

Fig. 13.5: Note pooling of fluorescein adjacent and inferior to scar

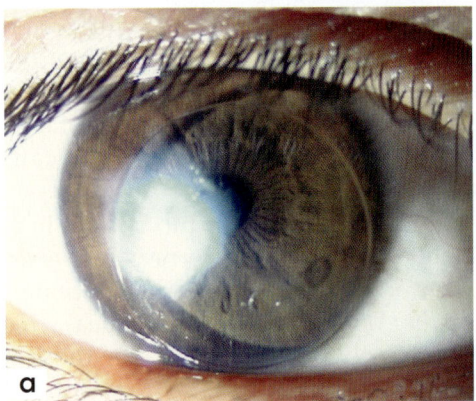
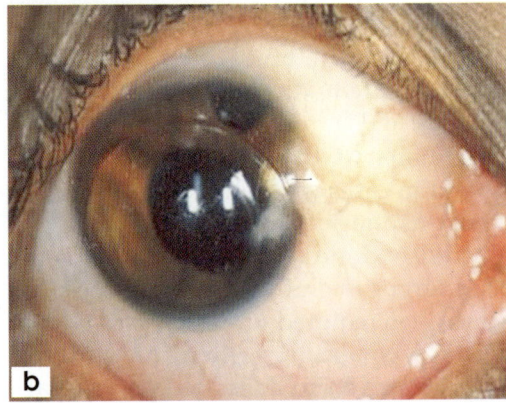

Fig. 13.6: (a) Decentered CL fitted on a leucomatous corneal opacity; (b) Decentered CL on an aphakic scarred eye with acceptable vision

are the usual remedial measures adopted while fitting corneas with scars/opacities.[8]

c. **Coexisting co-morbidities:** Presence of traumatic aphakia often requires use of soft lenses despite the suboptimal visual gain (Fig. 13.7). Since aphakia is most often uniocular, the patient is unable to adapt to presence of a heavy, down riding, RGP lens in one eye despite it providing a crisp visual gain.

However, there are instances where RGP lens fits well and remains centered in all cardinal ocular movements (Fig. 13.8). Such patients adapt to RGP lens wear and better quality of vision with this lens permits binocularity.

d. **Disturbed ocular surface:** A large scar disrupting ocular surface may not be amenable to successful RGP lens fit. For such patients other options like Rose K for irregular cornea or even miniscleral lens can be tried (Fig. 13.9).

An infrequent indication is use of lens in a patient awaiting keratoplasty for corneal dystrophy (Fig. 13.10). However, this is not recommended, as the dystrophic cornea can go into decompensation due to hypoxia generated with a contact lens *in situ*.

e. **Visual requirements:** Improvement in visual acuity with lenses over scarred corneas is sub-optimal. Increased central vision may not always accompanied by

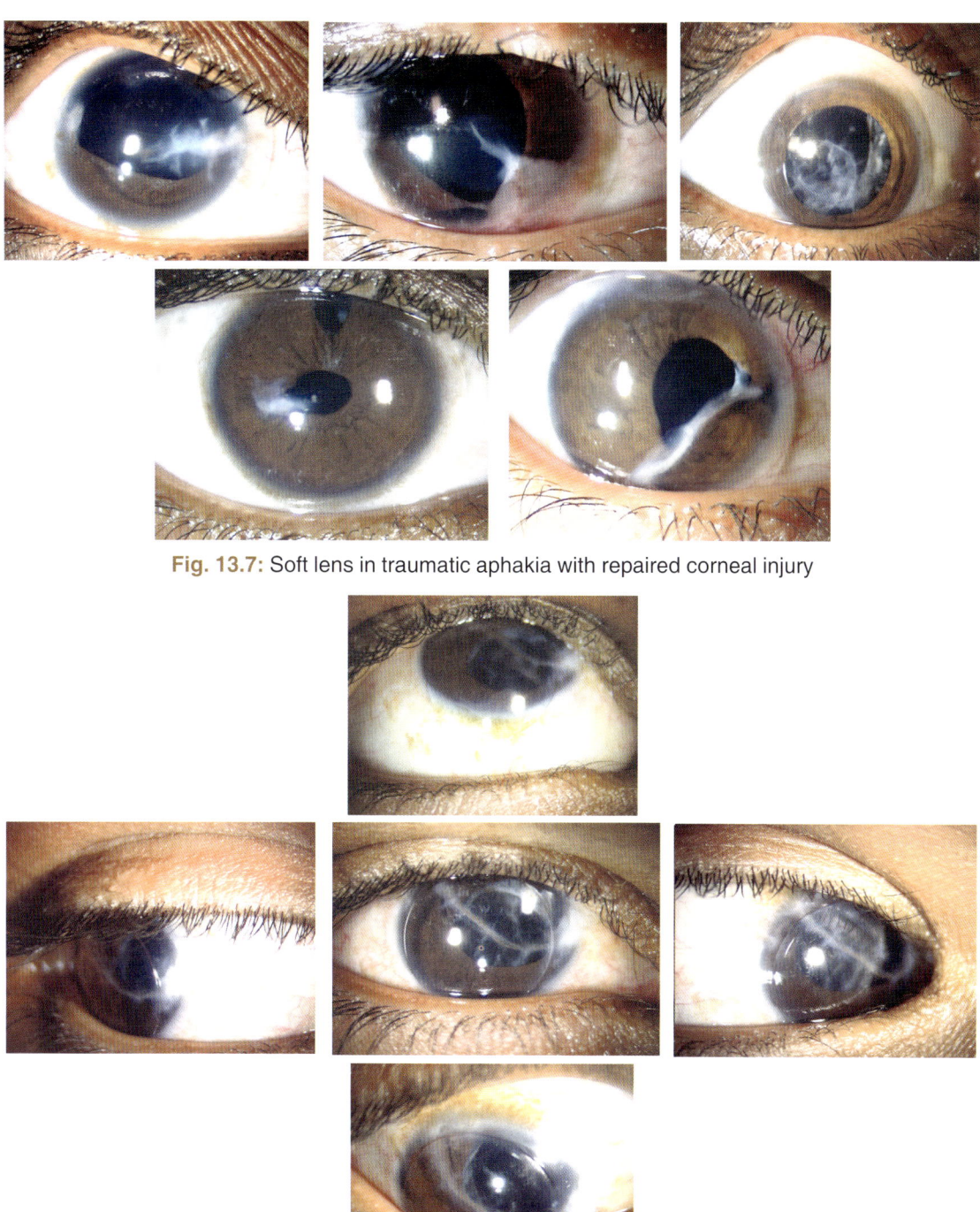

Fig. 13.7: Soft lens in traumatic aphakia with repaired corneal injury

Fig. 13.8: Aphakic RGP lens over repaired corneal perforation. Lens is centered well in all gazes, providing stable vision

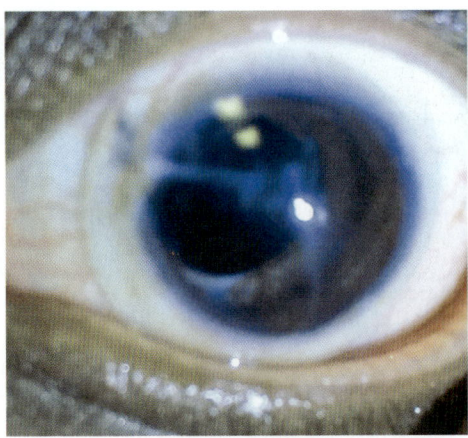
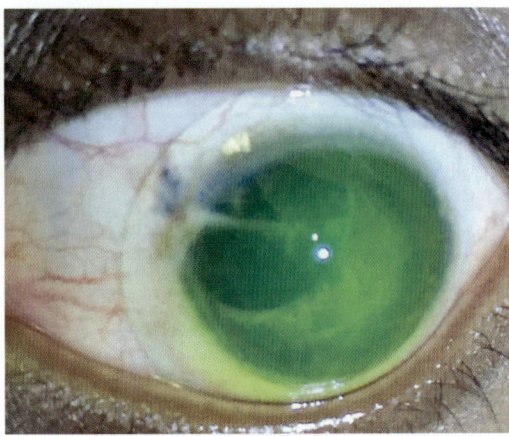

Fig. 13.9: Miniscleral lens over traumatic aphakia with repaired corneal perforation

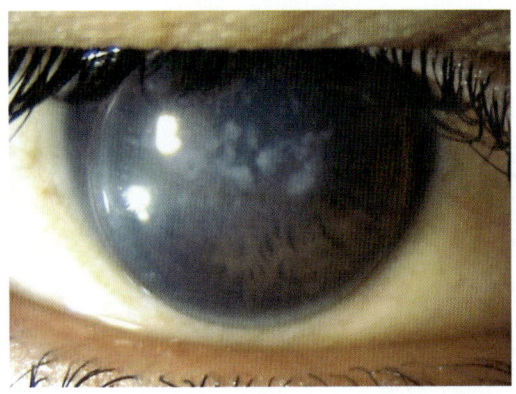

Fig. 13.10: RGP lens over granular dystrophy. Patient gained vision of 6/24

comparable improvement in contrast sensitivity especially in mesopic viewing conditions.[5] Thus the wearer must have realistic expectations about visual recovery. Despite contact lenses having a limited role in visually rehabilitating eyes with corneal opacities, they are worth pursuing as an option, since the alternative of surgical keratoplasty is not without dangers.[6] Firstly, the waiting period for keratoplasty is long especially in developing countries. Secondly, post-operative course of keratoplasty, both early and late, is turbulent; prone to complications and requires vigilant monitoring. Visual success after successful keratoplasty is never guaranteed with obstacles like surgical astigmatism, graft failure, glaucoma. Often contact lenses are still required for optimal vision after clear grafts.

Contact lens use can cause significant improvement in vision with restoration of patient's functionality and often avert the requirement of keratoplasty in scared and damaged corneas.[6]

REFERENCES

1. Smiddy WE, Hamburg TR, Kracher GP, Gottsch JD, Stark WJ. Contact lenses for visual rehabilitation after corneal laceration repair. Ophthalmology. 1989 Mar; 96(3):293–8.
2. McMohan T, Szczotka Flynn LB. Fitting the abnormal cornea. In Cornea, Krachmer, Mannis Holland, 1313–24.
3. Veys J, Meyler J, Davies I. Rigid contact lens fitting. In Essential Contact lens practice. A practical guide. Mumbai. Johnson & Johnson Vision Care Institute. 2002, 61–78.
4. Netto AL, Lui AC, Lui GA. Visual rehabilitation with contact lenses after ocular trauma. Arq Bras Oftalmol. 2008 Nov-Dec;71(6 Suppl):23–31.

5. Titiyal JS, Das A, Dada VK, Tandon R, Ray M, Vajpayee RB. Visual performance of rigid gas permeable contact lenses in patients with corneal opacity. CLAO J. 2001 Jul;27(3):163–5.

6. Singh K, Jain D, Teli K. Rehabilitation of vision disabling corneal opacities: Is there hope without corneal transplant? Cont Lens Anterior Eye. 2013 Apr; 36(2):74–9.

7. Grünauer-Kloevekorn C, Habermann A, Wilhelm F, Duncker GI, Hammer T. Contact lens fitting as a possibility for visual rehabilitation in patients after open globe injuries Klin Monbl Augenheilkd. 2004 Aug;221(8): 652–7.

8. McMohan T, Szczotka Flynn L. Fitting the abnormal cornea . In Eds Krachmer JH, Mannis MJ, Holland EJ. Cornea. Fundamentals, diagnosis and management Vol 1. 2nd ed, Elsevier Mosby, Philadelphia, 1313–24.

Reader's Note

CHAPTER 14

Contacts in Sports and for Therapeutic Cases

LENSES DURING SPORTING ACTIVITIES

To avoid perceived cosmetic blemish young people with mild refractive error often deny their poor vision and perform their daily activities without using spectacle correction. This undue emphasis on avoiding spectacles makes them do daily chores and work with suboptimal vision. Over a period of time eye fatigue ensues manifesting with headache, vision blur and lack of motivation to participate in activities requiring fine vision. The suboptimal distance vision also makes these young people avoid participating in sport activities. For those using spectacles, spectacle related fears of broken glasses, contact injury and limited field of vision again makes them avoid sporting activities. This ensures that these children dwell in their near world confines. This aspect is the genesis of the misconception that myopia occurs in those involved in excessive near activities, e.g. reading.

Contact lenses are extremely useful for such young adults and serve to correct the mild error, enhance visual and subsequent sport performance, without causing distress to such youngsters.[1,2] Contact lenses also allow a more natural, unrestricted field of vision with reduced peripheral, spatial distortion. For those with moderate to *high refractive error*, lenses provide a more real time and stable image of outside environment.

The privileges enjoyed by contact lenses over their spectacle cousins in this field are:

a. *Visual field*: In high/moderate refractive errors, spectacles reduce visual field by inducing both peripheral and spatial distortions (Fig. 14.1). Contact lenses, on

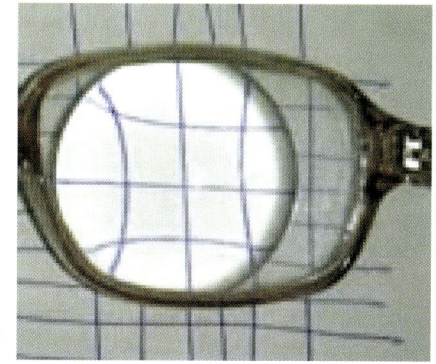

Fig. 14.1: (a) Barrel distortion seen through high minus lenses; (b) Pincushion as seen through high plus lenses

the other hand, enhance peripheral field by 15%, reduce and delete these distortions and improve hand body coordination.

b. *Size of image*: Image size with CL correlates better with 'real-world' size, because they provide lesser minification or magnification depending on myopic or hypermetropic error. This is very useful in sports where accurate assessment of size is important, e.g. cricket ball, tennis ball.

c. *Stability of vision*: Contact lenses remain *in situ* on the eye during active extraocular muscle movements and provide a more stable vision with enhanced depth perception because of no induced RSM (relative spectacle magnification) (*see* Fig. 11.1).[3] Spectacles, on the other hand, may get dislodged, decentered by physical exertions inherent to any sporting activity. Outdoor sports, water sports or sports during climate extremes fog up spectacle lenses with sweat, mist or water. In outdoor or night sports reflections and glare are associated with spectacles. All these problems are avoided with use of contact lenses.

d. *Stereopsis*: In refractive anisometropia depth perception is better with contact lenses but for axial anisometropia spectacles are optically the better option due to relative spectacle magnification (RSM). Any anisometropia of ≥0.50 D should be corrected for sportsmen since depth perception is crucial for fine vision required in most sporting activities.

e. *Risk of ocular injury* from broken frames or spectacle lenses is avoided in contact lens wearing sportsmen.

For most people using CL only during sports, soft lenses are a better option as they require minimal re-adaptation each time spectacle wear is substituted for lens wear. Disposable/frequent replacement programmes are ideal for such patients and invaluable in water sports.

The different types of sports requiring different lens types are detailed as follows.

Dynamic Sports

These sports involve active, strenuous body movement with examples being cricket, football, cycling, marathon racing, sprinting, lawn tennis, etc. Requirement of good contrast sensitivity to read subtle visual cues and stable vision during dynamic movements makes soft disposable lenses, lenses of choice for such sports.

To ensure stable vision a precise fitting which ensuring extra stability on eye is required, which is achievable with large diameter soft lenses. Smaller diameter rigid lenses with their poorer on-eye stability are liable to drop/pop out of the eye upon impact or during random unusual eye movement. In situations where RGP lenses cannot be avoided, large diameter lenses (9.2–10.5 mm) with lid attachment or minisclerals are preferred for their stability. It must be remembered that optic zone should be large enough (≥ 8.0 mm), to reduce flare subsequent to lens decentrations and pupil mydriasis induced by stress and sympathetic overdrive during sporting exertions. A slightly steep fit which avoids excessive edge lift, is preferred because of its stability. As lens induced dry eyes is exacerbated during sympathetic autonomic system predominant body milieu during sporting activities, concomitant use of lubricants is advised.

Water Sports

For swimmers use of tight, waterproof swimming goggles over contact lens is mandatory.[4] This not only protects the lens draped eye with contact from contaminated water but also allows clearer vision in underwater environment. If this is not feasible, the swimmers must be asked to close their eyes immediately prior to head immersion and while being underwater. Splashing of eyes with a re-wetting, sterile solution after cessation of water activities should be explained to all lens wearers.

Soft lenses, the usual lenses worn by swimmers, swell and tighten on the eye after being exposed to hypotonic fluid environment. This can cause red eye later on if appropriate measures like rinsing eye with re-wetting solution or sterile saline, immediately upon leaving water and/or lens removal is not done after cessation of water activities. Lens removal should be attempted only after use of lubricant drops has rehydrated such a swollen lens sufficiently to allow regaining of its mobility. As mentioned before, disposables are preferred option since the spectre of microbial contamination especially with dreaded acanthamoeba, always looms after exposure to swimming pool water.[5]

In fresh water sports (river swimming), a planned looser fit is aimed for as the lens tightens after immersion. The reverse of fitting a steeper lens in those doing sea/salt water sports is not advisable as it may cause hypoxic corneal damage over a period of time.[6]

The optics of underwater viewing also differ from terrestrial viewing conditions. Images underwater appear nearer and larger (requiring greater accommodation) and are made up almost exclusively of short wavelength end of visible spectrum.[5] Thus a presbyopic myope would need greater near add.

Winter Sports

Since winter sports are performed at high altitudes where atmospheric oxygen is reduced and temperatures are low, lenses with higher oxygen transmissibility are required to maintain corneal health. The additional physical elements detrimental for lenses are high speed winds, snow, and rarer atmosphere allowing ultraviolet exposure along with increased intensity of light. Ultraviolet absorbing contact lenses with additional sunglasses with sidepieces or polarized goggles have to be used as a precaution against ultraviolet keratitis due to light reflection off, snow covered surfaces.[7]

Another aspect is rapid lens drying due to low humidity in cold environs at reduced atmospheric pressure. This could cause alterations in optics specifically of high water content lenses. In such situations the less pliable, low water content lenses are preferred lenses. Again use of lubricating drops over lens helps in maintaining osmolarity and water content, thereby ensuring intactness of optical properties.

Type of Lens in Sports

This needs to be individualized as per sporting activity and wearer's refractive condition. Soft lenses score over RGP lenses in ease of insertion, stability on eye during all gazes, poor rate of dislodgement during intense physical activity/close contact with fellow players during sport activities.

- Soft toric lenses are preferred options for astigmatic patients over RGP lenses for those performing contact/dynamic/water sports, as they are less liable to be dislodged, thereby ensuring optimal vision at all times.
- If RGP lenses are to be used, then large diameter lenses (9.2 to 10.5 mm) with upper lid adherence or steeper fit with higher DK material are chosen to ensure lens stability. Large optic zone lenses of ≥ 8.0 mm are required in post-refractive surgery or keratoconus cases to minimizes flare during dim light conditions. The type of sporting activity also has to be considered while fitting such lenses. Centration in, down gaze is critical for chess players and centration in, up gaze is more important for cyclists who keep their head down while looking ahead.
- High water content lenses have to be used with caution as they are prone to dehydrating effects ensuing by reduced blinking associated with intense concentration. The reduced frequency of blinking allows more evaporation from lens draped ocular surface, during open eye period. Optics of a dehydrated lens get deranged leading to misty vision and errors of judgement. A thicker lens, with lower water content, is less susceptible to negative effects of

increased evaporation and is the preferred lens in such scenarios. This is more relevant in sports, where precise vision is crucial, e.g. archery, rifle shooting.

- Dark tinted contact lenses (70% absorption) are very useful alternatives in sports performed in bright sunlit conditions, e.g. skiing, yachting and marathon running. These lenses are also helpful in outdoor sports where wearing of protective sunglasses is not allowed.
- Color differentiating lenses, e.g. X chrome lenses are useful options in color deficient athletes, to enhance color discrimination.

Wherever feasible daily disposable lenses are preferred over other options. The sports pursuing lens wearer, must be asked to carry a spare pair of contact lenses or spectacles and re-wetting drops at all times.

THERAPEUTIC LENSES/BANDAGE CONTACT LENS (BCL)

Therapeutic lenses are used in pathologies where corneal epithelium is compromised, e.g. epithelial erosions or where epithelium integrity has been deliberately breached like post-refractive surgeries, collagen cross-linkage procedure. The placement of lenses in these conditions enhances epithelial healing, allows early covering of denuded cornea and protects from infections until the epithelium regenerates.

Indications

- As *structural reinforcement/tectonic support/splinting* in perforations or wound leak:
  - In small well-apposed, self-sealed corneal perforations of less than 2 mm, therapeutic lens allows opposition of wound edges and hastens healing by stopping aqueous seepage (Fig. 14.2). This is a viable alternative to surgical repair with the latter causing suture induced discomfort/astigmatism, and requirement of

a repeat surgical procedure for removal of sutures. In addition, resulting corneal scar post-suturing is often thicker and causes more visual disruption. Placing a bandage contact lens (BCL) with or without use of tissue glue as indicated, ensures healing and creates a thinner, less visually disabling scar (Fig. 14.3). Placement of a BCL also permits visualization of wound as healing is occurring. After placement of bandage lens stringent, meticulous follow up and use of antibiotics along with aqueous suppressants is needed. The BCL must be removed once wound integrity has been established, the process usually taking 2–3 weeks.

The option of BCL cannot be exercised in cases of iris tissue incarceration or other ocular injuries.

As a splint over tissue glue application, to prevent glue dislodgement subsequent to friction created by blinking lid movements.

- *Corneal epithelial abnormalities:*
  - Enhances healing of metaherpetic and/or atrophic ulcers. Bandage lenses are used in recurrent erosion syndrome where repeated epithelial breakdown occurs over an area of abnormal basement membrane. Therapeutic lenses promote healing, by ensuring firm adhesion of basal epithelium to underlying basement membrane and preventing constant shearing action on migrating epithelial cells by the blinking lid.
- *Surface/lid abnormalities:*
  - Temporary mechanical protection of disrupted/healing epithelium from external harm, e.g. trichiatic cilia/lid loss, before definitive surgery can be performed.
  - Exposure keratitis: Lid defects, exophthalmos, seventh nerve palsy or neurotrophic keratitis can cause exposure keratoapathy which is benefited with use of a BCL. This is a temporizing measure

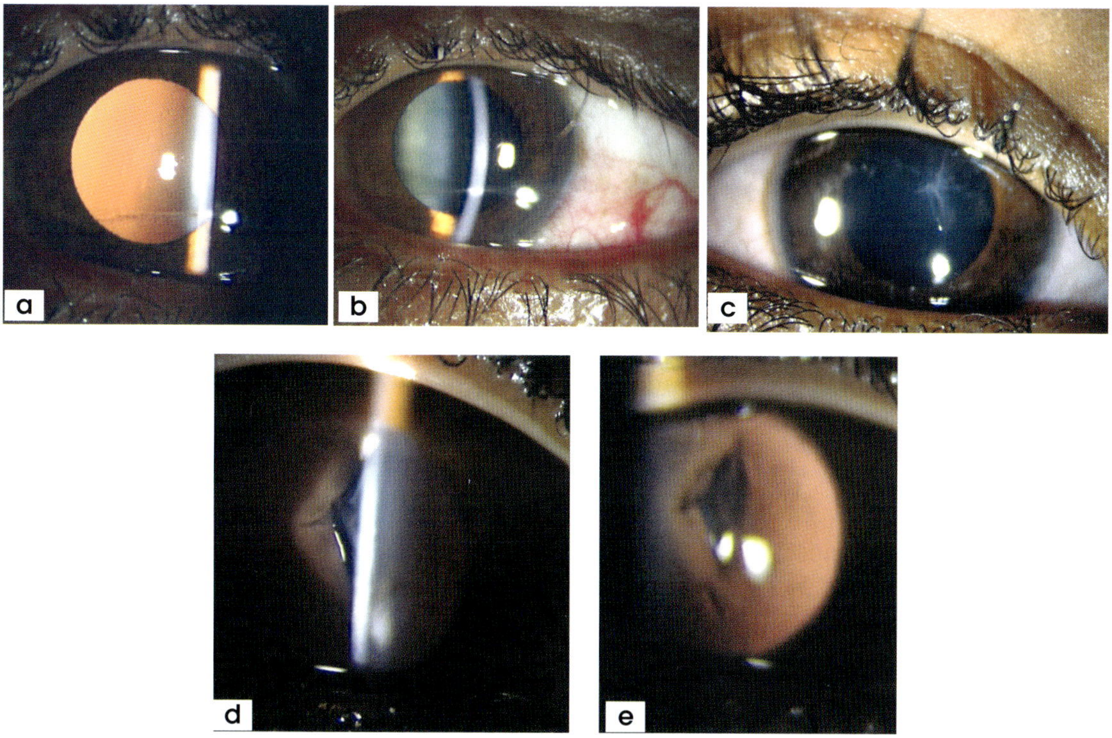

Fig. 14.2: Use of bandage lend to seal small corneal perforations: (a and b) Show a linear perforation effectively treated by using a BCL for 1 month along with antibiotics and anti-glaucoma medications; (c to e) show a larger jagged perforation, self sealed, with formed anterior chamber. During retro-illumination extent of perforation is easily visible.

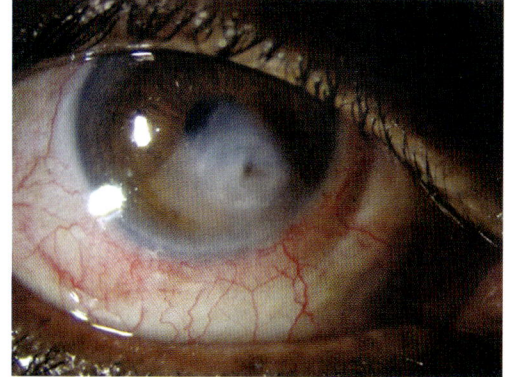

Fig. 14.3: A perforated corneal ulcer treated with cyanoacrylate glue and BCL

and ultimate relief occurs by taking care of the underlying pathology. Bandage lens should be used for maximum time of 4–5 weeks before it is replaced. Two to three replacements can be done, before definitive treatment is done or palsy resolves. A persistent non-resolving seventh nerve palsy or neurotrophic keratitis beyond this period would require a lateral tarsorrhaphy.

- *Pain relief:* Bandage lens provides pain relief in bullous keratopathy by flattening bullae, maintaining epithelial integrity by preventing rupture of bullae, dehydrating the oedematous epithelium and protecting exposed nerve endings from shearing action of lids. Reduction of all these ultimately provide comfort to the patient. Neutralization of irregular astigmatism by replacing irregular edematous cornea by the regular surface of BCL can also marginally improve visual acuity.

In filamentary keratitis, continuous shearing movement of lids during blinking moves filaments anchored to epithelium. This constant pull on filament causes severe piercing pain accompanied by reflex tearing, photophobia with subsequent poor vision. Often the symptoms are so incapacitating that the patient keeps his eyes voluntarily closed. A bandage lens relieves pain temporarily, until underlying condition of dry eye is treated and filament is manually removed.

- *Surgical adjuncts:* These lenses are useful in immediate post-operative period wherein they enhance epithelium healing, cell adhesion and reduce pain in cases where epithelial debridement has been done, e.g. post-refractive surgery/collagen cross-linkage/post-vitrectomy in diabetics. They may also be used to protect the cornea during some oculoplasty procedures.[8]

- *Vehicle for drug delivery:* Collagen shields soaked in antibiotic deliver a continuous flow of topical drugs while allowing epithelium to heal and provide early visual rehabilitation in cataract or retinal surgery cases. Such drug eluting contact lenses cannot be used in post-glaucoma surgery, as they would impair bleb filtration at limbus.

Advantages of this mode of drug delivery are: Prolonged contact at site of action, decreased requirement to instil topical drops, reduction of systemic toxicity arising due to nasal absorption of topical drugs.[9]

It must be remembered that therapeutic lenses cause corneal hypoxia and must be removed in one month's time, otherwise they can lead to persistent hypoxic induced corneal neovascularisation. In addition, they are prone to deposit formation, with intensity being proportionate to time duration of lens wear. The longer a therapeutic lens remains in the eye, higher is its pro-

pensity to get deposits. A deposit laden BCL serves as a nidus for microbial growth and causes infective keratitis in addition to ocular discomfort.

Altered Corneal Physiology with a Therapeutic Lens

a. *Induced corneal hypoxia:* In normal conditions oxygen demand of cornea is met by tears and partly by limbal diffusion. In open eye conditions partial pressure of dissolved oxygen in tear film is 155 mmHg, which is sufficient for corneal health. In closed eye conditions limbal vasculature and palpebral conjunctiva assume the role of primary suppliers of corneal oxygen at a reduced rate of 40–55 mmHg. Once a bandage lens is on the cornea, tear dissolved oxygen perforce must perfuse through lens to reach the eye. This situation is further exacerbated in closed eye conditions.

b. *Micro trauma:* Movement of therapeutic lens on cornea with blinking and eye movements causes microtrauma. This is exacerbated in conditions with irregular corneal epithelium, e.g. bullous keratopathy. The cornea responds to this repeated microtrauma with repair activity. This accelerated repair activity results in depletion of glycogen and ATP, increase in lactic acid and creation of an acidic milieu. Such an acidic pH causes tightening of therapeutic lens on eye.[3]

c. *Altered tear dynamics:* Tear exchange under a therapeutic lens is minimal which causes a stagnation of tear flow. This diminished tear circulation decreases effective flushing and cleansing action of tears. Thus concomitant use of lubricant and antibiotic eye drops over bandage lenses is advisable.

Types of Therapeutic Lenses

The nomenclature of bandage lenses depends on their water content and thickness. The three types of BCL are: High water content, medium water content and ultrathin lenses. Materials used are silicon hydrogels (e.g. lotrafilcon/balafilcon, senofilcon A, galyfilcon) and hydrogels (e.g. etafilcon).

a. *High water content* (70–80%) thick lenses (0.15–0.20 mm): The high water content confers high oxygen permeability to these lenses. These lenses are indicated in conditions where addition of a BCL can worsen the deranged physiology of a sick cornea, e.g. bullous keratopathy. In such situations the additional membrane of BCL reduces oxygen supply to a pathological cornea which is unable to tolerate the hypoxic insult and reacts by worsening decompensation. Such lenses must not be used in a "dry eye" state as they exacerbate symptoms by stealing tear fluid from ocular surface known as *steal phenomenon*.

b. *Medium water content lenses* (45–55%): These lenses are stiffer and serve as an adequate bandage in situations where minimal lens movement is beneficial, e.g. in corneal perforation or over/wound leak. High water content lenses in such situations would be too bulky.

c. *Ultrathin lens* (0.01–0.16 mm): These very thin membrane lenses have limited use as they are difficult to handle and are easily lost. However, they center well, provide better vision and dehydrate less in tear dysfunctional states. These lenses are useful in dry eye conditions.

Silicone hydrogels (0.10–0.15 mm) made of silicone rubber have the silicone conferred property of being highly oxygen permeable. The lack of water content, makes these lenses highly hydrophobic, non-wettable and therefore intolerable to ocular surface. They can only be used in the tear bathed milieu of eye, after special surface treatment to make them hydrophilic. The high oxygen permeability allows such lenses to be made *thicker* than poor oxygen permeability material lenses which depend on their thinness to transfer sufficient oxygen. This thickness makes such lenses easy to handle and reduces lens loss.[10] These lenses are preferred but are not always easily available.[11, 12]

Fitting Protocol

An irregular corneal epithelium is the main indication to fit a therapeutic lens. In such situations keratometry obviously cannot guide lens fitting. Fitting is thus performed by trial method or *one fit all* lens is used. The fit is checked after 20–30 minutes of wear as hydration and consequently fit alters while *in situ*. An excursion of more than 1 mm after 30 minutes of wear, constitutes an acceptable fit. High molecular weight fluorescein (Fluorexon) could be used to study the staining pattern, as regular fluorescein dye would stain the lens. Local anaesthetic drops should **not be used**, as they may mask the warning symptom of pain due to an ill fitting lens over the deformed epithelium.

Concomitant use of topical medications with therapeutic lens *in situ* would have an altered pharmacodynamics. Contact time between drug and cornea increases because of both, tear flow stagnation and lens acting as a reservoir. Preservatives present in drops build up in lens matrix and cause toxic epithelial damage. This is especially true with phenylephrine and epinephrine drops. The pH of the medication also affects lens fit by altering its hydration. Acidic pH medications cause lens dehydration with subsequent lens steepening, and alkaline pH causes lens flattening as a sequel to overhydration.

Removal of a Therapeutic Lens

Pinch method is applied to remove the therapeutic lens. The patient is asked to look up and the lens is pinched off from the inferior side. Use of lubricating drops 2–3 times before removal allows lens hydration and ensures easy removal.

REFERENCES

1. Rah MJ, Walline JJ, Jones-Jordan LA, Sinnott LT, Jackson JM, Manny RE, Coffey B, Lyons S; ACHIEVE Study Group Vision specific quality of life of pediatric contact lens wearers. Optom Vis Sci. 2010 Aug;87(8):560–6.

2. Walline JJ, Jones LA, Sinnott L, Chitkara M, Coffey B, Jackson JM, Manny RE, Rah MJ, Prinstein MJ; ACHIEVE Study Group. Randomized trial of the effect of contact lens wear on self-perception in children. Optom Vis Sci. 2009 Mar;86(3):222–32.

3. Mc Mohan T, Szczotka Flynn L. Fitting the abnormal cornea. In Eds Krachmer JH, Mannis MJ, Holland EJ. Cornea. Fundamentals, diagnosis and management Vol 1. 2nd ed., Elsevier Mosby, Philadelphia; 1313–24.

4. Wu YT, Tran J, Truong M, Harmis N, Zhu H, Stapleton F. Do swimming goggles limit microbial contamination of contact lenses? Optom Vis Sci. 2011; 88(4):456–60.

5. Brown MS, Siegel IM. Cornea-contact lens interaction in the aquatic environment. CLAO J. 1997 Oct;23 (4):237–42.

6. Josephson JE, Caffery BC. Contact lens consideration in surface and subsurface aqueous environments. Optom-Vis-science. 1991; 681: 2–11.

7. Ellerton JA, Zuljan I, Agazzi G, Boyd JJ. Eye problems in mountain and remote areas: prevention and onsite treatment—official recommendations of the International Commission for Mountain Emergency Medicine ICAR MEDCOM. Wilderness Environ Med. 2009 Summer; 20(2):169–75.

8. Dua HS, Cornes J, Singh A. Corneal epithelial wound healing. Br J Opthal 1994;78:401–8.

9. Campbell RC, Koch TO. Indications for contact lens use. In Eds Krachmer JH, Mannis MJ, Holland EJ. Cornea. Fundamentals, diagnosis and management Vol 1. 2nd ed., Elsevier Mosby, Philadelphia, 1309–11.

10. Veys J, Meyler J, Davies I. Contact lenses for therapeutic use. In: A practical guide. Essential contact lens practice. Eds. Vision Care Institute, Johnson and Johnson 2008; 155–168.

11. Martin R, de Juan V, Rodriguez G, Martin S, Fonseca S. Initial comfort of lotrafilcon: A silicone hydrogel contact lenses versus etafilcon: A contact lenses for extended wear. Cont Lens Anterior Eye. 2007 Mar; 30(1):23–8.

12. Gil-Cazorla R, Teus MA, Arranz-Márquez E. Comparison of silicone and non-silicone hydrogel soft contact lenses used as a bandage after LASEK. Refract Surg. 2008 Feb; 24(2):199–203.

Reader's Note

Reader's Note

CHAPTER 15

Scleral Lenses

Contact lenses are classified on the basis of bearing zone area as corneal, corneo-scleral and scleral lenses. Scleral lenses are those lenses which have a bearing zone on the sclera and large diameters ranging from 18 to 23 mm. These lenses by virtue of their surface area entrap a large tear reservoir, which property has been effectively used to aid corneal epithelial regeneration and protection.

HISTORICAL ASPECTS

The initial sclerals were made in 1880s from blown glass hemispherical shells to be used on an individual basis for keratoconus, irregular astigmatism and myopia by Eugene Kalt of France, Eugen Fick of Switzerland and August Müller of Germany respectively. August Müller while using it to correct his own high myopia of 15 D, reported a reduction of both minification and chromatic aberration compared to his spectacles.

Subsequently different materials were used by adopting Sir John FN Herschel's concept of impression moulding. The materials ranged from *plaster of Paris* by August Müller, *Negocoll seaweed* by Josef Dallos and reversible *hydrocolloid dental gels*. Lens insertion was facilitated by the topical anaesthetic cocaine, however, epithelial toxicity of this drug limited extensive use of these lenses.

After a hiatus of limited scleral lens activity, a lens renaissance occurred in late 1930s when

Theodore Obrig used Ophthalmic Moldite (cold, alginate material) to create scleral lenses by a technique of pouring the alginate into perforated acrylic impression trays with hollow tubular handles.[1] Wesley and Jessen refined this technique by introducing use of impression trays in making of these lenses. Commonest problem noted with use of sclerals was corneal oedema which was significant enough to be studied extensively by Sattler, who gave it the name of *Sattler's veil or Fick's phenomenon*. Sattler's veil defined as mistiness of vision accompanied by colored haloes during or after lens wear, led to lens intolerance and reduction of wearing time. Some astute observers realized that suboptimal lens fit (too flat or steep) and suboptimal corneal diameter (too large or too small) was linked to this edema. Another serendipitous observation in 1940s of air entrapment in post-lens tear film reducing this phenomenon, led to an era of ventilated or fenestrated lenses. Channels, perforations, slots and ducts in different positions and sizes were experimented with and finally a single fenestration, positioned interpalpebrally was found to be best tolerated. It was only in early 1950s that importance of oxygen for corneal metabolism and health was discovered and reason for Sattler's veil was attributed to hypoxia.

After development of the smaller corneal lens in late 1940s scleral lens were relegated to occasional use in advanced physical and pathological ocular conditions. Refinements in lens material and availability of computerized lathes has recently led to a resurgence in scleral lens usage.

Scleral/Haptic Lens Terminology

Figure 15.1 depicts the different parts of a scleral lens.

- Landing zone/scleral zone/haptic zone (Greek for 'to fasten/attach'): This is part of lens overlying sclera/conjunctiva.
- Optic zone or corneal portion: This is the central spherical or aspheric part of lens overlying cornea and limbus.
- Transition zone (TZ): It is the area of change in curvature/section between central optic and peripheral haptic. It determines the sagittal height of lens.
- Sagittal depth/apical height: This is the distance between flat and back surface of OZ. It depends on lens diameter, base curve, transition zone and corneal asphericity, shape of anterior sclera.
- Fenestration: Hole/s in lens to assist fluid exchange.
- Channel: Furrow on back surface of lens to enhance tear exchange.
- Preformed lens: A semi-finished stock lens constructed with a predetermined standardized back surface form/shape.
- Impression lens: A lens molded from cast of individual patient's anterior eye surface.
- Contact shell: Lens shape without optics.

Cosmetic (prosthetic) haptic lens: Lens designed to alter eye surface or hide disfigured eyes and impart optimal refractive correction. It can also be a haptic shell without optics which serves only to conceal damaged, disfigured anterior segments.

Indications for Scleral Lenses

A. Vision Improvement

These lenses are very useful in eyes with altered/irregular ocular surface where corneal lenses provide good optical correction but do not center sufficiently to provide stable vision. The common indications in this category are:

  i. Primary ectasias: Advanced keratoconic patients especially those with decentered cones, keratoglobus, pellucid marginal degeneration (PMD) alongwith coexisting ocular disorders like vernal catarrh (Fig. 15.2).[2–5]

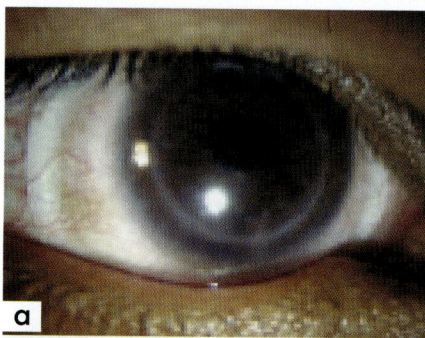

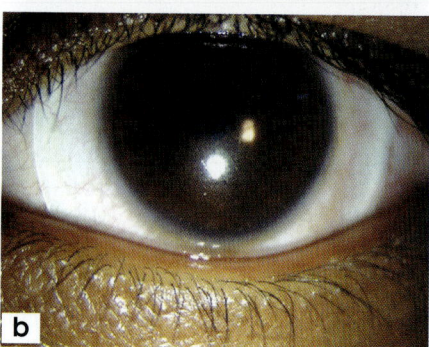

Fig. 15.2: Scleral lens fit in patient with keratoconus OU; (a) Right eye-operated graft; (b) Left eye-operated collagen cross linkage

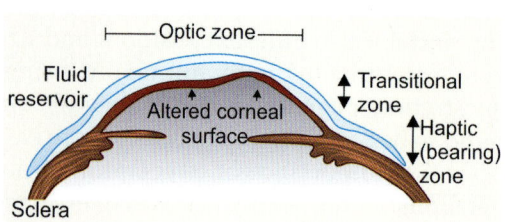

Fig. 15.1: Parts of a scleral lens. The diagram depicts fit over distorted cornea and function of fluid reservoir

ii. Secondary ectasia: Post-refractive surgery, post-keratoplasty.[2,4]

iii. Aphakia in extremes of age (infants, young children, elderly with hand tremors/arthritis) due to ease of handling/visibility and less lens loss compared to smaller corneal lenses. Patients, however, have a *steep learning curve*, during initial weeks of use to insert and remove these lenses.[2]

iv. Occupations involving work in dusty environments/using heavy machinery. The ability to remain *in situ*, not absorb contaminants, or alter its fitting characteristics makes sclerals lens of choice for such environs.

v. Sports: Dynamic vigorous sports, winter/water sports.

B. Corneal Protection

Sclerals aid corneal healing by generating a tear pool over corneal epithelium at neutral pressure which reduces both blink induced shearing action and evaporation. This fluid reservoir is depicted in Fig. 15.2.

i. Dry eye/altered corneal surface: Sclerals by covering most of anterior ocular surface help to protect cornea in addition to providing refractive correction. These conditions are: Post Stevens-Johnson, ocular cicatricial pemphigoid, graft versus host disease, neurotrophic corneal disease. Sjögren's syndrome and persistent epithelial corneal defects.[2, 6–9]

ii. Incomplete lid closure: Exposed globe situations post-trauma, post/burns, eyelid coloboma, exophthalmus, ectropion, nerve palsies and lid surgery causing dry eyes, fragile corneal epithelium and deformed ocular surface are helped by scleral lens wear.[10,11]

iii. Eyes with grossly decentered pupils, nystagmus and albinism.

C. Cosmetic

In damaged, scarred, shrunken blind eyes for recreating surface and in strabismic blind eye to create parallelism. It is also used by actors, models in achieving special effects.

D. Therapeutic

In ptosis where superior haptic of a scleral lens supports ledge of ptosis correcting crutch glass.[12]

A study of 1560 eyes fitted with scleral lenses found primary corneal ectasia, secondary ectasia, aphakia, myopia and ptosis to be the most common conditions benefited by scleral lenses with non-ventilated type being used most often.[2] The disadvantages of a scleral are its prohibitive cost, requirement of specialized learning and equipment, increased chair time and limited availability of the lens. However, use of this customized lens is sight saving in many conditions and a study evaluating cost effectiveness based on criteria of *quality adjusted life years (QUALY)* found it to be cost beneficial modality for visual rehabilitation.[13]

Fitting Technique

The preferred technique is by using preformed sclerals. In patients where this is not successful impression molding is resorted to which is labour intensive but very rewarding to the patient.

a. **Integrated fitting with preformed sclerals:** Preformed sclerals are lenses with precise reproducible specifications based on standard design of spherical haptic with transition curves of known dimensions. These lenses are thinner than moulded sclerals and adequate limbal/corneal clearance is easier to achieve. Both haptic and optic fitting are done using the same lens and patients can experience real time lens wear feel, prior to fitting of actual lens. However, these lenses designed for minimum clearance, are difficult to fit on highly toric or irregular eyes, due to presence of harsh bearing areas on the cornea. Trial in these situations can be done by smaller fenestrated lenses for optic measurements (FLOMs), to determine correct optical radius. Another problem with preformed lenses is requirement of a large inventory of fitting set, making this method an economically viable option only for practitioners with a large scleral practice.

b. **Impression/moulded scleral lenses:** For highly irregular distorted surfaces where preformed sclerals may be inadequate, lenses are fabricated after taking an impression of patient's eye, using a mould. Since the shape of anterior surface is precisely reproduced, such a lens has a better fitting. The impression retains its shape indefinitely, so a lens can be reproduced at any time. Such lenses are thicker than preformed sclerals (0.4 to 0.6 mm) and have decreased effective Dk/t value.

The **technique** involves two processes: Creating a negative mould or receptacle with the eye contour and preparing positive mould based on the negative impression.

i. **Negative mould***:* The first step involves preparing the material by mixing moulding powder with distilled water in a clean rubber bowl. The resultant mixture is drawn or placed into a syringe with help of a spatula. Drawing minimizes air bubble entrapment in mixture, is less messy and is preferred.

Patient preparation involves allaying of anxiety and instillation of topical xylo caine drops in eye to be moulded. The patient is placed in a reclining or supine position and asked to fixate on an intermediate distance target with the other eye to ensure centration of poor vision eye which has to be fitted. This method also minimizes any tropia. While patient looks down, upper lid is retracted and moulding shell (impression tray) is slipped beneath upper lid ensuring that nasal side of shell faces inner canthus. Subsequently patient is asked to look up, lower lid is retracted and lower part of shell inserted beneath

it. The prepared scleral material is squeezed via handle of moulding shell onto eye with help of the loaded syringe. Surplus material is allowed to flow out through perforations in tray by gently pressing the shell. The moulding mixture gels in about two minutes and achieves consistency of a hard-boiled egg. Once this occurs, the shell along with **negative** *impression* is removed and placed in water.

ii. **Positive mould:** Dental stone material is employed for making the positive impression and consists of plaster of Paris with water. It is prepared in a clean rubber bowl and all entrapped air bubbles are removed by allowing them to rise to surface and escape by tapping on sides of the bowl. The *negative impression* mould is removed from water, dried and placed upside down on a wide mouthed bottle. Dental stone mixture is poured into this negative mould from the side, allowing escape of entrapped air bubbles. The mixture is subsequently hardened for twenty minutes and a horizontal mark is drawn from inner to outer canthus with a marker pencil. Markings of N and T are made above this line to indicate nasal and temporal side with center labelled as R or L depending on eye cast. After an hour's setting, the positive is removed from negative mould and spherical lapping stones of specific radius are used to grind optic zone clearance and shape the back surface. Computer driven lathes then polish the mould and generate optical power by grinding an appropriate front surface radius onto the corneal zone.

Lens fit has to be assessed after several minutes of lens wear with scleral, corneal and limbal parts being evaluated separately.

The types of scleral lens fit are flush, sealed, semi-sealed and ventilated.

a. **Flush fit:** In this fit haptic lens is closely parallel and conforms to anterior eye contour.

b. **Semi-sealed fit:** This involves modifications like grooves, furrows, channels in haptic zone to allow egress of trapped post-lens tear film.

c. **Ventilated fit:** This fit employs fenestrations in areas of some clearance (typically limbal zone) to allow air entry into post-lens tear film for adequate corneal oxygenation.[2]

d. **Sealed fit:** This is the name given to snug fit with minimal lens movement which precludes tear exchange and is extremely harmful to corneal health.

Rubens Ideal Fit Criteria

Scleral part/haptic: Haptic is fitted with adequate corneal clearance based on adequate sagittal depth. This is done by aligning landing zone with anterior ocular surface and creating an adequate edge lift. Limbal clearance is crucial to permit tear exchange and flushing of debris. Tight fit is diagnosed by vessel blanching/crimping and creation of a lens imprint (conjunctival indentation) after lens removal. Loose fit is diagnosed by presence of excessive clearance and bubble formation.

Fenestrations if made are placed in corneal section, near corneo-scleral transition zone in interpalpebral area 1–2 mm below temporal margin of upper lid so that they get covered by upper lid. The diameter of these fenestrations is usually 1.0 mm.

Corneal part: Corneal part should depict a minimal 0.04–0.08 mm clearance over entire zone until 1–2 mm peripheral to limbus (Fig. 15.3). This clearance is sufficient to prevent corneal bearing and must be confirmed by instilling fluorescein in lens solution prior to insertion. Presence of a bubble is optional and if present, it needs to be mobile. Bubble is usually sausage shaped, seen over corneo-scleral junction with superior or temporal locations being preferred to prevent it from obscuring near vision.

Faulty Fit: Types and Features

a. Tight fit/areas: Localized areas of touch identified after a few hours of wear require corneal, limbal or haptic grindings for modification. *Cling effect* due to negative pressure generated beneath 'glove-like' fit of haptic must be avoided and can be diagnosed by difficulty in lens removal on application of suction cup.

b. Excess vaulting: Presence of a large bubble over central corneal area is diagnostic. The solution involves a 'haptic let-down' or uniform removal of lens material over entire haptic.

c. Bubbles: Presence of bubbles indicate excessive apical clearance, inadequate lens sizing and/or poorly conceived fenest-

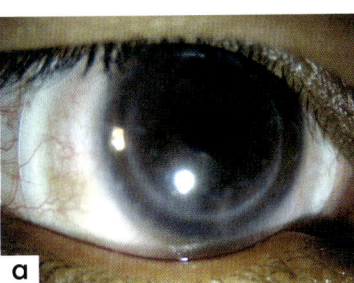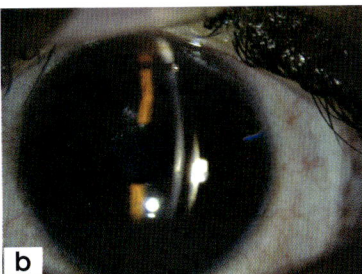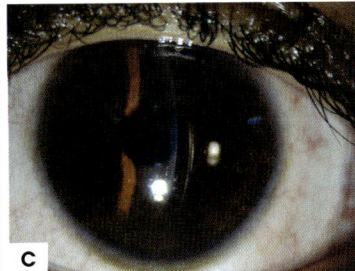

Fig. 15.3: (a) PROSE lens in postgraft eye; (b) Clearance/fluid reservoir thickness; (c) Clearance/fluid reservoir thickness =150 µ (magnified view)

rations. Sometimes bubbles are accompanied by a clicking sound and/or froth generation due to bubble traversing the inadequately sized or placed fenestration.

d. Fenestration related problems:
   – Large bubble preventing lens centration with corneal touch adjacent to bubble. This requires grinding of part causing the bearing. In cases with large bubble but no demonstrable area of touch, touch in haptic area peripheral to bubble is assumed and that area is then ground.
   – Large fixed bubble with well centered lens occurs due to excessive clearance on one side is relieved by a haptic 'let-down'.

e. Photophobia/tiredness or sleepiness while wearing lenses occurs due to inadequate tear exchange or insufficient limbal clearance causing corneal hypoxia.

f. Watery discharge/burning or stinging sensation/red eye is due to corneal bearing by poorly finished lens edge and inadequate tear exchange.

g. Blurred vision occurs due to poor tear wetting of front surface of lens causing appearance of dry spots.

h. Diplopia is due to misaligned optics, poor lens centration or presence of a large bubble.

Boston/PROSE lens

The prototype lens is Boston scleral lenses or PROSE (prosthetic replacement of ocular surface eco-system) is made from itafluorocon B, a fluro-silicon-acrylate polymer with Dk value 87 x10–11 units. This highly customized, proprietary, computer-assisted design uses topographic guided software linked to a manufacturing lathe, which has the capacity to alter lens fit parameters instantly. The posterior surface is lathed and residual refractive error is incorporated into frontal surface. Developed by Boston Foundation for Sight (BFS, Needham, MA), the Boston technology was granted FDA approval in 1994. It has been used extensively in complex corneal conditions including post-keratoplasty and children with ocular surface disorders (Fig. 15.3).[14,15]

Rose K XL Design

This lens is of Rose K series with an aspheric Back Optic Zone which decreases as BC steepens. The range available is from 5.80 to 8.40 mm BC, 13.60 to 15.60 mm OD, and powers from +30.00 to –30.00 D. The manufacturers offer edge lift (EL) options from 2.0 double flat, 1.0 standard flat, 0 standard, –1.0 standard steep and 2.0 double steep lift.

The material is Menicon Z, Lagado Tyro 97 or Boston XO. The trial set consists of 16 lenses with BC from 6.00 to 8.00 mm, of standard diameter 14.60 mm and 0 edge lift.

The fitting protocol as described by Dr Paul Rose is as follows:

• **Central fit:** The first trial lens is 0.2 mm steeper than average K's and central fit is assessed by altering BC flatter or steeper until a light feather touch is achieved at highest point on cornea.
   Once this fit is seen, a settling time of 20 minutes is given and fit is then re-evaluated (Fig. 15.4a).

• **Peripheral fit:** Peripheral fit is then looked at with optimal band being 0.8–1 mm wide (Fig. 15.4b). In case of wide band, lift off and bubbling at lens edge of lens with discomfort, the lift option used is decrease/steepen the lift. For narrow band, increased/flattened lift option is used. Irregular band is seen in cases of peripheral astigmatism. Edge lift is recommended as per corneal condition: 0.2 flatter than mean K for keratoconus, 0.6–0.7 steeper than mean K in PMD/postgraft/LASIK and 0.1 steeper than mean K in corneal rings. Ease of lens removal is a good reflection of sufficient EL.

• **Diameter:** For average cornea of 11.8 mm, lens should extend 1.3 to 1.5 mm outside limbus.

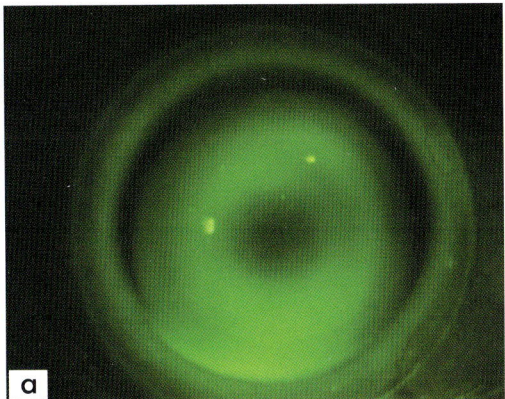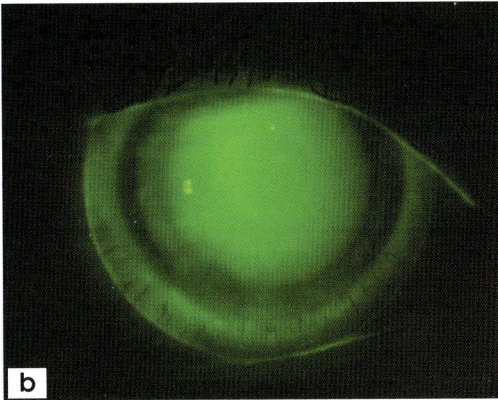

Fig. 15.4: Optimal fit of Rose KXL lens: (a) Central fit; (b) Peripheral fit

- **Location:** Lens should sit evenly around the limbus. Inferior location indicates decentered apex. In this situation increased OD lenses should be tried.
- **Movement:** A slight movement of less than 0.5 mm should be seen with blinking after settling in period. To assess movement patient is asked to look up and blink with the fitter looking at 6 o'clock position. Excess movement is rectified by decreasing EL, steepening BC and/or increasing OD. Decrease movement is rectified by increasing EL, flattening BC and/or decreasing OD.
- Power is verified by **over-refraction.**

Toric Sclerals

These can be front toric, back toric or bitoric lenses with examples being Maxim and Comfort (front toric), Medlens Innovations MSD, Essilor Contact Lenses, Inc., Dallas, TX and Jupiter (back toric), AVT, Dynana semiscleral and true-scleral (bi-toric).[3]

Fitting Technique of Preformed Sclerals

a. Lens insertion (Fig. 15.5)

- A sterile, bubble-free saline solution is used to fill the lens with fluorescein being added only if fit needs to be assessed.
- Patient is asked to bend head downwards parallel to floor.
- One hand of practitioner is used to raise patient's upper lid, and other hand to slide lens under upper lid while ensuring that solution remains in lens.
- Patient is subsequently asked to look down, while practitioner simultaneously

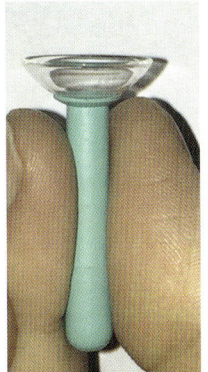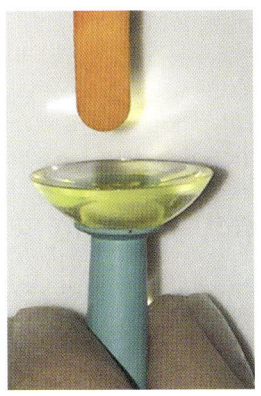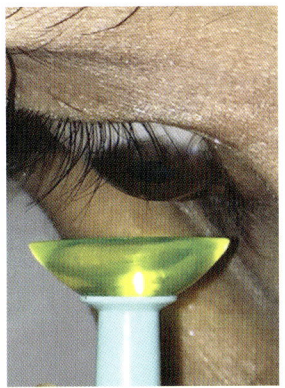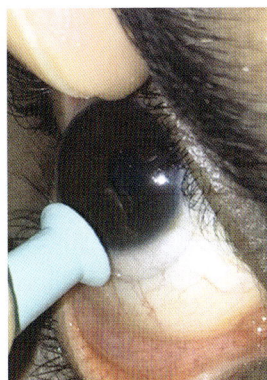

Fig. 15.5: Sequential fitting of a miniscleral lens

pulls down lower lid and slides lens completely in.

– Both lids are released and patient asked to raise his/her head.

A suction holder can also be used to insert the lens. Entry of a few bubbles can be ignored but excess bubbles impairing vision require lens to be re-inserted.

b. **Lens removal:** Patient is asked to look down and thumb of contralateral hand, e.g. left hand for right eye is swept beneath lash margin of upper lid from inner to outer canthus while raising upper lid above the edge of lens. During this manoeuvre slight pressure is exerted down and behind the lens, towards the globe. This disengages upper part of lens and allows lens to fall down into outstretched waiting ipsilateral cupped hand.

Alternatively a suction holder can be used. A clean and wet suction holder is held cup side up, it is pinched by middle by using thumb and index finger of dominant hand. A few drops of lens solution are put in upturned cup. Using middle fingers of the other hand pull and hold the upper lid margin firmly, against the upper orbital bone. Lower lid margin is pulled against the lower orbital bone, with middle finger of dominant hand while holding the pinched suction holder. Patents is as leed to look into a mirror and locate lower periphery of lens on eye. Subsequently cup of pinched wet suction holder is placed at **lower periphery** (6 o'clock) or temporal edge (never center) of lens surface and pinch is then released to capture the lens (Fig. 15.6). Lens is then peeled off by pulling outwards and across in an arc towards the nose. Suction between lens and cornea is broken.

Use of scleral lenses results in marked subjective improvement in quality of life of patients as a result of improved functional vision and pain relief.[4,16,17] These lenses have been a boon for patients where

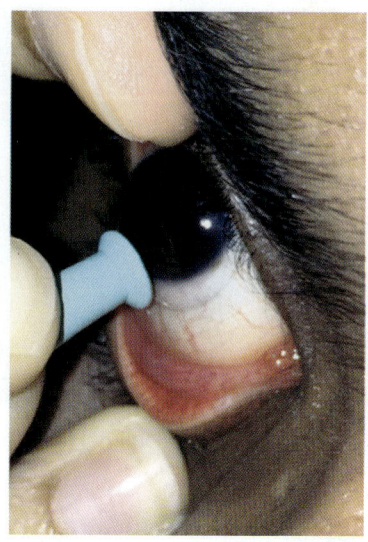

Fig. 15.6: Lens holder being used to remove the scleral lens from the eye

conventional contact lenses and medical treatment has failed to provide relief.[18] Documented wearing times have ranged from a few hours to 18 hours, with patients becoming heavily dependent on these lenses for daily living activities.[19,20] Often these lenses have averted requirement for definitive surgery in these subset of patients. Poor compliance with care regimens, however, can result in tear debris accumulation and microbial keratitis.[15,21]

Minisclerals

Recently a miniscleral design (MSD) has become available. The lenses have smaller diameter (15–18 mm) versus sclerals which have diameter ≥ 18 mm. These lenses should be tried as the first option is all conditions where sclerals are needed (Fig. 15.7a to e).[22,23] These lenses vault the cornea and limbus while resting evenly on sclera to achieve a semi-sealed state with partial tear exchange (Fig. 15.8). The lenses need to be filled with fluid (unit dose or non-preserved saline) prior to their application to prevent air bubble formation. They can be made in front surface toric firm or with toric periphery design in

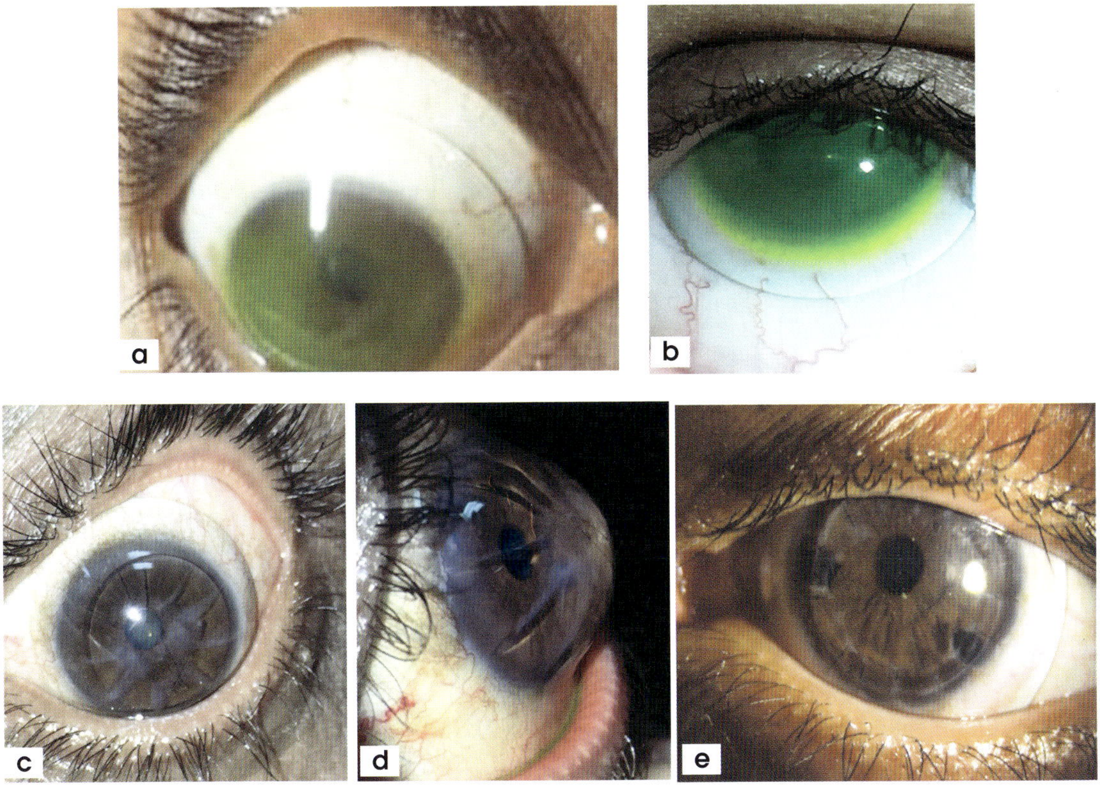

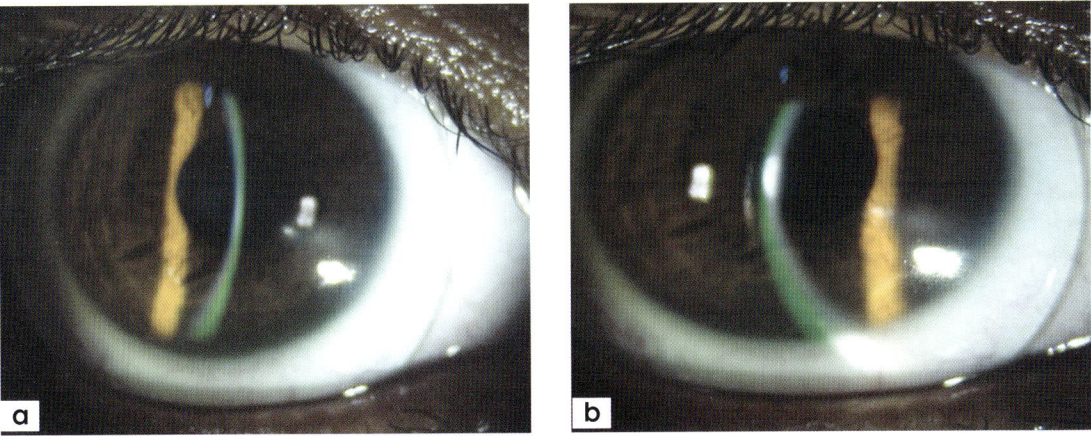

Fig. 15.7: Miniscleral lenses used for: (a and b) Advanced keratoconus; (c and d) Post-RK ectasia; (e) Post-keratoplasty

Fig. 15.8: (a) Miniscleral semi-sealed fit with partial tear exchange; (b) Fluorescein stained fluid reservoir adequate

conditions of residual astigmatism or highly toric sclera respectively.

Minisclerals are specified by either radii of curvature of central base curve and peripheral curves or by sagittal depth. Optimal fit should ensure that lens does not rest on limbus and achieve a tight realed state (Fig. 15.9). Despite use of highly oxygen permeable material (Boston XO), corneal hypoxic and limbal cell deficiency can occur. This needs to be monitred by looking for any signs of corneal neovascularization and/or loss of corneal transpauncy. The lens has the option of being made in quadrant specific to peripheral design. Available MSD options are Maxim, Jupiter. Boston MSD and MSD.

This fit needs to be checked in all gazes to ensure stability of vision (Fig. 15.10).

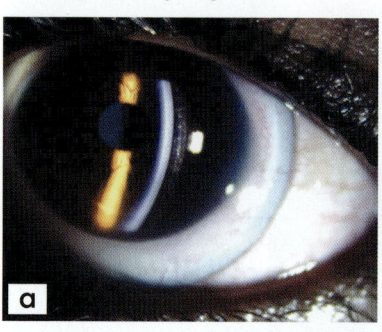
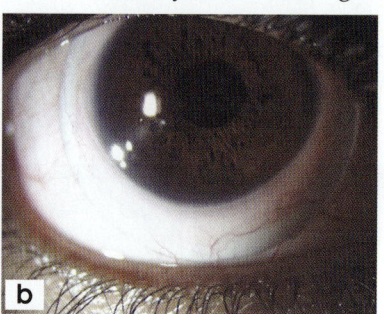

Fig. 15.9: Miniscleral lens fit: (a and b) Limbal flush seen

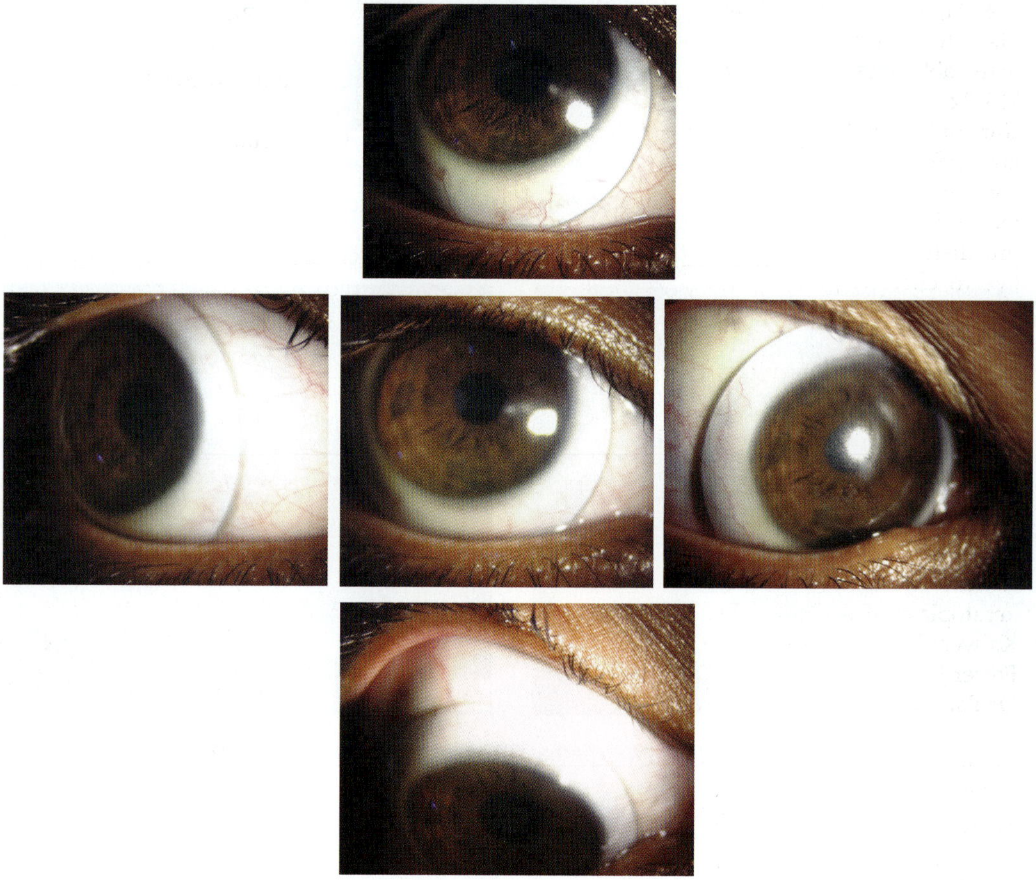

Fig. 15.10: Miniscleral lens, well-centered in all gazes

REFERENCES

1. Sclerals. IACLE. International Association of Contact lens educators. 2000 Module 9, Chapter 9.4, p.143, 1st ed. Sydney.
2. Pullum KW, Whiting MA, Buckley RJ Scleral contact lenses: the expanding role. Cornea 2005; 24:269–77.
3. Visser ES, Visser R, van Lier HJ, Otten HM. Modern scleral lenses part I: clinical features. Eye Contact Lens. 2007 Jan;33(1):13–20.
4. Segal O, Barkana Y, Hourovitz D, Behrman S, Kamun Y, Avni I, Zadok Scleral contact lenses may help where other modalities fail. Cornea. 2003 May; 22(4): 308–10.
5. Rathi VM, Sudharman Mandathara P, Vaddavalli PK, Dumpati S, Chakrabarti T, Sangwan VS. Fluid-filled scleral contact lenses in vernal keratoconjunctivitis. Cont Lens Anterior Eye 2012; 38: 203–6.
6. Kok JH, Visser R. Treatment of ocular surface disorders and dry eyes with high gas-permeable scleral lenses. Cornea. 1992; 11(6): 518–22.
7. Gungor I, Schor K, Rosenthal P, Jacobs DS. The Boston Scleral lens in the treatment of pediatric patients. J AAPOS 2008; 12:263–7.
8. Jacobs DS, Rosenthal P. Boston scleral lens prosthetic device for treatment of severe dry eye in chronic graft-versus-host disease. Cornea 2007; 26:1195–9.
9. Rathi VM, Mandathara PS, Dumpati S, Vaddavalli PK, Sangwan VS. Ophthalmology Boston ocular surface prosthesis: an Indian experience. Indian J Ophthalmol 2011; 59:279–81.
10. Rosenthal P, Croteau A. Fluid-ventilated, gas-permeable scleral contact lens is an effective option for managing severe ocular surface disease and many corneal disorders that would otherwise require penetrating keratoplasty. Eye Contact Lens 2005; 31:130–4
11. Kalwerisky K, Davies B, Mihora L, Czyz CN, Foster JA, De Martelaere S. Use of the Boston Ocular Surface Prosthesis in the management of severe periorbital thermal injuries: a case series of 10 patients. Eye Contact Lens 2012; 38:203–6.
12. Shah-Desai SD, Aslam SA, Pullum K, Beaconsfield M, RoseGE. Scleral contact lens usage in patients with complex blepharoptosis. Indian J Ophthalmol 2011; 59:279–81.
13. Shepard DS, Razavi M, Stason WB, Jacobs DS, Cohen M, Rosenthal P. Economic appraisal of the Boston Ocular Surface Prosthesis. Am J Ophthalmol 2009; 148:860–8.
14. Baran I, Bradley JA, Alipour F, Rosenthal P, Le HG, Jacobs DS. PROSE treatment of corneal ectasia. Cont Lens Anterior Eye 2012; 35: 222–7.
15. Rathi VM, Mandathara PS, Vaddavalli PK, Srikanth D, Sangwan VS. Fluid filled scleral contact lens in pediatric patients: challenges and outcome. Cont Lens Anterior Eye 2012;35: 189–92.
16. Siqueira AC, Santos MS, Farias CC, Barreiro TR, Gomes JÁ. Scleral contact lens for ocular rehabilitation in patients with Stevens-Johnson syndrome. Arq Bras Oftalmol 2010; 73:428–32.
17. Stason WB, Razavi M, Jacobs DS, Shepard DS, Suaya JA, JohnsL, Rosenthal P. Clinical benefits of the Boston Ocular Surface Prosthesis. Am J Ophthalmol 2010 ;149:54–61.
18. Rosenthal P, Cotter J. The Boston Scleral Lens in the management of severe ocular surface disease. Ophthalmol Clin North Am. 2003 Mar;16(1):89–93.
19. Romero-Rangel T, Stavrou P, Cotter J, Rosenthal P, Baltatzis S, Foster C. Gas-permeable scleral contact lens therapy in ocular surface disease. Am J Ophthalmol. 2000 Jul;130(1):25–32.
20. Tougeron-Brousseau B, Delcampe A, Gueudry J, Vera L, Doan S, Hoang-Xuan etal. Vision-related function after scleral lens fitting in ocular complications of Stevens-Johnson syndrome and toxic epidermal necrolysis. Am J Ophthalmol 2009; 148:852–9.
21. Zimmerman AB, Marks A. Microbial keratitis secondary to unintended poor compliance with scleral gas-permeable contact lenses. Eye Contact Lens. 2014 Jan;40(1):1–4.
22. Dalton K, Sorbara L. Fitting an MSD (mini scleral design) rigid contact lens in advanced keratoconus with INTACS. Cont Lens Anterior Eye. 2011 Dec; 34(6):274–81.
23. Alipour F, Behrouz MJ, Samet B. Mini-scleral lenses in the visual rehabilitation of patients after penetrating keratoplasty and deep lamellar anterior keratoplasty. Cont Lens Anterior Eye. 2015 Feb;38(1):54–8.

Reader's Note

CHAPTER 16

Prosthetic Lenses and Tints

TINTED

Tinting of lens is done so as to enable the wearer to easily locate and identify lenses. Since the reason for lens wear is poor vision, patients often have difficulty in locating the thin lenses and historically tinting was done to aid the poor vision wearer in identifying lens against white background of lens case. In earlier times it was done with vegetable based food dyes for hydrogel lenses.[1] Current expanded indications of tinting include optical and cosmetic reasons. The two main types of tints used are **transparent and opaque.** Transparent tinted lenses have large-diameter tint area approximating visible iris diameter, whereas opaque tints incorporate artwork or images that block light. Hydrogel lenses can be tinted easily but RGP lenses tinting requires a specialized process.

Physiology of Eye Color

Visible eye color is largely dependent on iris color with lighter colors (blue/green/hazel) being a result of absorption of longer red wavelength of light and reflection of shorter blue wavelengths due to lesser compact iris stroma, over a posterior pigmented iris epithelium—the *Rayleigh phenomenon*. Dark color (black/brown) is a result of absorption of both long and short wavelengths with no reflection of light, along with increased melanin content in iris epithelium and iris stroma, especially the anterior border layer.

Types and Indications for Tinted Lenses

A. *Handling tints*: These serve to make contact lens conspicuous and aid in its location and handling.

B. *Cosmetic*: Cosmetic soft lenses are used to enhance or alter iris colors by actors, models and those whishing to alter their eye color. Colored or tinted rigid lenses are used by actors (front mirrored) and by scientists employed in performing psychophysical experiments to monitor eye position/movement.

C. *Prosthetics*: These are used to hide/conceal, disfigured cornea. The nomenclature is often interchangeable between cosmetic and prosthetic.

D. *Therapeutic*:

    i. Reduce light transmission: This aspect of tints is utilized in patients of albinism, aniridia, iris colobomas and traumatic mydriasis to reduce glare. These patients suffer from disabling photophobia in sunlight/brightly-lit environment and tinted lenses by eliminating para-axial rays from entering exposed retina, permit functional vision.

    ii. As an alternative to occlusive patches in treatment of amblyopia and intolerable diplopia.

iii. Red green color impregnated lenses, e.g. X chrome lenses are used to differentiate between colors by color defective individuals.[2,3]

A. Handling Tints

Light tints incorporated in RGP/hydrogel/scleral lenses serve to enhance lens visibility when off the eye, which helps poor vision wearer in identifying and handling the lens. They also aid in locating lens in palm of hand, in storage containers and/or to differentiate between right and left lenses by using different tints for two eyes. These *visibility tints* present across entire lens diameter are of low density with high transmittance and luminous transmission factor of about 95% (Fig. 16.1). If darker tints are to be used, then *clear pupil zone* feature is employed, to minimize potentially adverse effects related to full pupil coverage tints. These adverse events result from reduced illumination in night time outdoor activities like driving, altered perception of visible spectrum leading to altered hues of lightly colored objects in mesopic light. The problem with *clear pupil zone tinted lenses* is visibility of natural iris color under the lens, during pupil miosis or oblique viewing conditions, creating artificial heteochromia. Hydrogels with

their minimal excursions over the iris, ensure a realistic color change. Tinted RGP lens, on the other hand, with their obvious movement may result in tinted portion overlying white sclera, giving rise to a perilimbal colored crescentic halo appearance.

B. Cosmetic/Opaque Tints

i. **Opaque hydrogels** are used for cosmetic reasons like altering iris color or for therapeutic reasons like concealing corneal scars (Fig. 16.2). Normal iris color arises from wavelengths reflected from back of iris with melanin present in stroma giving it a *depth*. Thus in situations where color is imparted by contact lens anterior to natural iris plane (source of true eye color), the look is unnatural due to lack of depth (Fig. 16.3).

Most cosmetic lenses have a fixed-diameter clear pupil zone which has a sharp cut-off/tapering-off edge with variable color density, depending on dot size used in artwork (Fig. 16.4). Despite the clear pupil zone being larger than mesopic pupil, ghosting resulting from decentration of artificial pupil/clear zone relative to actual pupil is a common complaint

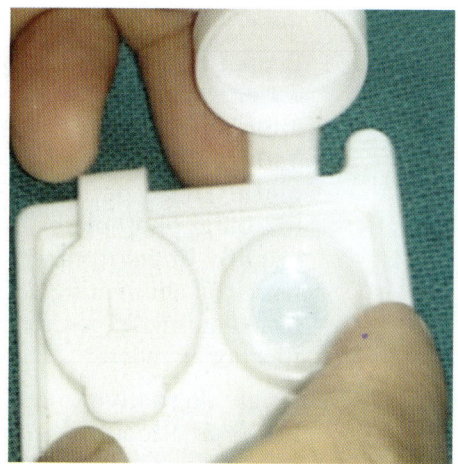 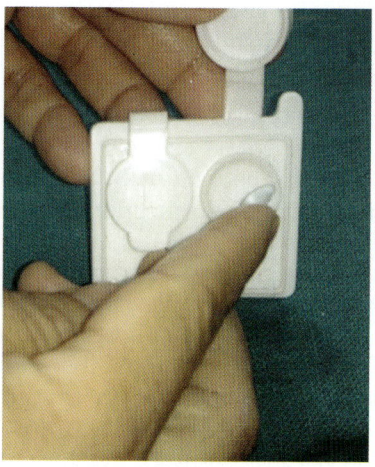

Fig. 16.1: Handling tint makes lens easily visible and easier to remove from case

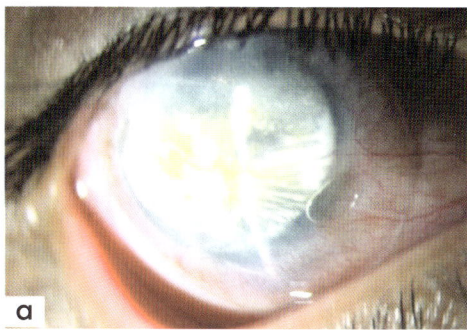 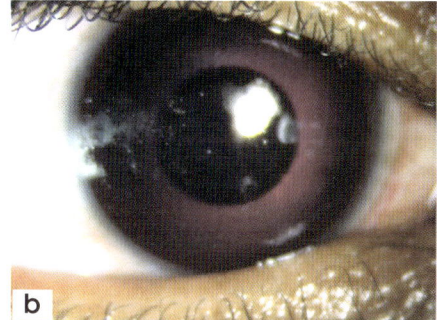

Fig. 16.2: Prosthetic lens concealing corneal scar (pre and post)

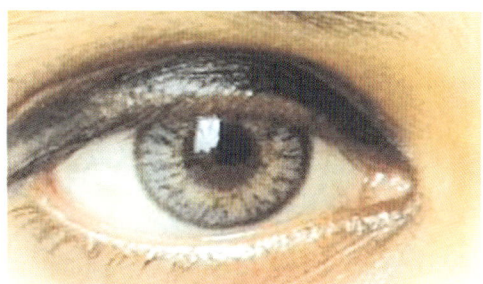 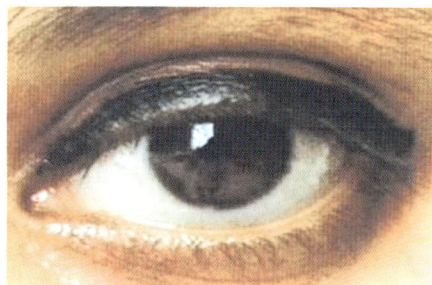

Fig. 16.3: With cosmetic contact lens in right eye. Note lack of depth in color gives an artificial appearance to right eye versus normal look of left eye (not wearing a cosmetic lens)

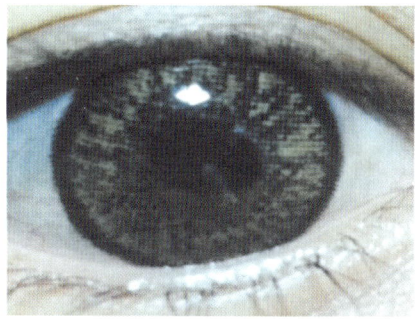

(Fig. 16.5). Visual field is also restricted from minimal to significant extent depending on tinting technology, sharpness of artificial pupil edge and diameter.[4] Figures 16.6 and 16.7 depict

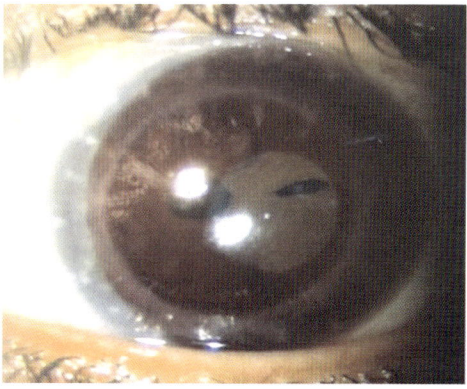

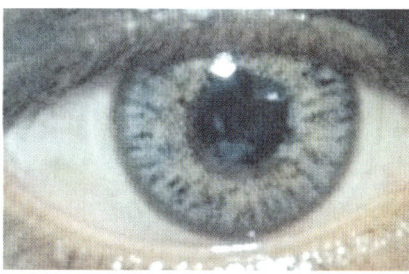

Fig. 16.4: Variable color is proportionate to dot size used

Fig. 16.5: Cosmetic contact lens with clear pupil showing decentration. As pupil edge is being bisected by optical zone, patient would complain of visual blur and ghosting

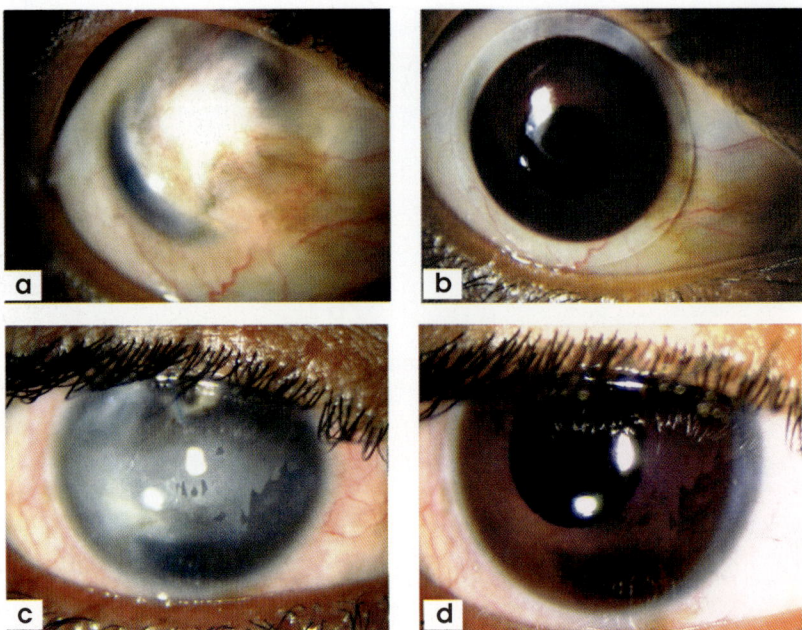

Fig. 16.6: Prosthetic contact lens, *pupil opaque* (pre-lens—a, c, post-lens—b, d). In situation (b) with band-shaped keratopathy (BSK), posterior lens surface may get abraded by the calcareous deposition, thus it is advisable do EDTA chelation of cornea prior to prescribing the lens

pupil opaque and pupil clear types of prosthetic contact lenses respectively used to conceal disfiguring scars and eyes.

ii. **Scleral (haptic) lenses** are used to conceal a disfigured eye and gross strabismus not amenable to surgery (Fig. 16.8). The lenses with opaque centers eliminate the visual image, provide acceptable cosmesis and relieve intractable diplopia.[5] For blind eyes with distorted/eccentric pupil or strabismus, eccentric positioning of artwork is required on the lens to impart a realistic look of orthophoria (Fig. 16.9). Such prosthetic lenses may be iris painted alone or have both iris and sclera images. The pupil may be opaque if used for cosmetic purposes and clear if used for optical purposes, e.g. in albinos. Such artwork is done by hand painting or photomechanical reproduction.

Since large diameter sclera/miniscleral lenses are by nature immobile, the tinted area remains appropriately positioned for distance and near viewing. Color matching is done by comparing with the contralateral eye in both photopic and mesopic lighting conditions.

Cosmetic shells differ from cosmetic CL in being thicker, larger and covering entire palpebral aperture and come in differing thickness. They are used to cover disfigured eyes and impart volume to atrophic/phthisical eyes. A microphthalmic eye may benefit cosmetically by fitting a scleral lens or a high plus soft lens with a standard cosmetic tint.

C. Therapeutic tints

   i. **In color vision defectives (CVD):** Appropriately tinted contact lens can enhance discrimination between confusing colors by inducing a brightness

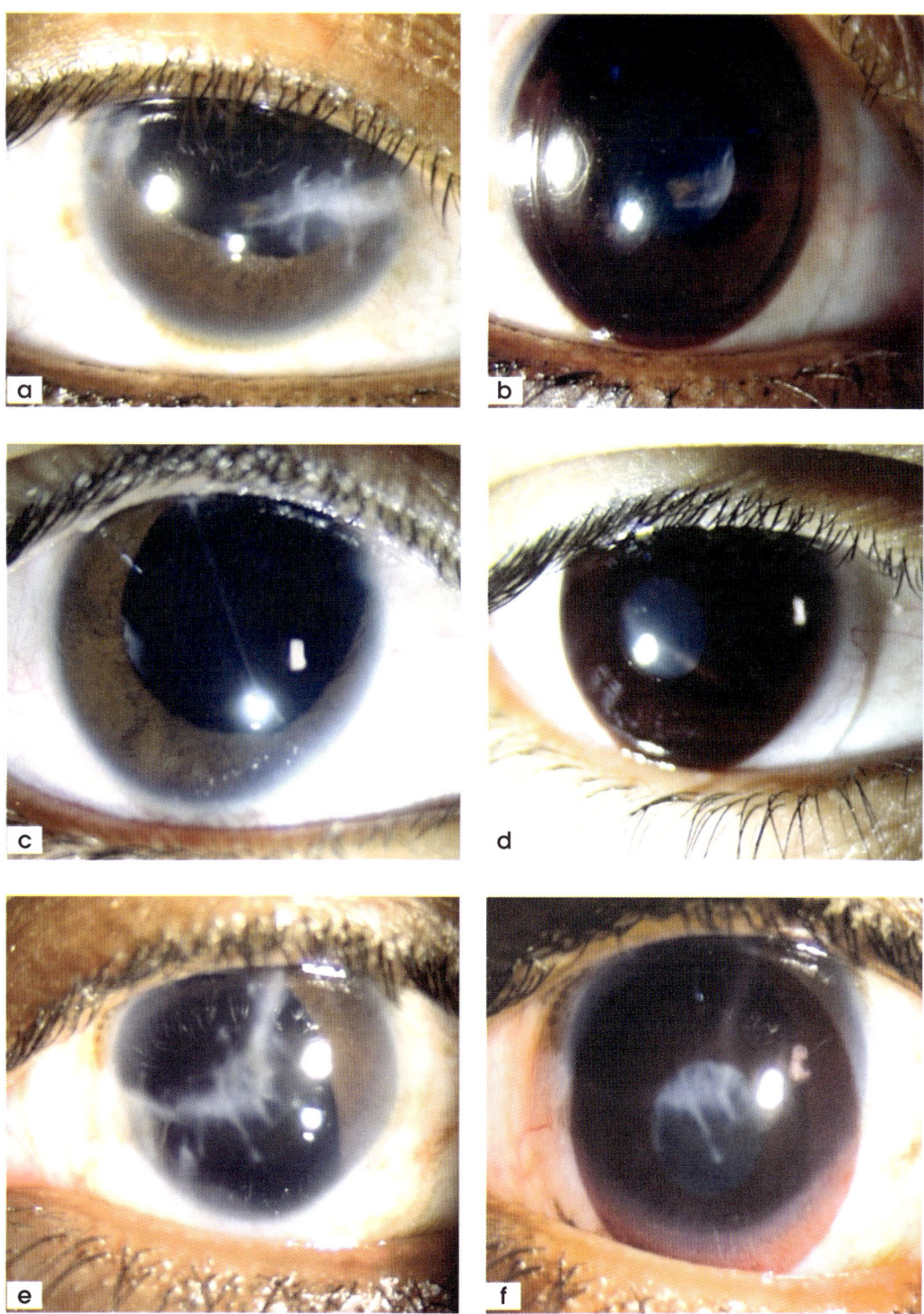

Fig. 16.7: Prosthetic contact lens, *Pupil clear* (pre-lens–a, c, e, post-lens–b, d, f)

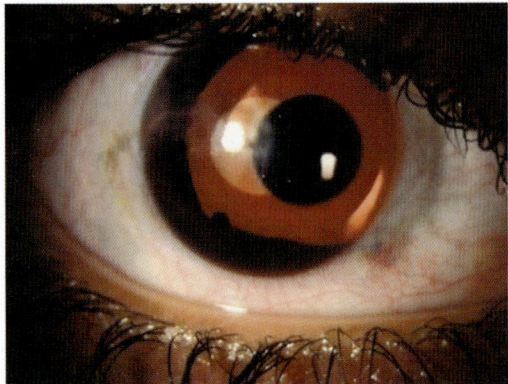

Fig. 16.8: Cosmetic lens over a patient with decentered prosthetic IOL with retinal detachment (blind eye)

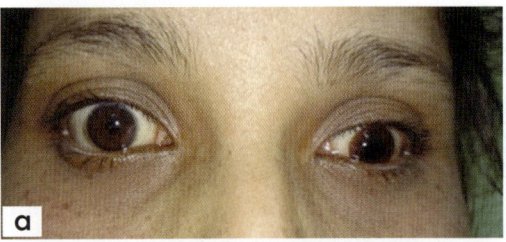

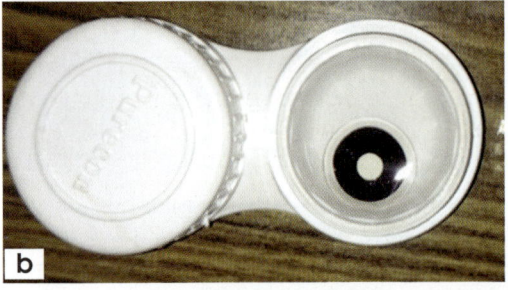

Fig. 16.9: Prosthetic lens inserted into left blind eye. Note that sensory exodeviation of LE becomes more evident once CL is on

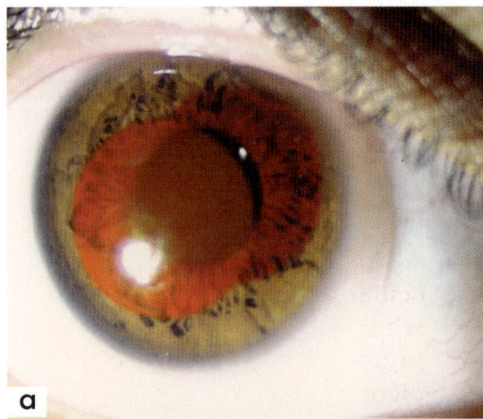

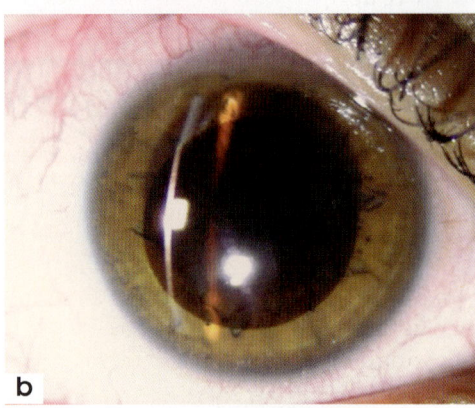

Fig. 16.10: X-chrom lens: (a) Red color vision defective; (b) For green color vision defect

difference between these colors. For example, X-chrom lens is a red or green tinted contact lens which aids in red-green deficiency, according to protanopia or deuteranopia element predominating (Fig. 16.10). Made of PMMA or hefilcon material, it is used in one eye of the patient. In conditions of gross color deficiency like achromatopsia, a red tint lens is able to improve the achromat's ability to discriminate objects by intensifying red-colored objects.[6–8]

The flip side of these lenses is blurred vision, reduced stereopsis and obvious cosmetic blemish.[6] It can also affect color perceptions detrimentally with increased reaction time seen with red green color deficient individuals wearing aqua, amber, blue and green transparent tinted lenses.[7] Use of these lenses may impair ability to detect red signals under challenging situations like mist or light rain and could be detrimental for commercial vehicle drivers or marine navigators. Unlike popular misconception, normal traffic light viewing is not so much a problem in CVD, due to standardized protocol of positioning red light always placed at top of a stop signal, so any light at top is equated with red color.

ii. **Albinism aniridia:** Albinism is an ocular or oculocutaneous condition where melanocytes of posterior pigmented iris epithelium lack pigment. This results in a translucent eye appearance with a red glow arising from light reflected off the retinal vessels. Transparent tinted lens or iris-occluding design with clear pupil are used for these patients so as to reduce entry of excessive light and decrease photophobia and glare. This enhances vision quality by allowing functional vision indoors and improved comfort outdoors.[9] In cases of iris coloboma, a tinted lens with clear pupil enhances quality of vision significantly only if the condition is not associated with retinal coloboma. Another therapeutic use of tinted lens is in conditions of aniridia especially post-trauma (Fig. 16.11). Often such patients are also aphakia and use of tinted, aphakia lens restores functional vision.

iii. **Amblyopia:** Occlusion therapy is the cornerstone of amblyopia. Often children resent and resist placement of occluding patch over their better seeing eye due to associated stigma or peer ridicule leading to depression and anger. Such children may benefit by use of opaque/dark contact lens in lieu of occlusion.[5] This method of occlusion is more difficult to dislodge accidentally or remove intentionally, thereby improving compliance. These lenses can also be employed in conditions of skin allergy/excessive sweating which can cause discontinuation of patching.

Another type of lens used as an alternative to occlusion is high plus power lens, which works as a *fogging device*. This method for "occlusion" uses *defocus* for its effect, while retaining light perception and some degree of peripheral vision.

Ultraviolet Absorption by Transparent Tints

Most lenses incorporate a UV blocker which blocks lower (violet) end of visible spectrum. However, this UV blocking is not completely effective and wearers need to be advised of the need for additional UV blocking sunglasses when exposed to conditions requiring

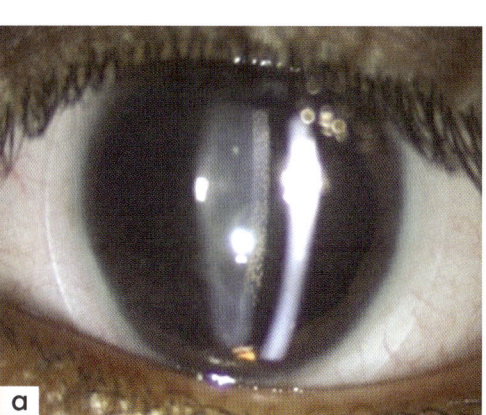
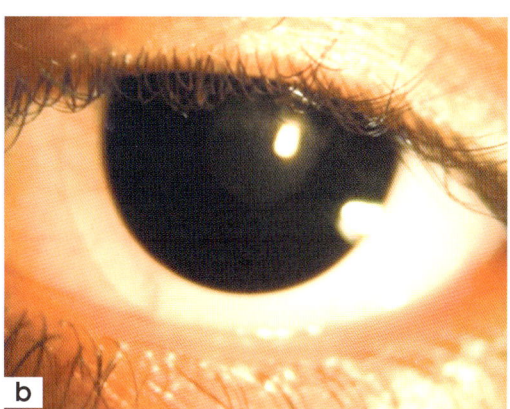

Fig. 16.11: (a) Traumatic aniridia; soft lens tinted; (b) Cosmetic pupil clear lens

ultraviolet protection, e.g. during mountaineering, skiing, yachting and river rafting.

Specific Issues During Prescription and Follow Up

a. **Visual performance with lens *in situ***: The visual performance with transparent tinted lenses should ensure no significant decreases in vision, contrast sensitivity, glare testing and color discrimination.[10] Tinted lenses with a luminous transmittance less than 85% should not be dispensed to patients who intend to use them at night.

Laminated full-coverage opaque tinted lenses are thicker than transparent lenses with resultant decreased oxygen transmissibility, which can cause corneal hypoxia.

b. **Loss of tint**: Leaching of tint occurs with use of chlorine-based cleaning systems, hydrogen peroxide, chlorinated swimming pools and eye drops containing organic peroxides.[11] Frequent replacement schedules are required to minimize this aspect.

c. **Deposits and crazing**: Tinted surfaces are more susceptible to scratching, spoilage, crazing and deposits necessitating frequent replacement schedules.

d. **Iatrogenic lens tinting**: This occurs due to inadvertent use of sodium fluorescein dye with hydrogel lenses *in situ*. Use of henna, hair dyes or use of Holi (festival of colors celebrated in India) colors while wearing hydrogels also causes permanent lens discoloration.

REFERENCES

1. Newcomer PC, Janoff LE. Methods of tinting Soflens contact lenses. Am J Optom Physiol Opt. 1977 Mar;54(3):160–4.

2. Welsh KW, Vaughan JA, Rasmussen PG. Aeromedical implications of the X-Chrom lens for improving color vision deficiencies. Aviat Space Environ Med. 1979 Mar;50(3):249–55.

3. Schlanger JL. The JLS lens: an aid for patients with color vision problems. Am J Optom Physiol Opt. 1985 Feb;62(2):149–51.

4. Lee DY, Jurkus JM, Sun Ma. Effect of the opaque, colored dot-matrix contact lens on visual field. International Contact Lens Clinic 1990: 17(7–8): 188–91.

5. Burger DS, London R. Soft opaque contact lenses in binocular vision problems. J Am Optom Assoc. 1993 Mar;64(3):176–80.

6. Hartenbaum NP, Stack CM. *Color vision deficiency and the X-Chrom lens.* Occup Health Safety. 1997: 66(9): 36–40.

7. Pun HW, Brown M and Lui R. Tinted contact lenses slow reaction time in color defective observers. Clinical and Experimental Optometry 1986; 69(6): 213–8.

8. Siegel IM. The X-Chrom lens. On seeing red. SurvOphthalmol. 1981 Mar-Apr;25(5):312–24.

9. Abadi RV, Papas E. *Visual performance with artificial iris lenses.* J Brit Cont Lens Assoc. 1987; 10: 10–5.

10. Hovis JK, Sirkka D. *Color discrimination of deutan and protan observers through tinted soft contact lenses.* IntCont Lens Clin. 1990;17(6): 287–95.

11. Janoff LE. *The effect of thirty cycles of hydrogen peroxide disinfection on Ciba Softcolor lenses.* IntCont Lens Clin. 1988; 15(5): 155–64.

Reader's Note

Reader's Note

CHAPTER 17

Orthokeratology

Orthokeratology (OK) is the name given to a technique of programmed application of specially designed contact lenses which reshape the cornea to temporarily reduce or modify myopia. Such a lens application causes a reversible, temporary refractive correction over a narrow range of refractive errors.

Historical Perspective

An observation in 1962 by George Jensen, that rigid PMMA lenses modify corneal shape and thus refractive status, was the genesis of orthokeratology. Initially programmed application of "conventional geometry' (back peripheral curves progressively flatter than central curve) contact lens was done to modify the prolate elliptical cornea to an oblate (flatter centrally) shape. A series of contact lenses were used to cause progressive flattening of cornea and on achieving target vision, a schedule of 'retainer' lens wear was initiated which maintained the visual gain. This retainer-lens usage was reduced by decreasing both duration and frequency of lens wear. These early lenses were conventionally flat-fitting, rigid lenses which induced significant with-the-rule corneal toricity subsequent to decentration, commonly occurring with the use of such lenses.[1,2]

The renaissance for orthokeratology (OK) occurred after two decades with the development of highly oxygen permeable lens material like Boston XO and modification in lens design from conventional to reverse geometry. This special design, *reverse-geometry* lens established orthokeratology as a safe, viable procedure in late 1980.[3–5] A *reverse geometry* design is flatter in center (to flatten corneal apex) and steeper in periphery (to aid lens centration). It is the reverse of a 'conventional' RGP lens design, where peripheral curves radii are *flatter* than BOZR. Over years this lens evolved to a three zone design with steeper peripheral curves for better lens centration along with minimization of unwanted induced irregular or with the rule astigmatism. The current lenses have 4–5 zones which enable them to offer a large treatment zone, thereby ensuring rapid effect with maximum change occurring over a single night wear.[6] This 'accelerated orthokeratology' design ensures full effect within a few days which is retained for minimum 6 hours to throughout the working day of "*no wear*" of lens.[7,8]

Indications of Orthokeratolgy

- Mild to moderate myopia (−1.00 D to −6.00 Ds): Use of OK lenses has resulted in 84–92% reductions in spherical equivalent of mild myopia.[9,10]
- Astigmatism: Use of OK lenses corrects up to −2.00 Dc with-the-rule corneal astigmatism or till −0.75 Dc against-the-rule astigmatism.
- LASIK patients with refractive surprise.

Contraindications

- Any active acute or chronic ocular disease including dry eyes, recurrent epithelial erosions.
- Irregular corneal shape, e.g. keratoconus.
- Factor limiting good lens centration, like ATR astigmatism, deep-set eyes, reduced lid tonus
- Pupil >4.0 mm in normal illumination or > 6.0 mm in low illumination. This is because large pupil size would causes flare during mesopic conditions, post OK lens use.
- Significant lenticular astigmatism
- Severe limbus-to-limbus corneal astigmatism
- High eccentricity

Principle and Design of the Lens

The reverse geometry OK lens designed with a flatter central base curve generates positive pressure on central cornea, achieving sphericalization of prolate cornea resulting in reduction of myopia. The principle is generation of high pressure points at central and peripheral zones of bearing and low pressure zones at areas with no direct lens bearing. The steeper secondary curves entrap an annular tear pool, which in turn generates negative pressure leading to mid-peripheral thickening (Figs 17.1 and 17.2).[6,11,12] Mucin component of tears helps secondary curves to trap an adequately thick tear film, by creating a seal under lens edge. Lid blinking generates positive pressure on this entrapped tear meniscus which hydraulically shears and redistributes epithelial cells tangentially from center to periphery.[4] The end result is thinning of central corneal epithelium accompanied by thickening of mid-peripheral stroma at edge of the flattened zone.[11] The amount of epithelial tissue displaced is calculated by *Munnerlyn's formula* which links corneal sagittal height to diameter of treatment zone and dioptric correction. A 20 μ reduction in corneal epithelial thickness (normal being

50–60 μm) has been documented over a 3-month period of OK lens wear.[8]

Factors Determining OK Effect

- Tear film : A minimum tear film thickness of 3–5 μ is essential for generated hydraulic forces to be effective.
- Corneal asphericity: Completely spherical corneas (e = 0) are not amenable to ortho-keratology.
- Corneal topography: Curvatures in range of 40.00 D (8.44 mm) to 45.50 D (7.42 mm) are best suited for OK effect.
- Treatment zone generated by steeper secondary curve: Smaller the spherical treatment zones higher is the correction. However, this is limited by pupil diameter, since treatment zones smaller than mesopic pupil diameter would give rise to visual blur, as mentioned previously in contraindications of OK use.
- Age: The OK response is faster and more predictable for younger people.[13]

The OK lens is made of a very high Dk material (> 85), e.g. Boston XO, which allows sufficient oxygen transmission during overnight lens wear and prevents corneal hypoxia. Refractive endpoint reached with seven to eight hours lens-wearing protocol, occurs within 7 to 10 nights.[6]

Different parts of this reverse geometry lens are shown in Fig. 17.1.

- *Central Back optic zone radius (BOZR):* Radius of curvature of this zone is calculated as flat K minus desired amount of correction, minus the compression factor of 0.75 D.

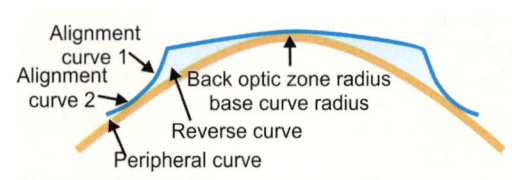

Fig. 17.1: Diagrammatic depiction of a five-curve reverse geometry lens

- *Reverse curve 2nd Curve*: This steep reverse curve aligns back surface of lens with cornea.
- *Alignment curve or 3rd and 4th Curve*: This 1.0 to 1.5 mm wide bearing zone is made flatter than reverse curve, thereby allowing close alignment to peripheral cornea. This curve helps in centering lens and enhancing the orthokeratology effect.
- *Peripheral curve.* This aids lens lift, ensures adequate tear exchange and helps in lens removal.

Fitting Technique

The algorithm of OK lens fit is given below:

1. **Evaluating corneal shape:** Corneal topography is performed to determine corneal size, flat-K value and eccentricity. Flat-K value determines central radius of curvature and corneal eccentricity determines radius of curvature for periphery (Table 17.1).

   - **Corneal Eccentricity "e"**, is defined as the rate at which cornea flattens from central to peripheral area. High "e" value implies rapid corneal flattening towards the periphery and "e" value of zero implies a spherical shape.[14] The OK effect is proportionate to "e" value with effect being higher in corneas with higher "e" values. This "e" value also determines adequacy of fitting of alignment curve, as it rests on corneal mid-periphery and subsequently dimensions of the OK trial lens.

Table 17.1: Eccentricity values in comparison to trial lens and power adjustment required

Eccentricity value	Trial lens BC
0.30 – 0.39	0.50–0.75 D steeper than flat K
0.40 – 0.45	0.00–0.25 D steeper than flat K
0.46 – 0.54	On flat K
0.55 – 0.60	0.25–0.50 D flatter than flat K
0.61 – 0.65	0.50–0.75 D flatter than flat K
0.66 – 0.70	0.75–1.00 D flatter than flat K

- **Corneal size (visible iris diameter)** determines part of cornea coming in contact with alignment curve. Normal corneal size of equal to or greater than 11.6 mm requires a 10.6 mm sized diagnostic OK lens.

2. **Trial lens calculation:** Trial lens is placed after application of a drop of lignocaine to minimize lacrimation and lid spasm. The initial lens is based on **adjusted flat K**. Adjusted flat k implies adjustment with eccentricity "e" as per table provided (Table 17.1). For eccentricity values ranging between 0.46 and 0.54, flat K value does not require any adjustment.

3. **Evaluate fit:**

   i. *Ensure centration*: After a few minutes of lens settling, fluorescein is instilled and centration is checked. Centration is critical to achieve desired ortho-k effect. Decentered lenses not only fail to produce desired myopia reduction, but also distort the cornea and cause visual blurring. A steep fit is diagnosed by a small central bearing zone usually accompanied by bubbles and a flat fit by a decentered lens, (usually superior), resulting in a larger central bearing area, not aligned on pupil.

   ii Static fit is then observed by evaluating fluorescein pattern (Fig. 17.2). An ideal fit pattern is a *bull's eye pattern*, with a 3.5–4.0 mm central zone of light touch under main bearing zone of lens. In this *touch* area, a thin viscous mucin layer is present between lens and epithelium. This central zone is surrounded by a wide midperipheral ring of fluorescein pooling, or 'tear reservoir', under steeper secondary curve and a peripheral circular band of alignment/touch tapering off to an 0.2 – 0.4 mm wide edge lift. A well-fitted lens must depict a movement of 1 mm with blinking.

4. **Assess immediate OK effect:** After one hour of lens wear under supervision, in office, lenses are removed and patient's

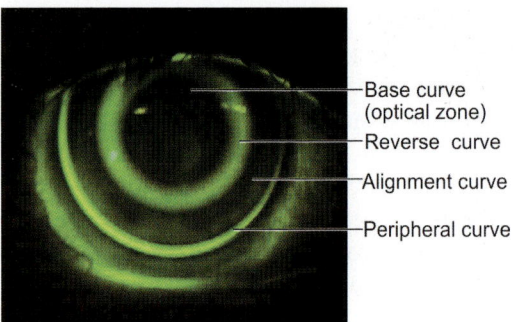

Base curve
(optical zone)

Reverse curve

Alignment curve

Peripheral curve

Fig. 17.2: Five curves, reverse geometry lens depicting ideal "bull's eye" fluorescein pattern

visual acuity checked. Due to accelerated OK effect, some amount of improvement in vision can always be elicited. If no improvement is seen, then fit requires re-evaluation. In case of reasonable visual improvement, lens with similar parameters is prescribed. This is called the *treatment lens*.

5. **Treatment phase:** Subsequently patient is advised to wear *treatment lens* every subsequent night for a fortnight, until desired end point of unaided 20/20 (Snellen 6/6) vision is attained. End point may also be defined as no further myopia reduction with stable unaided vision. This *marks the completion of treatment phase.*

6. **Maintenance phase:** The "treatment lens" is now used part-time (for minimum time)

to 'retain' the OK effect and is now called the *retainer lens.* After overnight use of *retainer lens* and subsequent removal, unaided vision should be maintained during the day at 20/20, with minimal diurnal fluctuation.

Wearers with minimal regression, can switch to alternate night *retainer lens* wear or even less frequently. For myopia of <4.0 D, alternate night wear to 2 days a week suffices. Delay in use of *retainer lenses* leads to corneal 'recovery' (regression/reversion of myopia).

7. **Failure end point:** If end point has not been reached by one week, a lens with a BOZR 0.2 mm flatter than original lens can be fitted and evaluated for any enhancement of effect on corneal shape. If this also does not achieve the desired refractive change, then it is assumed that orthokeratology is unlikely to be successful for this patient.

Topographical patterns achieved with ortho K effect are:

a. Bull's eye pattern: Implies optimum centration and optimum effect (Fig. 17.3a).
b. Central island appearance: Implies sub-optimal lens fitting (Fig. 17.3b).
c. Smiley face or frowny face appearance: Implies sub-optimal lens fitting (Fig. 17.3c and d).

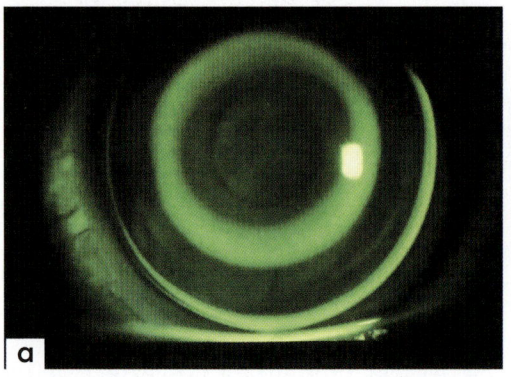

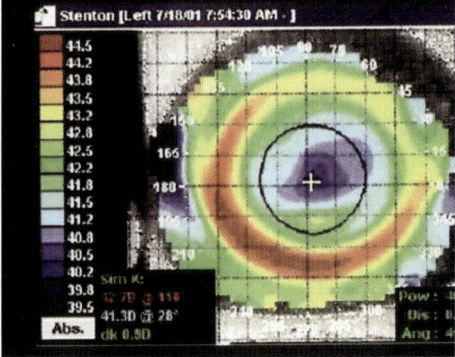

Fig. 17.3a: "Bull's eye" optimal fit and well centered OK lens. Subsequent topography also reveals a "bull's eye pattern"

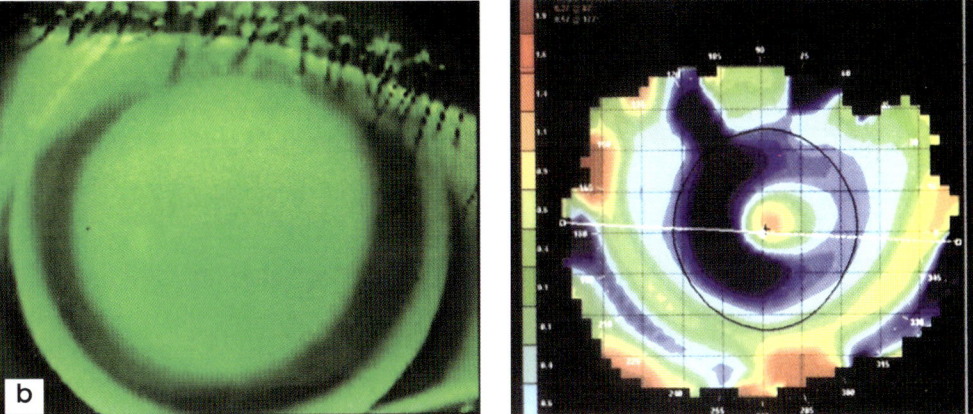

Fig. 17.3b: " Central island" pattern due to steep fit. Subsequent topography shows the central island

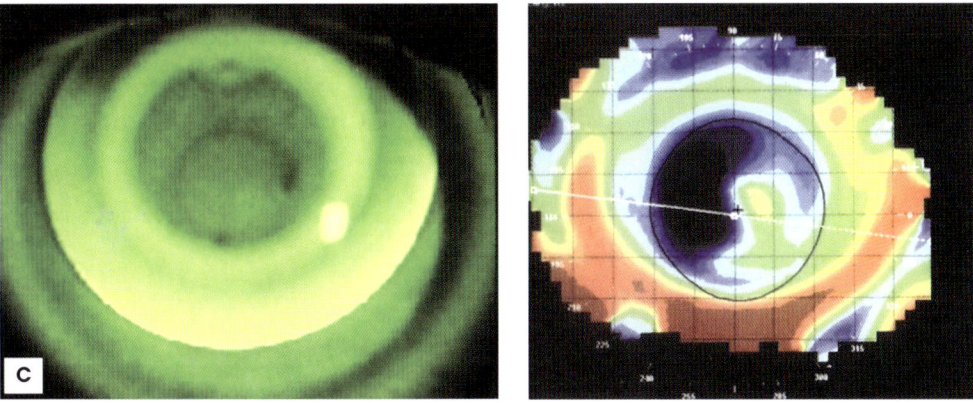

Fig. 17.3c: High positioning OK lens fit. Subsequent "smiley face" topography induced

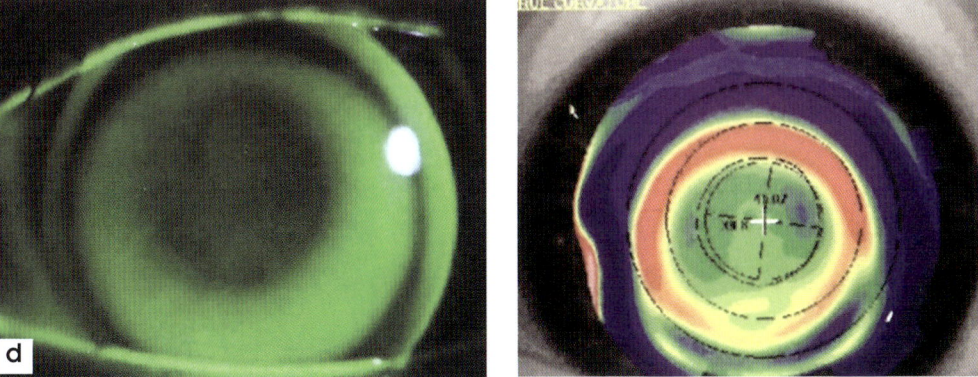

Fig. 17.3d: Frowny face appearance due to low positioning OK lens. Subsequent topography shows "frowny face" pattern. Figures reprinted with permission from Bausch & Lomb: *A guide to overnight orthokeratology*

The following figures depict certain illustrative examples of Ortho k fit:

A. *Good centration:* A well-centered lens exhibits quick lens movement of around 1 mm with a base curve zone touch of 4–6 mm. Both the reverse curve zone (green-colored ring) and alignment zone (black part) have equal widths. Figures 17.4 and 17.5 represent topography of a well-centered lens depicting central flattening followed by a mid-peripheral ring of steepening.

Continuous OK wear causes sequential central flattening or the OK effect (Figs 17.6 and 17.7).

B. *Poor centration (steep fit):* A steep lens moves less than 1 mm, often rides low, with a narrow (<4 mm) base curve zone touch. Under the reverse curve zone, a thick ring or air bubble is seen and alignment zone is broad. In this situation BC is altered till an ideal fit is demonstrated, as shown in Fig. 17.8.

C. *Poor centration (flat fit):* The movement of a flat fit lens is excessive, greater than 1.0 mm, the base curve zone is wide (>5 mm), reverse curve zone has an irregular width and alignment zone is narrow (Fig. 17.9).

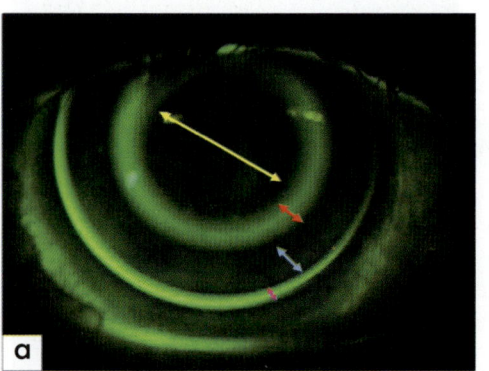 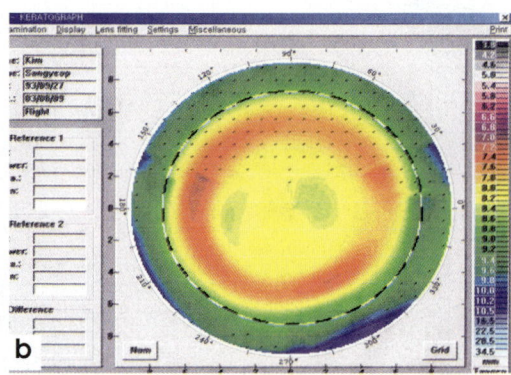

Fig. 17.4: (a) Yellow zone: Base curve zone touch; Orange zone: Reverse curve zone touch (tear reservoir): Green blue zone: Alignment zone; Pink arrow depicts peripheral curve; (b) Post OK fit. Topography depicting central flattening followed by a mid-peripheral ring of steepening

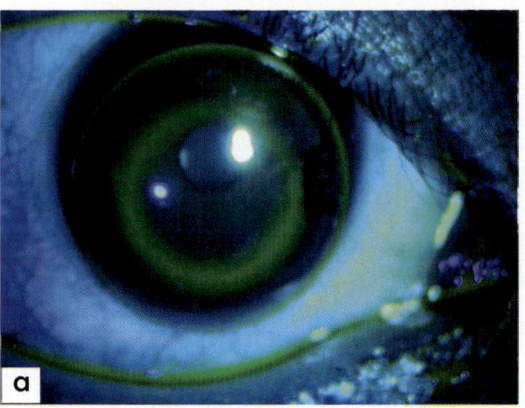 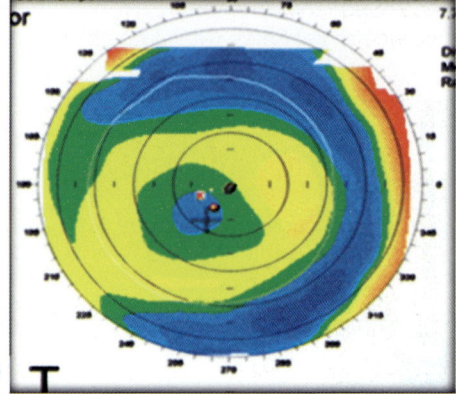

Fig. 17.5: (a) Post-fit topography in a good fit with bull's eye fluorescein pattern; (b) Topography confirmed central flattening is seen after use of this lens

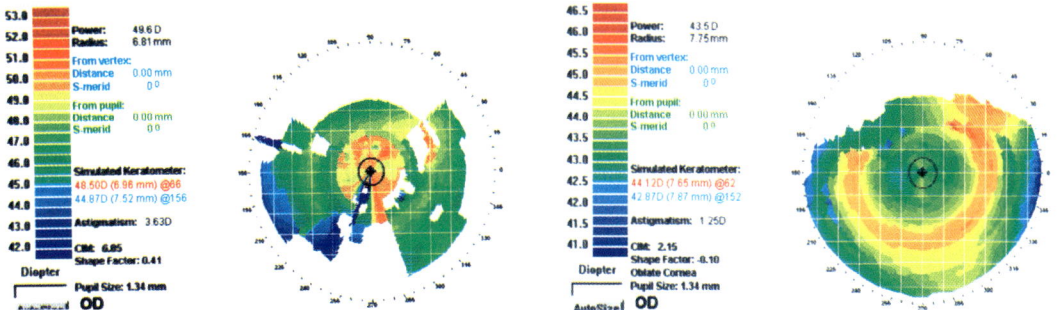

Fig. 17.6: Sequential corneal topography demonstrating OK effect of central flattening and mid-peripheral steepening

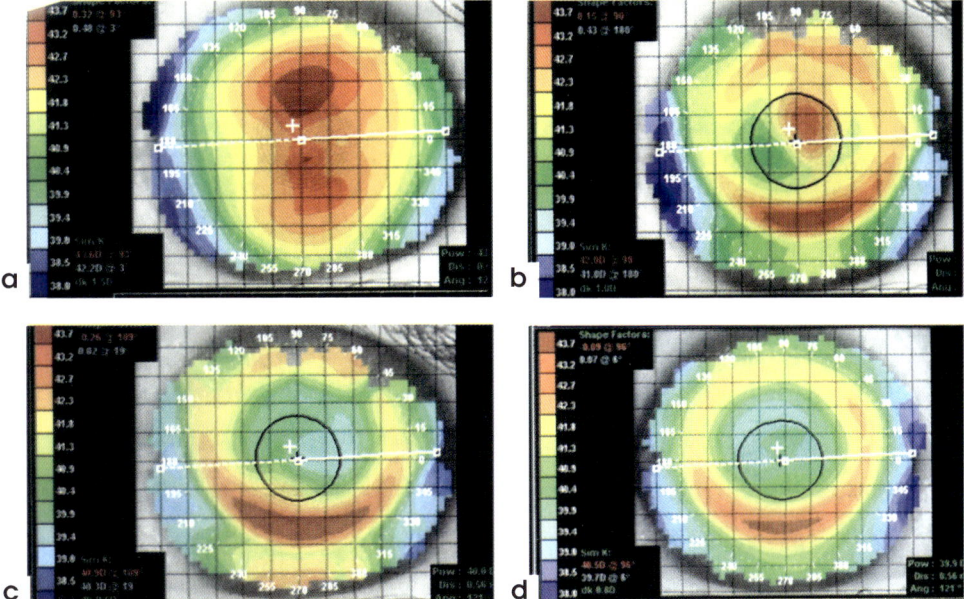

Fig. 17.7: Sequential topography alteration post OK lens use. (a) Pre-treatment (b) Day 1; (c) One week; (d) Two weeks (reprinted with permission from *A guide to overnight orthokeratology* by Bausch & Lomb)

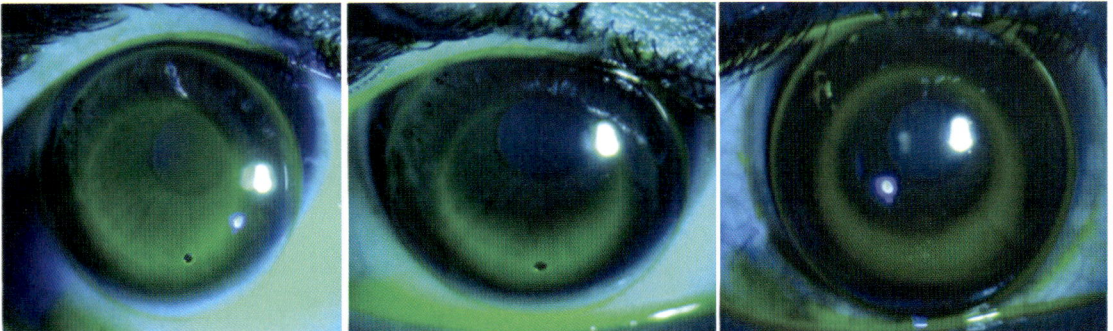

Fig. 17.8: Sequential fitting from steep fit to ideal fit during trial fitting of an OK patient

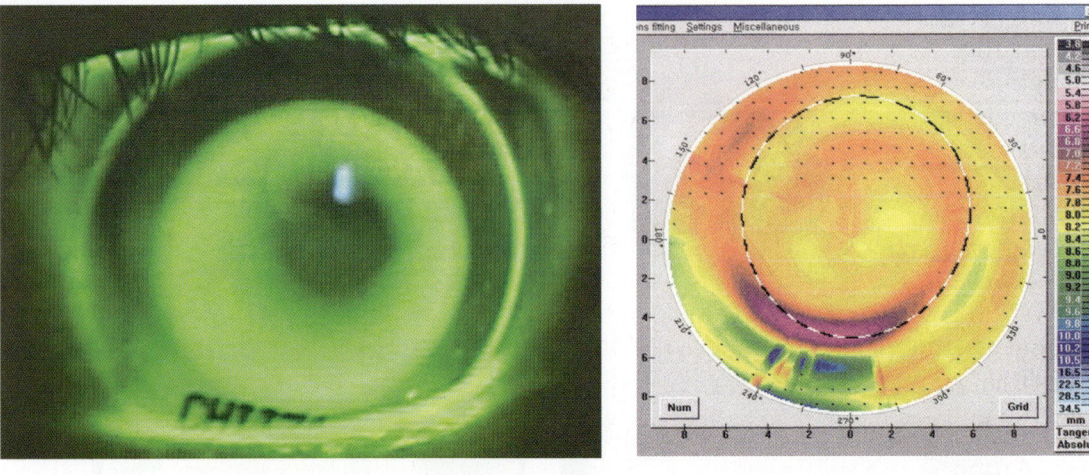

Fig. 17.9: Fluorescein pattern and topography in flat fit Ortho K lens

The following example highlights technique of fitting.

A 21-year-old female with –3.50 D myopia has keratometry values: (Rh): – 7.48 mm, (Rv): –7.61 mm, and eccentricity value of – 0.49. Since the "e" value falls within 0.46–0.54 range, there is no need to adjust for flat-K value (Table 17.1). The trial lens selected thus would be = 7.61 BC/–3.5 Ds/10.6 mm. After lens insertion fluorescein pattern is evaluated for lens centration, alignment, movement, tear meniscus size and shape. If lens adheres/or air bubbles are noted in reverse curve zone then central bearing needs to be changed and fit made steeper. *Ortho-K effect* is evaluated after removing lens, after 1 hour of wear.

Unaided visual acuity is checked, slit lamp examination is done for corneal staining and corneal topography may be performed. Subsequently over-refraction is done to determine final lens' target power. In this example, the patient's *visual* acuity changed from 0.08 to 1.0 (Snellen 6/6) after 2 hours of lens wear (Fig. 17.10).

Selection Criteria

The decision to proceed for OK and its success is highly influenced by selection criteria. The main criteria are enumerated below:

- Motivated patient. This is the pre-requisite as a motivated patient will comply with proper lens usage. However, the expecta-

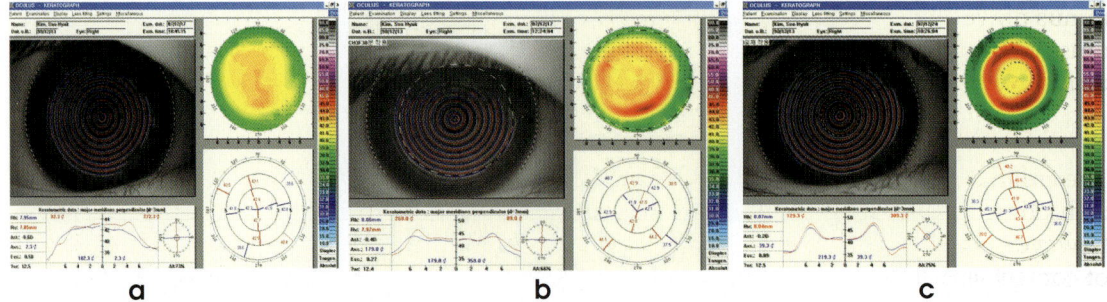

Fig. 17.10: Sequential topography changes in a patient with Ortho K lens wear; (a) Pre-fit; (b) Post 1 hour wear (c) Post 3 days of wear

tions of patient should be realistic regarding timeframe and amount of ametropia that can be corrected.

- Refractive errors greater than 5 D may not achieve full correction and patients must be made to realize that their unaided vision will not reach the ideal 6/6. However, most high myopes are happy to achieve functional vision, with the option of using low-powered spectacle prescription for optimal vision.
- Residual astigmatism may remain in cases with high astigmatism.

Effect Graph

Maximum effect occurs within first month of wear and gets reinforced over next 3 months. After 3 months of wear the effect stabilizes and OK effect lasts throughout the day with a few authors even documenting a reduction of effect by 0.50 to 0.75 D.[4] The completeness of effect varies with amount of myopia, with one week of wear sufficing for mild myopia.[8] After cessation of OK lens wear vision regression occurs rapidly within 2 weeks, however corneal topography takes longer (4–12 weeks), to return to baseline level.

Sometimes after long period of OK lens use, the effect wanes off due to progressive flattening of peripheral cornea. The explanation for this is that the initial flat, central cornea becomes relatively steep again which negates the OK effect. Another cause for waning of effect, is posterior corneal flattening which *decreases* contribution to minus power. Thus a check on posterior float must be kept during the follow up of OK lens usage.

Effect on Myopia Progression

The credo of OK lens is to cause a permanent reduction or arrest of myopia. Literature, however, is ambivalent on this beneficial effect of contact lens wear on arresting or retarding myopia progression. A few authors have documented stabilizing effect of conventional RGP lens wear in retarding progression of myopia.[12,16]

Since myopia progression after puberty is usually due to axial elongation, biometric measures of axial length are an effective way to assess effectivity/failure of OK lenses.[17] Such a stabilization of axial length has been effectively documented by LORIC (longitudinal orthokeratology research in children) study and ROMIO (retardation of myopia in orthokeratology) study on children wearing OK lenses versus spectacle wearing controls.[18,19] There is substantive evidence that orthokeratology is an option for slowing myopic progression but the multifactorial etiology of myopia makes predictability and validity of this technology still unpredictable.[18]

Complications

1. **Decentration of lens** during overnight wear: This is the commonest complication and direction in vertical or horizontal axis depends on amount of myopia, astigmatism and lens design. Decentration leads to a reduction in orthokeratology effect and can cause diplopia or glare problems.[20] This complication is more common with excessively tight or loose fitting lens wear. Corneal topography is used to diagnose the cause and specific patterns attained are:

   a. *Central steep island:* Indicates insufficient flat curve of the BOZR of the OK lens leading to suboptimal central compression of corneal epithelium (Fig. 17.3b).

   b. *Smile pattern*: The **smiley face** pattern occurs due to a superiorly decentered lens which creates a flat zone in superior cornea with a partially steeper zone inferiorly in a ring fashion (the smile) (Fig. 17.3c).

   c. *Frown pattern*: A **frown pattern** showing a relatively steeper zone superiorly with a flat zone inferiorly is a result of inferiorly decentered lens, too steep a lens or a lens with a small diameter.

d. *Ring Jam*: These are local topographical irregularities and present as crowding of rings, incomplete or irregular rings.

2. **Corneal staining:** This common side effect occurs in almost 50% cases and is caused by lens overwear, flat/decentered lens, entrapment of debris, lens deposits/scratches or lens adherence. Improper lens removal technique, pre-existing tear problems and inadequate lid closure during sleep also contribute to corneal staining. The intensity ranges from mild to severe, with the latter occasionally causing corneal pigmented arcs.[21] Mild staining can occur as part of adaptive response of cornea to overnight lens wear and requires no intervention. Incomplete inferior or mid-peripheral rings can occur within a few weeks of OK lens wear which progress to complete rings if undiagnosed and untreated. Ring location of staining coincides with margins of 'bull's eye' map and needs to be differentiated from thick mucus on epithelium, following removal of an adherent OK lens. Mucus build up would dilute over a few minutes post-lens removal and the epithelium normalize, whereas staining would persist.

Reverse geometry back surface design of an OK lens, encourages deposit build up and makes digital cleaning difficult. These deposits in turn cause epithelial staining. The remedy is to adopt more stringent cleaning techniques, like use of cotton buds soaked in cleaning solution, use of lubricants after lens insertion *in addition* to regular cleaning regimen.

3. **Vision problems:**
   - Size of OK treatment zone versus pupil diameter is crucial for adequate effect. A treatment zone smaller than pupil diameter would cause ghost images, flare and haloes, with these signs being more problematic in mesopic viewing.
   - Astigmatism : Both irregular astigmatism and WTR astigmatism can occur.[22]

- Increased higher-order wave-front aberrations like spherical aberration and decreased contrast sensitivity for high spatial frequencies are also seen after OK lens use, leading to reduction in quality of vision.[23,24] These aberrations are proportional to magnitude of myopic correction and are fully reversible after discontinuation of OK lens. A patient unable to adjust to these aberrations should be advised to abandon this technology.

4. **Lens adherence/binding:** This occurs due to thinning of post-lens aqueous tear film with an increase in its viscosity during the overnight wear. An overly 'aggressive' orthokeratology design or dry eyes is the usual reason. In case of adherent lens, wearer is instructed to use lubricants along with digital manipulation of lens edge through lower lid margin to allow tear entry. This is followed by continued gentle digital manipulation until lens movement is detected. Prophylaxis includes use of lubricants or fenestrations in lens at tear reservoir region.

Lens overwear can result in lens binding in addition to inducing hypermetropia. The latter can be corrected by reducing lens wear time and/or by slightly steepening the BC.

5. **Refractive regression following lens removal:** The amount of regression following lens removal has been documented to be less than 0.5 D over an 8-hour period and is usually seen after three months of OK wear.[4] Diagnosis of regression requires change in retainer lens or increase in wear time.

6. **Corneal oedema:** Design of an orthokeratology lens requires a thick lens which automatically reduces oxygen transmission (Dk/t) to the cornea. Despite the material being of very high Dk values, oxygen supply to cornea is sometimes inadequate and can result in stromal

oedema. To pick up evidence of edema, aftercare visits should be scheduled as early in morning after OK lens wear as possible.

7. **Microbial keratitis:** The incidence of microbial keratitis in OK wearers has been postulated to be 7.7 per 10,000 patient years which is equivalent to any extended lens wear schedule but much higher than daily rigid lens wear of 1.2 per 10, 000 wearers.[25-27] The keratitis is more often documented in children and organisms involved are often the aggressive ones like *Pseudomonas aeruginosa* or *Acanthamoeba.*[28-30]

Lens cases have been found to be major sources of contamination with lens hygiene being implicated as the cause. Compliance with lens case care instructions and/or regular replacement, hand hygiene, frequent case replacement, a strict **no to tap water** use, avoidance of eye rubbing while sleeping with OK lens are some beneficial strategies in preventing this serious vision threatening complication.[31]

REFERENCES

1. Kerns RL. Research in orthokeratology. Part VIII: results, conclusions and discussion of techniques. *J Am Optom Assoc* 1978;49:308–14.

2. Binder PS, May CH, Grant SC. An evaluation of orthokeratology. *Ophthalmology* 1980;87: 729–44.

3. Swarbrick HA, Alharbi A. Overnight orthokeratology induces central corneal epithelial thinning. *Invest OphthalmolVis Sci* 2001;42:S597

4. Mountford J. An analysis of the changes in corneal shape and refractive error induced by accelerated orthokeratology. *ICLC* 1997; 24:128–44.

5. Lui W-O, Edwards MH. Orthokeratology in low myopia. Part 1: efficacy and predictability. *Cont Lens Anterior Eye* 2000;23:77–89.

6. Swarbrick HA. Orthokeratology (corneal refractive therapy): what is it and how does it work? Eye Contact Lens. 2004; 30(4):181–5.

7. Rah MJ, Jackson JM, Jones LA, Marsden HJ, Bailey MD, Barr JT. Overnight orthokeratology: preliminary results of the Lenses and Overnight Orthokeratology (LOOK) study. Optom Vis Sci. 2002; 79(9):598–605.

8. Soni PS, Nguyen TT, Bonanno JA. Overnight orthokeratology: visual and corneal changes. Eye Contact Lens. 2003;29(3):137–45.

9. Cheung SW, Cho P, Chui WS, Woo GC. Refractive error and visual acuity changes in orthokeratology patients. Optom Vis Sci. 2007; 84(5):410–6.

10. Chan B, Cho P, Cheung SW. Orthokeratology practice in children in a university clinic in Hong Kong. Clin Exp Optom. 2008;91(5):453–60.

11. Alharbi A, Swarbrick HA. The effects of overnight orthokeratology lens wear on corneal thickness. Invest Ophthalmol Vis Sci. 2003 Jun;44(6):2518–23.

12. Walline JJ, Holden BA, Bullimore MA et al. The current state of corneal reshaping. Eye Contact Lens. 2005 Sep;31(5):209–14.

13. Jayakumar J, Swarbrick HA. The effect of age on short-term orthokeratology. Optom Vis Sci. 2005 Jun;82(6):505–11.

14. Joe JJ, Marsden HJ, Edrington TB. The relationship between corneal eccentricity and improvement in visual acuity with orthokeratology. J Am Optom Assoc. 1996 Feb; 67(2):87–97.

15. A guide to overnight Orthokeratology. Polymer technology. Bausch & Lomb, North America edition 2004.

16. Perrigin J, Perrigin D, Quintero S, Grosvenor T. Silicone-acrylate contact lenses for myopia control: 3-year results. Optom Vis Sci. 1990; 67(10): 764–9.

17. Walline JJ, Rah MJ, Jones LA. The Children's Overnight Orthokeratology Investigation (COOKI) pilot study. Optom Vis Sci. 2004 Jun; 81(6):407–13.

18. P. Cho, SW Cheung, and M Edwards. "The longitudinal orthokeratology research in children (LORIC) in Hong Kong: a pilot study on refractive changes and myopic control," *Current Eye Research*, 2005, 30(1):71–80.

19. Cho P, Cheung SW. Retardation of myopia in orthokeratology (ROMIO) study: a 2-year randomized clinical trial. Invest Ophthalmol Vis Sci 2012: 53: 7077–85.

20. Yang X, Zhong X, Gong X, Zeng J. Topographical evaluation of the decentration of orthokeratology lenses. Yan Ke Xue Bao. 2005 Sep; 21(3):132–5, 195.

21. Cho P, Chui WS, Cheung SW. *Reversibility of corneal pigmented arc associated with orthokeratology.* Optom Vis Sci. 2003; 80(12): 791 – 5.

22. Kohnen T. Overnight orthokeratology induces irregular corneal astigmatism. J Cataract Refract Surg. 2004 ;30(7):1389.

23. Hiraoka T, Okamoto C, Ishii Y, Okamoto F, Oshika T. Recovery of corneal irregular astigmatism, ocular higher-order aberrations, and contrast sensitivity after discontinuation of overnight orthokeratology. Br J Ophthalmol 2009;93(2):203–8.

24. Hiraoka T, Okamoto C, Ishii Y, Kakita T, Okamoto F, OshikaT. Time course of changes in ocular higher-order aberrations and contrast sensitivity after overnight orthokeratology.

25. Bullimore MA, Sinnott LT, Jones-Jordan LA. The risk of microbial keratitis with overnight corneal reshaping lenses. Optom Vis Sci. 2013; 90(9):937–44.

26. Watt KG, Swarbrick HA. Trends in microbial keratitis associated with orthokeratology. Eye Contact Lens. 2007; 33(6 Pt 2):373–7.

27. Stapleton F, Keay L, Edwards K, Naduvilath T, Dart K, Brian G, Holden BA. The incidence of contact lens-related microbial keratitis in Australia. Ophthalmology. 2008;115(10): 1655–62.

28. Swarbrick HA. Orthokeratology review and update. Clin Exp Optom. 2006 ;89(3):124–43

29. Van Meter WS, Musch DC, Jacobs DS, Kaufman SC, Reinhart WJ, Udell IJ. Safety of overnight orthokeratology for myopia: a report by the American Academy of Ophthalmology. Ophthalmology. 2008; 115(12):2301–13.

30. Shehadeh-Masha'our R, Segev F, Barequet IS, Ton Y, Garzozi HJ. Orthokeratology associated microbial keratitis. Eur J Ophthalmol. 2009;19(1):133–6.

31. Taun Tran, Chameen Samarawickrama, Constantinos Pestoglou, Stepahnie Watson. Recent cluster of childhood microbial keratitis due to orthokeratology. Clincal and Experimental Ophthalmol 2014, 42(8);793–4.

Invest Ophthalmol Vis Sci. 2008 Oct; 49(10):4314–20. Epub 2008 May 23.

Reader's Note

Reader's Note

CHAPTER 18

Dry Eyes Scenarios

DRY EYES

For optimal optics of a contact lens continual lubrication by healthy tear fluid is essential. The success of lens wear is dependent on tear flow and adequate moistening of the lens on the eye. There exists a reluctant yet delicate symbiosis between the foreign body in the eye read contact lens and natural warriors plus nourishers of eye read tear film. A well-fitted contact lens floats on a tear cushion and is enveloped with tears while on the eye. This tear film gets replenished with each blink, the act being proportional to lens mobility. Presence of this foreign element of lens impedes both cleansing action of tears in removing debris and nutritive action of supplying oxygen. Its adverse effect on blinking, tear spread combined with enhanced evaporation contributes to development dry eye syndrome (**DES**).[1-3] The altered tear film in turn initiates events which compromise quantity and quality of lens wear, partly due to altering the water content of soft hydrogels. This innocuous chain of events build up to dry eyes which is one of the commonest reasons for contact lens intolerance and its discontinuation. It is euphemistically known as CLIDES (contact lens induced dry eyes symptoms).[4]

Dry Eyes in Relation to Lens Type

Water content of a hydrogel lens is of extreme importance in determining its oxygen permeability with a linear equation existing between the two. A 100% water content lens has a Dk value of 80 barrers.[5] Higher water content lens also permits the lens to be made thinner and therefore more pliable, whereas low water content lenses are invariably thicker. Alteration of water content of a lens *in situ* on wearer's eye alter its mechanical and optical properties, the effect being more pronounced in high water content lenses. Such alteration of lens parameters affects lens fitting, optical performance and patient comfort. From these facts it is evident that adequate amount and function of tears is critical for good performance of a soft lens.

The story differs for a rigid lens whose optical and mechanical properties are relatively independent of tear content. Adequacy of tear film has a different role in RGP fit by permitting lens movement, preventing dry spots/deposits on lens surface, replenishing tear lens and providing stable vision.

Factors causing "on eye" drying of lenses and dry eye syndrome (DES):

- **Environment related:** Dryness due to alterations in temperature, humidity and wind speed.[6]
- **Patient related:** Older age and female gender is associated with increased incidence of dry eye. Women under influence of hormonal changes subsequent to pregnancy, oral contraceptives, menopauses

are more prone to develop dry eye. Blink efficiency and rate are the other patient related factors influencing DES.

– *Time related*: Over a period of time, lens wear causes a decrease in number of functional meibomian glands leading to intensification of DES.[7]

– *Tear related*: **Systemic diseases like** rheumatoid arthritis, diabetes, thyroid disorders or use of **systemic medications** like antihistamines, decongestants, antihypertensive drugs, antidepressants reduce tear production. **Ocular conditions** like chronic blepharitis, meibomianitis also contribute and need thorough treatment, before prescribing a contact lens.

• **Work related:** Inadequate tear resurfacing due to decreased blink efficiency/rate, increased lens wearing time, work profile requiring precise visual attention all adversely affect tear resurfacing. Reduced blinking is characteristic of people engaged in near or distance visual tasks requiring concentration. This in turn enhances tear evaporation by widening exposed ocular surface area.[8–10] Inadequate mucous and lipid distribution, as well as tear thinning overexposed lens surface further increases tear break-up and evaporation. This accelerated tear evaporation leads to increased tear osmolarity and gives rise to symptoms of discomfort.

The near tasks requiring concentration are often associated with work at computer terminals. In current times tasks performed on computers for long hours, in cramped, poorly ventilated environs exacerbate negative effect of reduced blink frequency. Re-circulating air from air conditioners often laden with cigarette smoke and stale breath is the genesis of the well recognized, *sick building syndrome*. In such a scenario contact lens hydration, more for soft and less for RGP lens, takes a beating.

• **Lens related:** High water content, thinner lenses and ionic hydrogel are more vulnerable to dehydration.[11] These lenses can exacerbate dry eye due to an effect known as *"Steal phenomenon"*. Higher water content lenses have a tendency to absorb fluid from its environment to maintain its hydration. This property causes such lenses to absorb fluid from tear fluid, thereby worsening the DES. In such a scenario changing the lens type to silicone hydrogels (hioxofilcon or omafilcon A) or using lower water content lens can help.[12,13] Remember lower water content lenses usually have lower oxygen transmission.

Poor lens cleaning or deposit on lenses cause inadequate tear resurfacing and exacerbate symptoms of dry eye. Prolonged wear of such deposit laden lenses induced lid changes like contact lens induced papillary conjunctivitis (CLPC), which in turn again initiates the dry eye cycle (Fig. 18.1).

Clinical Features

All soft lenses dehydrate to some extent when placed in the eye, the situation becomes pronounced in previous dry eye sufferers. Symptoms vary from foreign body sensation, itchy/red eye, ocular fatigue to blurred vision occurring after work involving intense concentration. Signs vary from dry looking lens surface, punctate corneal staining in lower quadrant of cornea—the so-called *Smile stain* (Fig. 18.2).

Diagnosis

The diagnosis of DES is based on clinical features and tear quantity measures by tests like inferior tear prism height, Schirmer test, tear break up time (BUT) and phenol red test. Blink frequency often gives a clue to the cause, with incomplete and/or frequent ineffective blinking being common in CL wearers.

Treatment

a. Blink efficiency: Improving blink efficiency with concomitant use of lubricant or

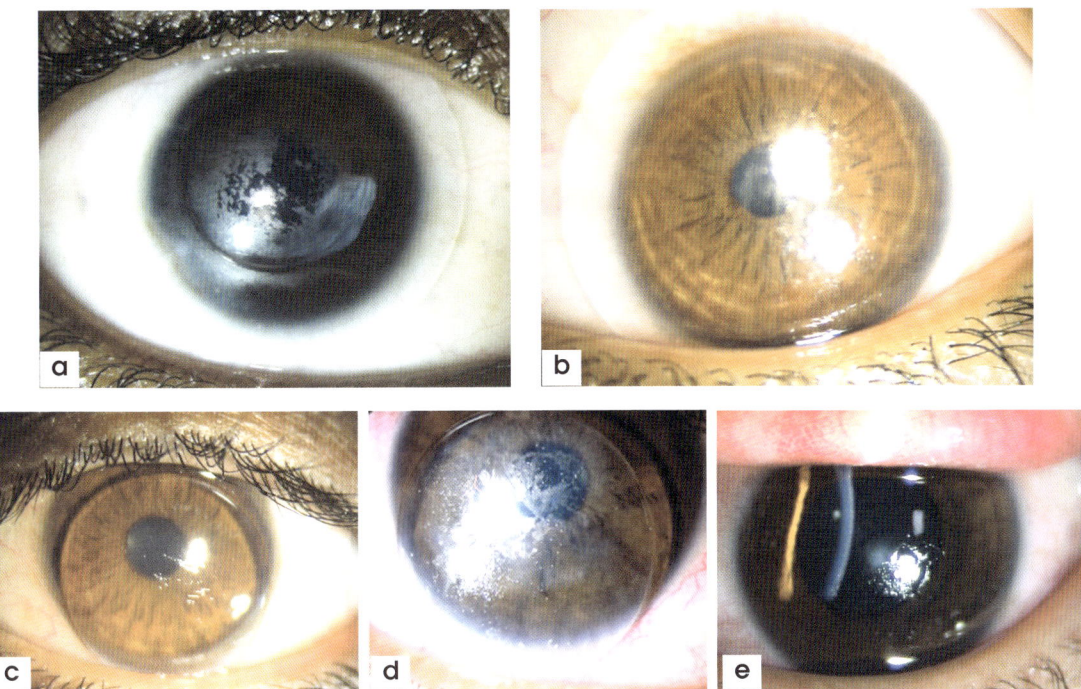

Fig. 18.1: (a to d) Deposit laden lenses in dry eye syndrome (DES) contribute to; (e) CLPC

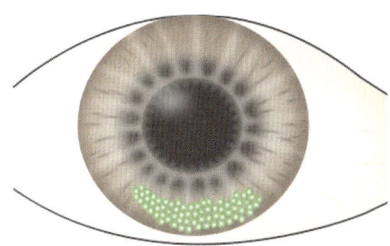

Fig. 18.2: Smile stain: Punctuate staining in inferior half of cornea due to excessive lens dehydration

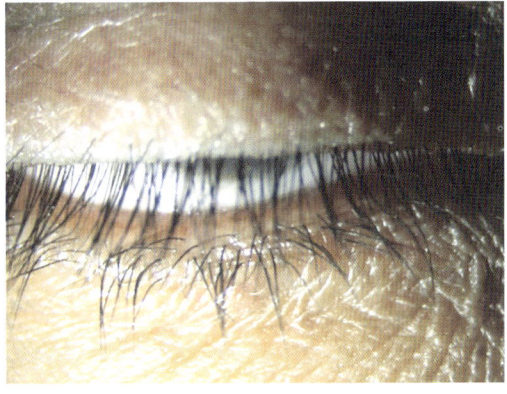

Fig. 18.3: Incomplete lid closure

rewetting drop instillation often suffices for mid to moderate dry eye patients. Complete blinking must be taught to patient and incomplete blinking discouraged. Since most people do not realize that they are blinking adequately, they must be made to practice proper blinking in front of mirror till they do it fully (Fig. 18.3).

b. Lens/solution related: Surfactant action in some cleaning solutions could cause dry eyes and altering cleaning solution alone

would solve the problem for such cases. Certain special hydrogel lenses purported to reduce symptoms of dry eyes are Proclear lenses (Cooper vision), Extreme H_2O (Hydrogel Vision) and Safigel lenses (incorporate hyaluronate polymer). These high water content lenses have properties of attracting and retaining their water content through entire wearing period, with manufactures claiming that by absorbing body heat, these lenses release tear wetting polymers.[14]

c. Treating the cause of dry eye, e.g. blepharitis, use of antihistaminics.

d. Environment modification: Air draught current from fans, air coolers and heat from room heaters increase tear evaporation and should be avoided. Use of humidifiers in workplace or at home environs may benefit dry eye due to these causes.

EXTENDED WEAR (EW) LENSES

It is the term used for overnight soft lenses wear and is approved by FDA from 7 to 30 nights. Advocated by de Carle in 1970, these lenses were initially only approved for therapeutic uses and in aphakia.

The types of extended wear lenses as elaborated by Donshik PC et al are:

a. High water content: These lenses with a water content of 70–80%, have high oxygen transmissibility. These lenses are, however, more fragile in addition to being deposit prone.

b. Low water content: With water content of 38–45% water, these lenses are very thin and cause handling difficulties.

c. Medium water content: These lenses have water content of 48–69%.[15]

Complications Seen with Extended Wear

• Corneal infections: Hypoxia induced by EW lens increases corneal binding of bacteria and alters microbial flora with an increase in gram-negative organisms being documented. This has been known to increase risk of microbial keratitis by 5 times, especially for *P. aeruginosa*, since EW wear reduces IgA specific for *Pseudomonas aeruginosa* alongwith decreased inflammatory mediators like interleukin 8 and 12 HET.[15]

• Discomfort, dry and red eyes

• Noninfectious complications: CLARE (contact lens induced acute red eye), GPC, peripheral corneal infiltrates, SEAL (superior epithelial arcuate lesions) (Fig. 18.4).

Risk of complications led to the approval for extended wear to be reduced from 30 days to 7 days of continuous wear. The fear of infections also became the incentive for introduction of disposable lenses and frequently replaced lenses.

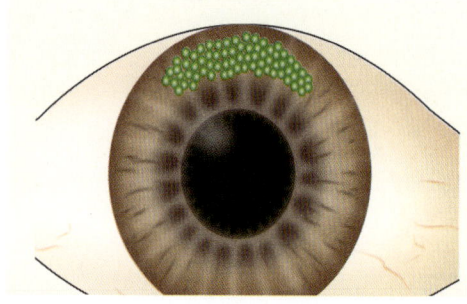

Fig. 18.4: Superior epithelial arcuate lesions (SEAL) due to inadequate tear resurfacing

REFERENCES

1. Chuprov AD, Kudriavtseva IuV, Zhukovskaia IN. The clinical and functional characteristics of the course of the dry eye syndrome associated with soft contact lens wear. Vestn Oftalmol. 2010 May–Jun;126(3):31–4.

2. Guillon M, Maissa C. Contact lens wear affects tear film evaporation. Eye Contact Lens. 2008 Nov;34 (6):326–30.

3. McMonnies CW. Incomplete blinking: exposure keratopathy, lid wiper epitheliopathy, dry eye, refractive surgery, and dry contact lenses. Cont Lens Anterior Eye. 2007 Mar;30(1):37–51. Epub 2007.

4. Richdale K, Sinnott LT, Skadahl E, Nichols JJ. Frequency of and factors associated with contact lens dissatisfaction and discontinuation. Cornea. 2007 Feb;26(2):168–74.

5. Jones L, Kathy Dumbleton K. Contact lens fitting today Silicone hydrogels Part 1: Technological developments Optometry Today 2005 Nov; 23–9.

6. Wolkoff P, Nøjgaard JK, Troiano P, Piccoli B. Eye complaints in the office environment: precorneal tear film integrity influenced by eye blinking efficiency. Occup Environ Med. 2005 Jan;62(1):4–12.

7. Arita R, Itoh K, Inoue K, Kuchiba A, Yamaguchi T, Amano S. Contact lens wear is associated with decrease of meibomian glands. Ophthalmology. 2009 Mar;116(3):379–84. Epub 2009 Jan 22.

8. González–Méijome JM, Parafita MA, Yebra-Pimentel E, Almeida JB. Symptoms in a population of contact lens and noncontact lens wearers under different environmental conditions. Optom Vis Sci. 2007 Apr;84(4):296–302.

9. Toda I, Yoshida A, Sakai C, Hori-Komai Y, Tsubota K. Visual performance after reduced blinking in eyes with soft contact lenses or after LASIK. J Refract Surg. 2009 Jan;25(1):69–73.

10. Chalmers RL, Hunt C, Hickson-Curran S, Young G. Struggle with hydrogel CL wear increases with age in young adults. Cont Lens Anterior Eye. 2009 Jun;32(3):113–9. Epub 2009 Feb 7.

11. Ramamoorthy P, Sinnott LT, Nichols JJ. Contact lens material characteristics associated with hydrogel lens dehydration Ophthalmic Physiol Opt. 2010 Mar;30 (2):160–6.

12. Schafer J, Mitchell GL, Chalmers RL, Long B, Dillehay S, Barr J, Bergenske P, Donshik P, Secor G, Yoakum J. The stability of dryness symptoms after refitting with silicone hydrogel contact lenses over 3 years. Eye Contact Lens. 2007 Sep;33(5):247–52.

13. Riley C, Chalmers RL, Pence N. The impact of lens choice in the relief of contact lens related symptoms and ocular surface findings. Cont Lens Anterior Eye. 2005 Mar;28(1):13–9. Epub 2004 Nov, 13.

14. Vyes J, Meyler J, Davies I. Assessment of the tear film. In : A practical guide : Essential contact lens practice. 2008. Johnson & Johnson Med Ltd. Mumbai, 37–48.

15. Donshik PC. Extended wear contact lenses. In Ophthalmology Clinics of North America Contact Lenses 16(3) : 2003, 305–9.

Reader's Note

Complications and Care

Reader's Note

CHAPTER 19

Complications Seen in Contact Lens Practice

The optical, occupational, sporting and cosmetic advantages of contact lenses make them a favored option for refractive correction with estimated global prevalence of 125–140 million contact lens wearers.[1,2] Given this large population of contact lenses wearers, even complications with a low incidence affect a significant number of individuals. In addition, the value of worldwide contact lens market at $7 billion plus puts a question mark on the reliability and veracity of manufacturers in reporting any adverse complications.[3] Therefore, it is mandatory on part of the lens fitter to be aware of epidemiology of lens related disease with reference to lens types and wearing patterns, common complications accruing out of lens wear and their contributory factors so as to make an informed choice for lens modality, wear schedule and hygiene regimes to be prescribed.[2] Out of global estimates of 125–140 million lens wearers, complications related to lens wear range from 6 to 50%.[4,5] These vary from mild discomfort and dry eye to serious vision threatening keratitis, the latter accounting for 1 out of every 500 lens users per year.[6] Complications depend on type of lens, prior ocular co-morbidity, socioeconomic and educational status of patient. In the former category it is rigid gas permeable (RGP) lenses and daily disposable hydrogels which account for the least complications.[5,7]

Complications with lens wear can be divided into those inherent with lens use, those occurring subsequent to poor fit and poor maintenance and those which are primarily accidental. Since second category is most commonly seen and is also preventive, remedial measures for complications are eminently feasible.

Inherent reasons for contact lens complications are:

- Contact lenses compromise normal cleansing action of ocular surface by inhibiting and altering tear film flow.
- The lens being a foreign element in close proximity to ocular surface is a source of micro-organisms especially in cases with poor hygiene.
- Mechanical abrading effects of lens moving on epithelium further compromise effectivity of epithelium as a barrier.
- Contact lens shape changes due to ocular surface interaction occur on a temporary (flexure) or permanent basis (warpage).

For sake of understanding we could divide complications occurring due to CL in the following categories.

I. Ocular Discomfort

The commonest complication reported by patients is **ocular discomfort.** This may translate into reduced wearing time to cessation of lens wear, with symptoms varying from grittiness to burning sensation, hot scratchy eyes, puffy lids, watering and sore eyes. A thorough history including type of discomfort, laterality of discomfort and diurnal variation if any gives a clue to the etiology. The common complaints and causes are depicted in Table 19.1.

Table 19.1: Contact lens induced ocular discomfort: Manifestations and management			
Type of discomfort	*Probable cause*	*Laterality*	*Treatment*
Gritty	Foreign body/chipped lens Fig. 19.1a	Unilateral	Change lens/remove FB and disinfect lens
Itching	Inflammatory response, e.g. GPC/CLPC	Bilateral, may be asymmetric	Discontinue CL/substitute with disposable or RGP/use anti-inflammatory drugs and lubricants
Sore/tired eyes	Convergence issues in those switching to CL after spectacle wear, altered refractive status	Bilateral	Self limited if convergence issues/recheck refraction, if persists
Dry/burning eyes	Lens deposits/dry eyes Fig. 19.1b	Unilateral/ bilateral	Clean, change lens, lubricants, blinking exercises
Puffy red eyes	Overwear/early infection	Unilateral/ bilateral	Refit with high DK lenses, lens discontinuation along with antibiotic use in case of infection

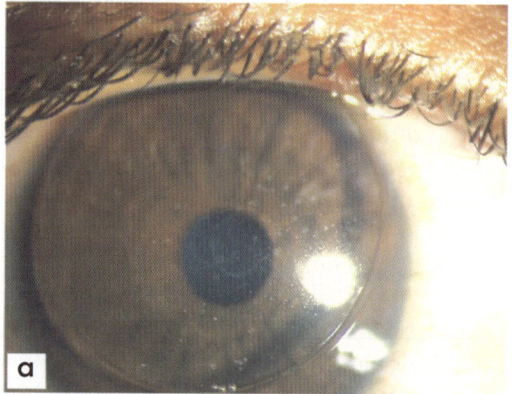 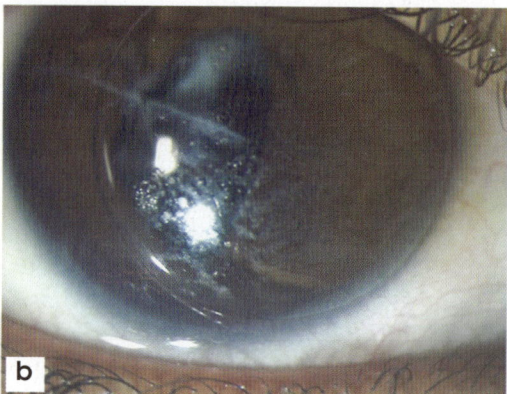

Fig. 19.1: (a) Shows zigzag track marks left by a foreign body trapped under lens; (b) Dirty lens with deposits and scratches

II. Effects due to Inadequate Blinking
Dryness

This is the most common complaint of CL users especially at end of a working day. Tear insufficiency due to reduced blink rate and/or poor tear film quality due to presence of 'on eye' lens is the usual reason. A dry looking lens coupled with poor break up time points to the diagnosis. Incomplete or reduced blinking is more common with those working on computers and living in dry or air conditioned environs. Reduced tear exchange as a consequence of incomplete blinking, causes uneven tear distribution and *3 and 9 o'clock* staining. Corneal signs range from punctate staining, epithelial erosions, dellen formation and neovascularization. *Dellen* is a localized depression in limbal cornea due to localized dryness as a result of poor tear resurfacing. The ensuing loss of corneal hydration causes compaction of corneal lamellae, which manifests as a depression on peripheral cornea with intact epithelium (dellen) (Fig. 19.2).

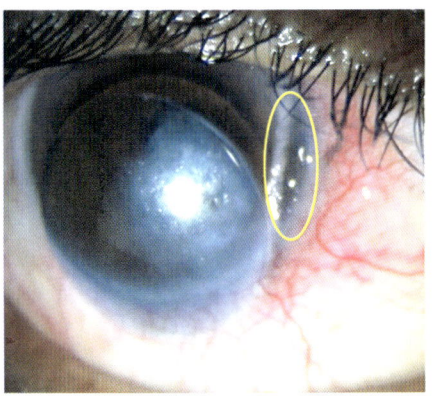

Fig. 19.2: Dellen at 3–4 o'clock meridian at limbal area due to poor lens fit

Lens deposits are a common association, with them being both the cause and effect of inadequate blinking. These are also a result of poor cleaning practices and/or disturbed tear film or lid resurfacing. Figure 19.3 depicts some different types of lens deposits.

Treatment involves use of preservative free lubricant, refitting with a lower water content lens in case of dry eye (to prevent steal phenomenon) or switching to disposable lenses. Lens cleaning/replacement depending on extent of deposits and reducing wear time are other options. Blinking exercises need to be taught where wearer is asked to practice frequent blinking of more than 10 blinks/minute. In addition, complete blinking must be taught (Fig. 19.4).

- **Tight lens syndrome/lens adhesion:** Lens adhesion occurs due to inadequate wetting of cornea. For hydrogels excessive evaporation or lens overwear, causing fluid loss leading to lens desiccation is the usual

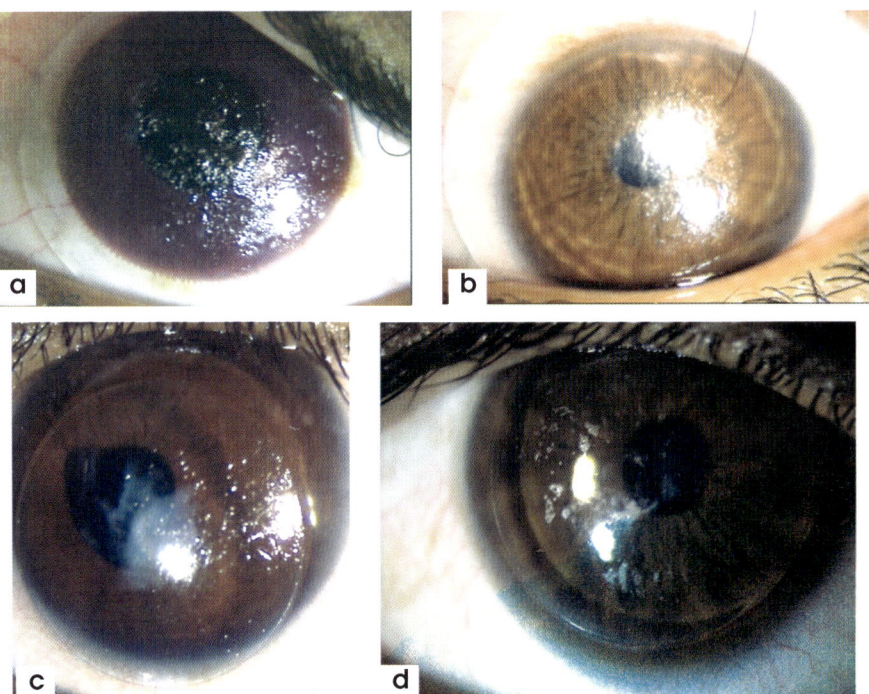

Fig. 19.3: (a) Cosmetic lens with mulberry deposits; (b) Soft lens with filamentous deposits; (c) RGP lens with lipid deposits; (d) RGP lens with calcareous deposits

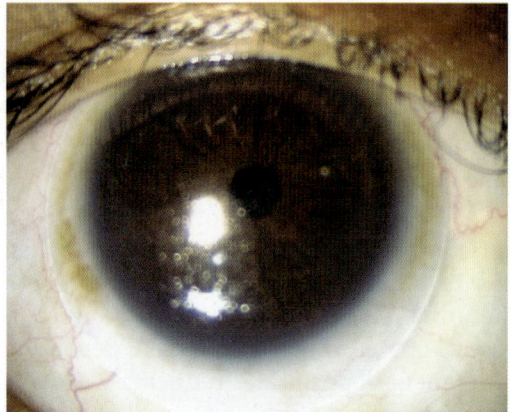

Fig. 19.4: Dry lens. Patient requires to do blinking exercises and put lubricants

sequence. This drying causes steepening of base curve, subsequent tightening and adhesion of lens on cornea. The usual causes for soft lenses are overwear, sleeping or swimming with lens on and for RGP lenses it is usually poor fit. The end point is thinning of tear film, creation of mucinous tear film without adequate aqueous moiety leading to sticking of lens. This causes lens to get *"glued on"* the corneal surface, in an eccentric position. The binding force of *stuck on* lens creates a compression ring, which persists for a few hours post lens removal (Fig. 19.5).

The patient of tight lens syndrome presents with symptoms of photophobia, blurred vision and discomfort occurring within a few hours of lens fit. Circumcorneal congestion, arcuate corneal staining in peripheral cornea, minimal lens movements, epithelial infiltrates, and kinking of blood vessels under lens edge is evident. Rarely anterior chamber inflammatory reaction may be seen in severe cases. Treatment includes wetting of the tight lens with copious instillation of lubricant drops followed by gentle lens removal. Subsequently lens wear is discontinued, cycloplegic antibiotic combination prescribed and patient refitted with a higher Dk, flatter lens with adequate peripheral clearance. These aspects must be again verified *after a few weeks of lens* wear, since parameters often change after initial wear.

III. Adverse Effects due to Corneal Hypoxia

These can present as acute hypoxia or chronic hypoxia.

a. *Acute hypoxia* occurs due to lens overwear or tight lens syndrome and is typified by pain, lacrimation, blurred vision, photophobia leading to lens intolerance. Patient

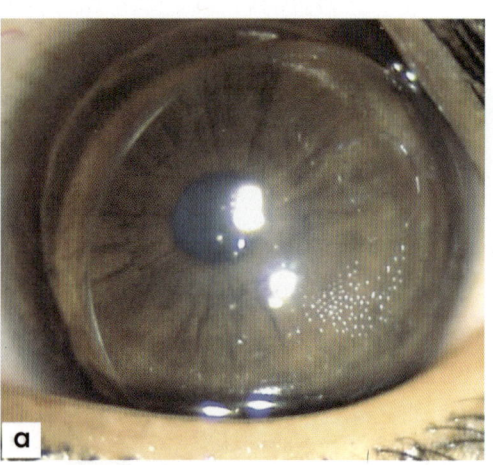

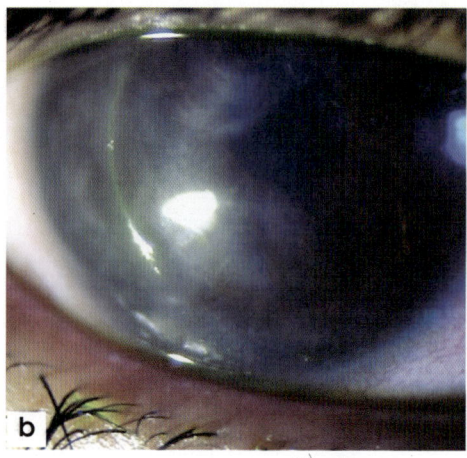

Fig. 19.5: (a) Tight lens with dimple veiling; (b) Fluorescein pattern after removal of a glued on CL, depicting compression ring visible from 7 o'clock to 10 o'clock position

presents with ciliary congestion, diffuse epithelial staining and blurred vision similar to a *tight lens syndrome* (Fig. 19.6).

b. ***Chronic hypoxia*** can manifest in the following ways:

- *Corneal folds/striae:* Folds occur due to buckling of Descemet's membrane and/or corneal endothelium. They are seen once corneal edema exceeds 8%, with lesser amounts of edema manifesting as *corneal striae*. The advent of more oxygen permeable materials has made these complications infrequent in current times.

- *Microcystic epithelial edema/Sattler's veil:* Intercellular fluid accumulations in corneal epithelium occur after exposure to reflex tearing or hypertonic lens solution. Asymptomatic small irregular inclusions (microcysts) in basal layers of epithelium occur after a lag period of 1–3 months of CL wear (Fig. 19.7). Rarely these microcysts break through anterior corneal surface and can be stained. Best diagnosed on *retroillumination* or *sclerotic scatter,* microcystic epithelial oedema causes blurred vision and colored halos. Gradual increase of lens wearing time over first few weeks allows adequate adaptation time to cornea and avoids this complication.

- *Stromal edema*: Seen with extended wear lenses, daily lens overwear and after periods of extended lid closure, this edema is a result of hypertonic tear film (Fig. 19.8). Another cause is depletion of stromal keratocytes, stromal thinning and corneal exhaustion consequent to chronic lens wear.[8] Daily wear lenses cause stromal oedema of 2–7% only.

- *Endothelium:* Acidic milieu and hypoxia induced hypercapnia causes initial transient blebs in corneal endothelium which become visible as black holes.

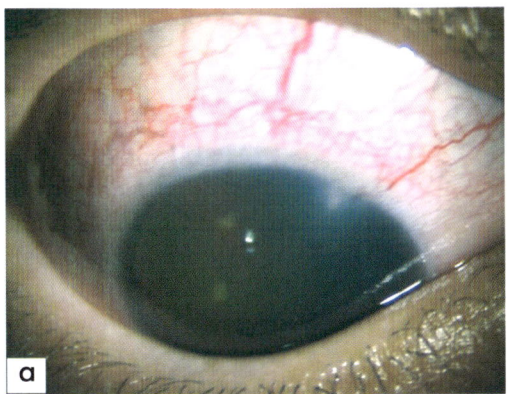

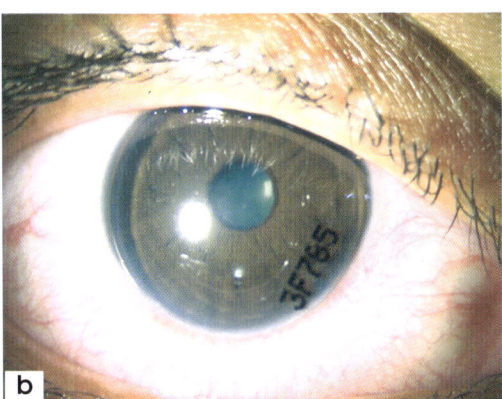

Fig. 19.6: (a) Lens overwear with dimple veiling, seen after lens has been removed. Note steamy cornea and circumcorneal congestion; (b) Mild congestion seen after a few hours of steep lens wear

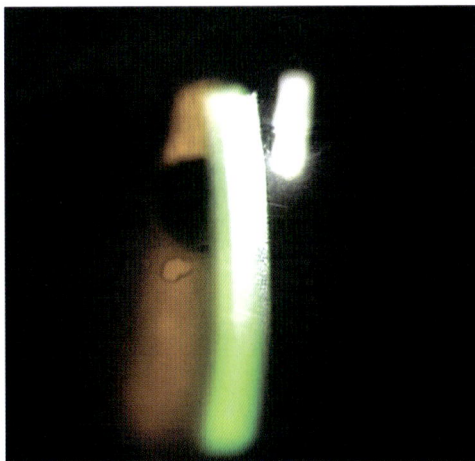

Fig. 19.7: Epithelial edema visible after lens removal. Note epithelial microcyst at central part of cornea at 8.30 clock position

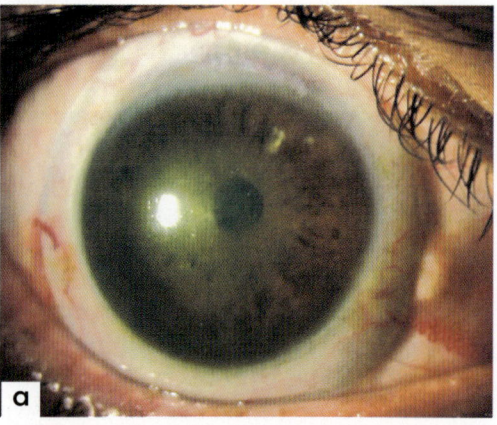
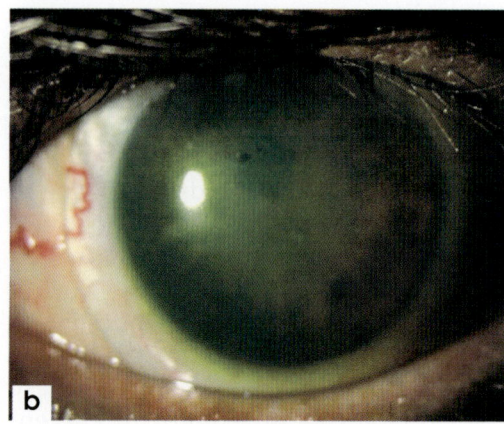

Fig. 19.8: (a) Lens overwear, depicting digging in lens edge from 1 o'clock to 6 o'clock; (b) Lens overwear showing epithelial and stromal edema under soft lens *in situ*

This phenomenon occurs in un-adapted wearers and diminishes in intensity with time. A self-limiting phenomenon, it requires no treatment but in cases with intense bleb activity, a refit with higher Dk lens is advisable.

Chronic endothelial stress manifests with polymegathism (increase in endothelial cell size). This may be partly genetic as a more intense response has been noted by some researchers in Asian races.[9]

- *Neovascularization at limbus*: Superficial and deep neovascularisation at limbus mimicking a pannus can occur in chronic hypoxia. Deep vascularisation and/or vessels extending beyond 2 mm are an indication to refit with a higher Dk lens.

- Myopic creep: This reversible, obsolete complication was documented as a refractive change with a 0.5 D increase of myopia.

Treatment for all these manifestations involve discontinuation of lens, use of lubricants and low dose steroid antibiotic combination followed by fitting with flatter and/or higher Dk lens.

IV. Mechanical Adverse Effects

- **Corneal abrasion:** Corneal abrasion is a discontinuity of corneal epithelium involving superficial cells or full thickness epithelial layer. It can occur due to lens imperfections, foreign bodies/dust entrapped beneath the lens and clumsy insertion/removal technique (Fig. 19.9). Even a well-fitted lens induces sufficient hypoxia to make corneal epithelium more fragile and vulnerable to damage.

An abrasion results in a painful, watering eye, blurred vision with intolerance to lens wear. Treatment involves removal of CL, washing out foreign body using antibiotic solution, instilling antibiotic drops and patching eye for 24 hours. The lens needs to

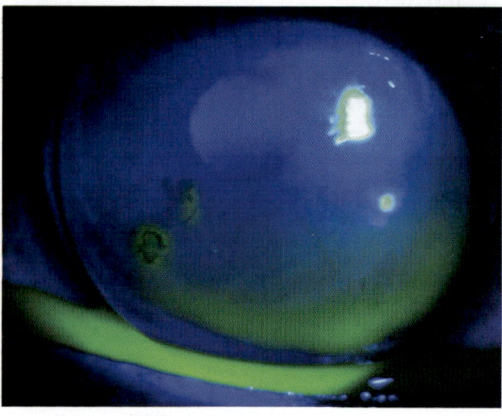

Fig. 19.9: Corneal abrasion resulting from entrapped particles under RGP lens

be discontinued for a week after epithelial healing; to prevent *slipping off* of fragile new epithelium under mechanical effect of lens wear intensified by blinking. If a chipped/broken or dirty lens is the cause, lens needs to be replaced, if poor handling is the etiology then wearer has to be re-instructed in correct methodology of lens usage.

- *Lens binding/adherence*: Refer to page 148 and 243.
- *Lens Deposits:* The lens deposit types may be organic, inorganic or mixed.
  - *Tear-related deposits* arise from lyso-zyme, lipids, albumin, mucin, immuno-globulins (A, G and E), lactoferrin, fibronectin and calcium. Lysozyme gets deposited on lens once tears evaporate, subsequently mucin adheres and a deposit build up starts from this nidus.
  - *Non-tear related deposits* from environ-ment are rust, kajal, mascara, perfume, fungal, mercurial or tobacco residues. Extended wear, aphakia, high water content lens, ionic lenses, poor hygiene, dry eyes, improper blinking all serve to increase deposits on the lens (Fig. 19.10).
  - *Protein deposits*: Sheets of denatured lens proteins appear as flat, film-like deposits or as jelly bumps (**mulberry spots barnacles**) and are more often seen with high water content hydrogels and aphakic lenses. **Jelly bumps** appear as gelatinous amorphous, translucent mulberry-like deposits in inferior exposed parts of lens (Fig. 19.10). Discomfort and enhanced lens awareness caused by protruding deposits usually results in cessation of lens wear. If wearer continues to wear these deposit laden lenses, then problems like CLPC, GPC and even lens flexure can ensue. Removal of deposits is impossible as their base lies within the lens matrix and forced removal would create a lens pit which often acts as a nidus for rapid re-growth of deposit. The solution is replacement with a new lens, preferably a low water content one. Recurrence of deposits in subsequent lenses may require change to frequent replacement or disposable schedule.
  - *Lipid deposits*: These often appear as greasy, smooth and shiny adherent films, with a fingerprint like incomplete tear film being characteristic (Fig. 19.11). Inherent thick oily tears, lid conditions like chronic blepharoconjunctivitis/meibominitis, exposure to environmental pollutants and poor quality eye cosmetics are risk factors. Prevention involves use of alcohol-based surfactant cleaners, water-based cos-metics/skin preparations and frequent replacement schedule lenses.

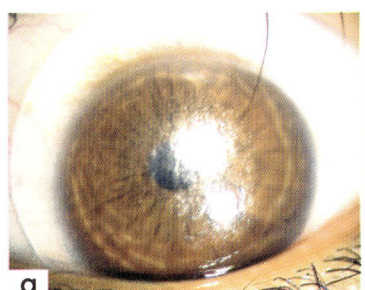 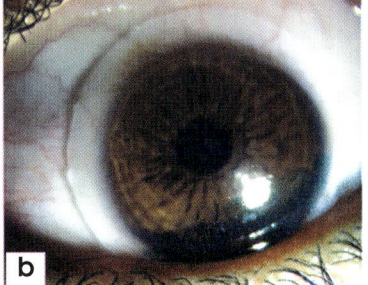 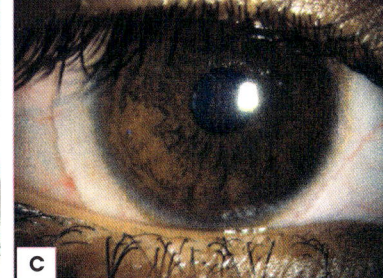

Fig. 19.10: Deposits on soft lenses (a) Mulberry and filamentous deposits on RGP lens; (b) Filmy membrane like deposits on soft lens (c) Gelatinous deposits visible at nasal margins of lens edge

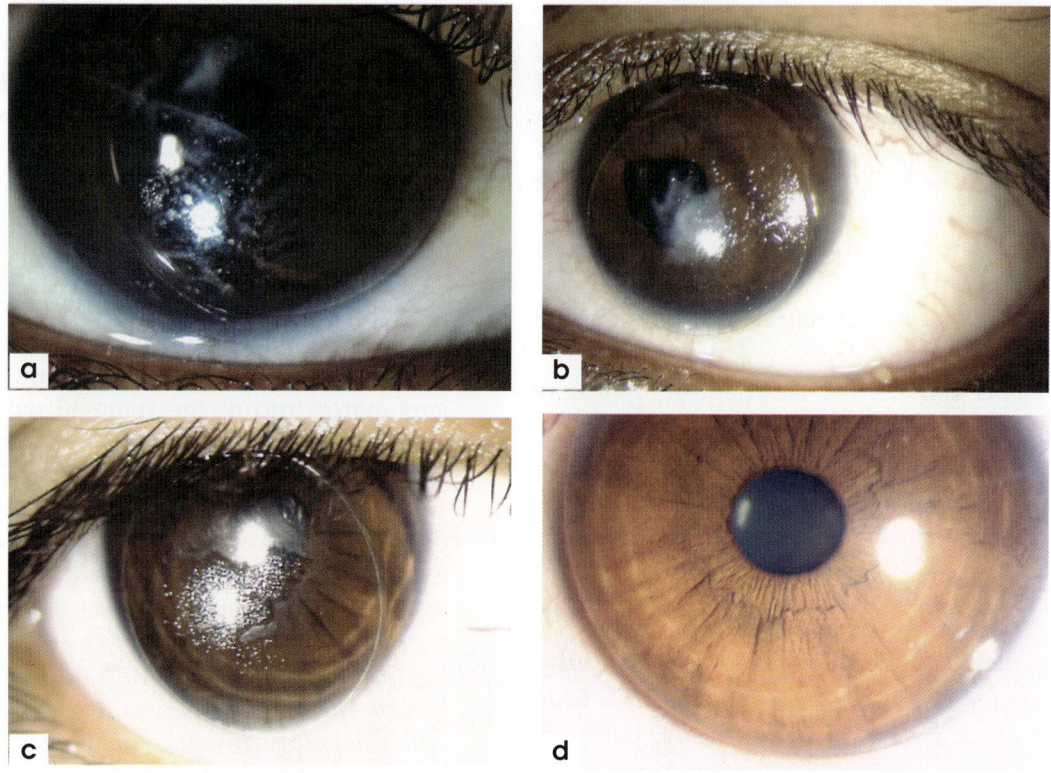

Fig. 19.11: Deposit on RGP lenses (a, b, c and d) shows same lens as (c) after ultrasonic cleaning

– **Inorganic films/salts:** These white crystalline specks on lens surface/matrix may form a film or occur as localized spots. Arising from precipitation of calcium carbonate or phosphate from tears onto lens surface, these specks evolve rapidly within days/weeks and get covered by a protein film rendering rough surfaces smooth. Such deposits are frequently seen with aphakic high plus lenses and in patients with dry eyes (Fig. 19.12). As is the case with most deposits, incomplete blinking facilitates their growth. These small crystals are difficult to remove with chemical disinfection systems, but can be easily dissolved with thermal disinfection. Removal leaves pits on lens surface thus replacement is again a better option. Non-phosphate buffered saline and saline with chelating agents (calcium inhibitor) must be used to store the new lenses.

– *Filamentous/film deposits*: These deposits occur in patients indulging in intermittent wear with prolonged storage of lens in cases leading to contamination of lens case/solution. Fungal or bacterial contamination is common which can invade lens matrix (Fig. 19.13). Patient presents with discomfort and signs of corneal toxicity. Lens along with lens case should be replaced.

Deposits reduce surface wetting, impair vision and cause discomfort. They initiate an immune response which manifests as GPC. Proper cleaning, **"rub and rinse"** methodology with surfactant solutions, occasional use of enzymatic cleaners can go a long way in preventing this problem.

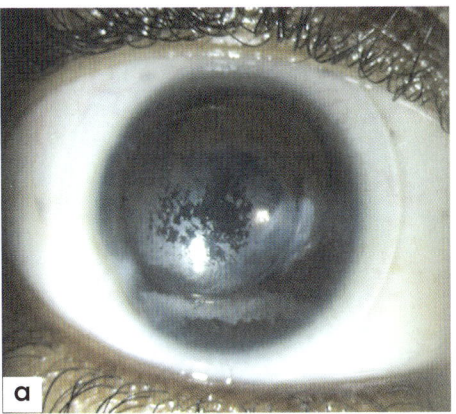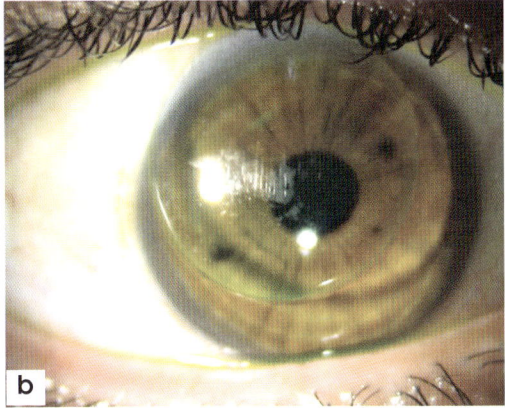

Fig. 19.12: Crystalline deposit on; (a) Soft hydrogel lens; (b) RGP lens

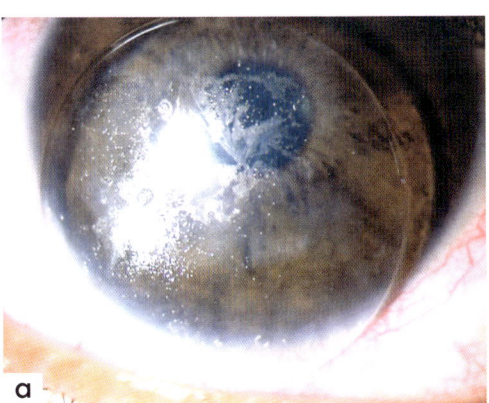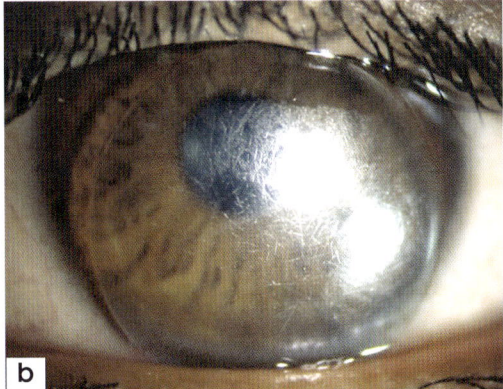

Fig. 19.13: Filamentous deposit on RGP lenses

V. Inflammatory Adverse Effects

These adverse effects manifest with conjunctival hyperaemia, vascularization, corneal infiltration, dry eyes. The effects have been given interesting abbreviations which are detailed below.

- *CLPU (Contact lens induced peripheral ulcer):* This term is used to describe sterile, small (<1.5 mm), sub-epithelial and anterior stromal ulcers occurring as a result of immune response mounted by eye to either lens material or to its cleaning solutions. Hypoxia induced by extended wear lens (EW)/lens overwear is also a known trigger. The condition must be differentiated from infective etiology with the latter being more symptomatic, larger in size and associated with increased anterior chamber reaction. Treatment includes discontinuation of lens, use of broad spectrum topical antibiotic like fluoroquinolones followed by low dose steroids after a 24-hour period. The infiltrates respond rapidly, but patient should be re-fitted with daily wear lenses if extended wear was the culprit.

- *SEAL (Superior arcuate epithelial lesions):* This term denotes arcuate lesions seen between 10 and 2 o'clock positions in limbal/paralimbal area (Fig. 19.14). They occur as a result of mechanical chaffing of limbal vasculature by lens edge during blinking movements. The condition is

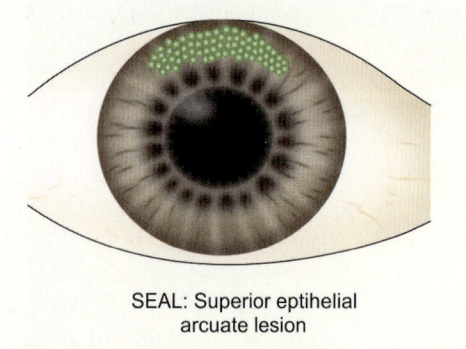

SEAL: Superior eptihelial
arcuate lesion

Fig. 19.14: SEAL diagram

aggravated by tight fit and poor wettabilty of lens. Superior limbic keratoconjunctivitis may also be seen with use of preservatives like thiomersal in cleaning solutions (Fig. 19.15). Treatment involves discontinuation of CL with use of frequent lubricant drops. The patient is then refitted with a new lens and cleaning solution is altered. Sometimes disposable lenses may be required if condition persists.

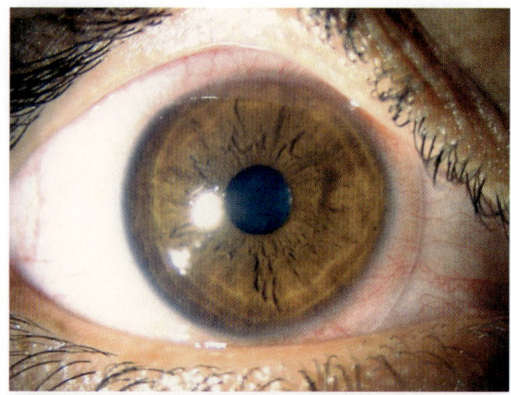

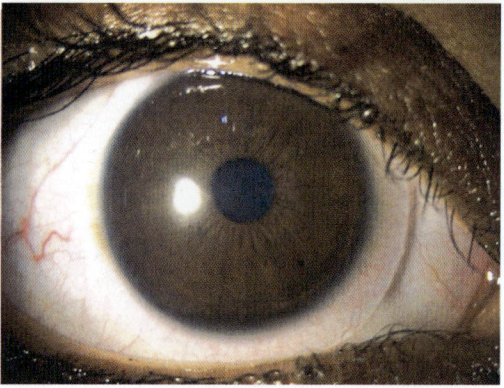

Fig. 19.16: *Contact lens induced red eye* with tight fitting lenses

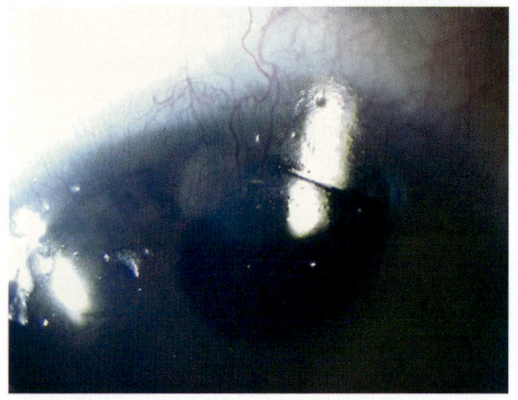

Fig. 19.15: Superior vascularization and scarring in an aphakic patient fitted with convex hydrogel lens

- *CLARE (contact lens induced red eye):* As the name suggests CLARE implies acute red eye with corneal infiltration and occurs with extended wear lens usage or lens overwear (Fig. 19.16). Toxins from bacteria present in EW lenses cause peripheral stromal infiltrates, conjunctival injection and anterior chamber reaction. The condition resolves completely on discontinuation of the lens, but can recur on reintroduction of another EW lens.

- *GPC/CLPC (giant papillary conjunctivitis/contact lens induced papillary conjunctivitis):* This very common condition occurs after a few months of lens wear. More frequent with soft lens use it manifests with ocular discomfort, gritty sensation, itching, foreign body sensation, mucoid discharge and lens intolerance after a few hours of use. On everting the upper lid multiple, enlarged conjunctival papillae larger than 0.3 mm are seen. The tarsal conjunctiva is hyperaemic with loss of vascular pattern (Fig. 19.17a to c). Active GPC stains with fluorescein as depicted in Fig. 19.17d. Diffuse GPC as a result of immune response to lens deposits needs to be differentiated from localized GPC which is due to mechanical trauma with faulty lens edge design or poor lens fit.

Treatment depends on extent of GPC. If mild, temporary lens discontinuation, use of mast cell stabilizer, olopatidine and lubricants suffices. It is important to ensure that patient is blinking adequately and frequently. If, however, on reusing lens GPC recurs, then lens needs to be discarded, lens wear discontinued for a few weeks and medications mentioned above used for a period of 4–6 weeks. Subsequently patient can be fitted with a new lens. For cases with recurrent GPC despite these measures, refit with either disposable lenses or RGP lenses is the solution.

VI. Infectious Adverse Effects

Contact-lens-related microbial keratitis (CLMK): It is a severe and potentially blinding condition requiring urgent treatment to contain damage and to improve prognosis.[10–12] It is often associated with poor hygiene, delayed lens replacement and smoking.[12] Afflicting almost 5 in 10,000 wearers it can result in corneal scarring, visual impairment and even blindness if neglected.[13] Symptoms include blurred vision, pain especially on exposure to light (photophobia), redness with or without discharge and foreign body sensation.

Infective keratitis may occur due to bacterial, viral (herpetic), fungal causes and specifically acanthamoeba organisms in lens

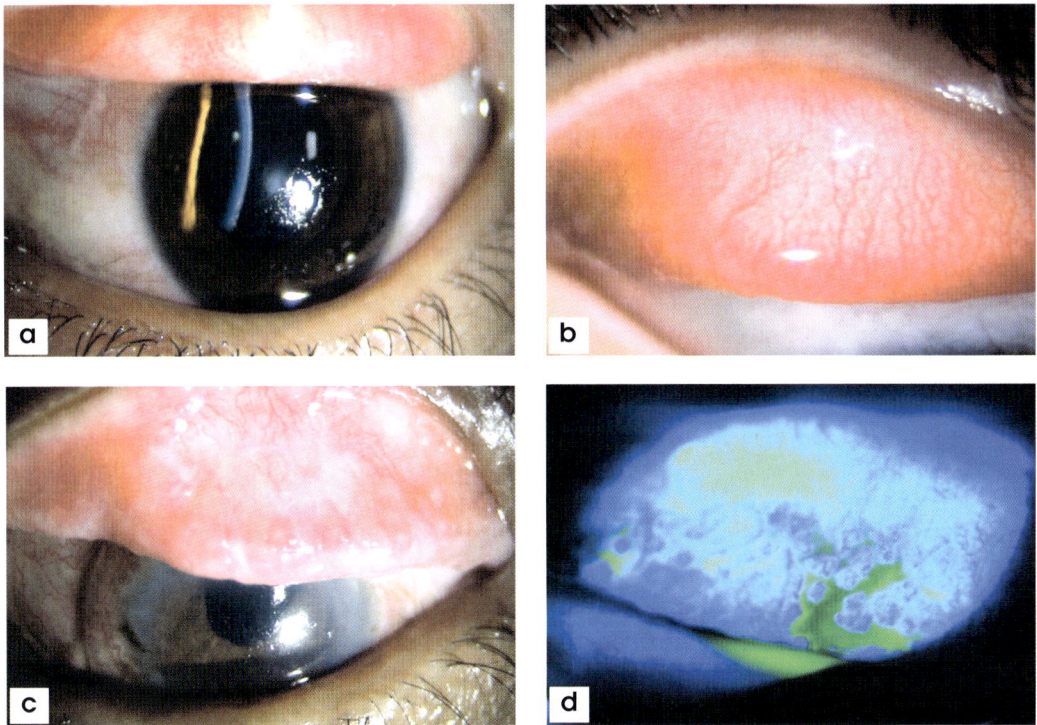

Fig. 19.17: Figure shows grades of contact lens induced papillary conjunctivitis: (a) Mild; (b) Moderate; (c) Advanced over pre-existing trachomatous Arlt's scar; (d) With active staining papillae

users. Bacterial keratitis represents the overwhelming majority and fungal etiology is usually associated with traumatic corneal injury, especially from vegetable matter (Fig. 19.18). The common pathogens isolated in CLMK are bacteria like staphylococcus or pseudomonas.[11,14,15] Fungal ulcers are uncommon and present typically, as dry elevated lesions with feathery borders, often surrounded by satellite infiltrates. Viral keratitis occurs due to reactivation of latent herpes simplex virus-1 (HSV-1) migrating down the axon of nasociliary nerve (trigeminal). The classic lesion is extremely symptomatic, stain positive, dendritic/geographic ulcer with terminal bulbs and decreased corneal sensation.[16,17]

Acanthamoeba keratitis manifests as an extremely painful ring-shaped infiltrate associated with use of unpreserved contact lens solution/homemade saline or tap water, swimming with lenses on and/or poor hygiene (Fig. 19.19). The condition presents as central or paracentral haze, ring infiltrate, radial perineuritis which is responsible for pain being disproportionate to signs.[16,17] The condition needs to be differentiated from bacterial and herpetic keratitis. Prompt diagnosis and treatment has to be initiated to save vision from this virulent infection. Treatment is with propamidine isethionate, chlorhexidine, miconazole nitrate, and

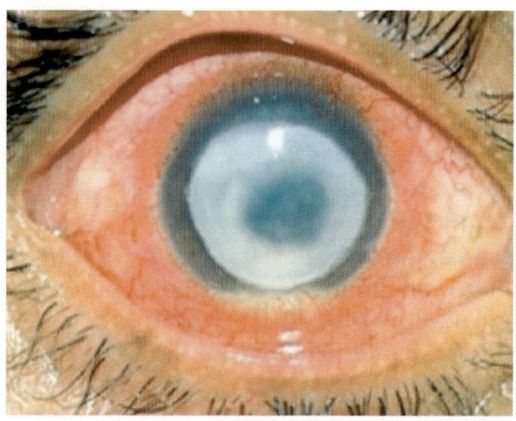

Fig. 19.19: Acanthamoeba keratitis with ring inflitrate and hypopyon (*Courtesy:* Dr Neera Aggarwal)

neomycin. Most patients present late, with history of keratitis not responding to multiple antibiotics often requiring keratoplasty. On clinical suspicion corneal scraping specimen and a piece of contact lens is cultured on sheep blood agar plate with *E. coli* overlay. Acanthamoeba if present would ingest the bacteria, leaving a clear patch on plate around lens/specimen area.

Treatment

CLMK is assumed to be bacterial until proven otherwise and empirical treatment covering both gram-positive and gram-negative organism is started after appropriate corneal scraping and culture. The initial treatment

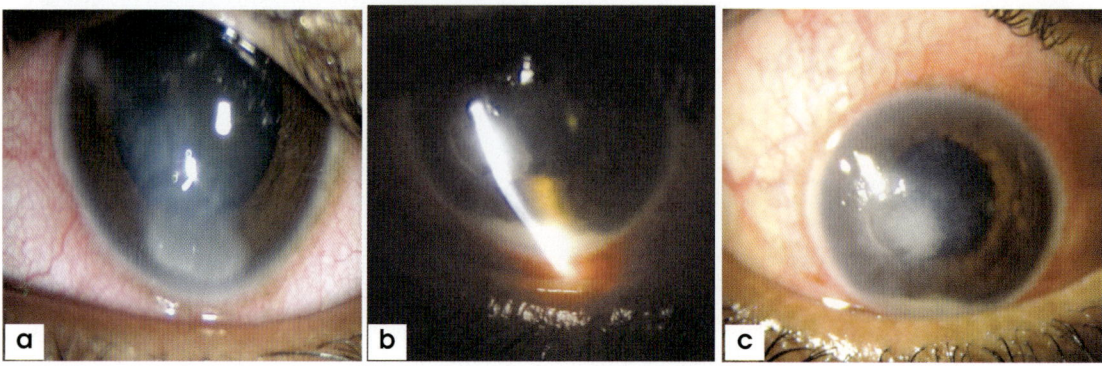

Fig. 19.18: Contact lens-related microbial keratitis: (a) Healing corneal ulcer; (b and c) Hypopyon keratitis

consists of combination with fortified cefazolin 5% and tobramycin 1.3% drops.[17] Alternately monotherapy with second generation fluoroquinolones (Ciprofloxacin or Ofloxacin) or third generation fluoroquinolones (Moxifloxacin or Gatifloxacin) is initiated.[18–20]

Antibiotic frequency is 2 hourly for first 2–3 days and on attaining a response, it can be, tapered to four hourly and then four times a day till ulcer resolution. Relief of pain, photophobia and reduction of epithelial defect, infiltrate size and anterior chamber reaction indicate efficacy of treatment. Additional use of ciprofloxacin/tobramycin ointment at bedtime and cycloplegic drugs are useful adjunctive therapies.[16,21] Minimal or partial response, disproportionate pain and immuno-compromised status should indicate a fungal aetiology or Acanthamoeba infection.

In all situations lens use must be immediately discontinued and lens along with samples from lens case should be sent for culture sensitivity. Systemic antibiotics are rarely used but can be considered for severe infections.[21] Keratoplasty needs to be considered when aggressive microbial keratitis does not respond to medical therapy.

- *Marginal keratitis:* Marginal keratitis occurs as a response to staphylococcal exotoxins and presents with multiple subepithelial, stain positive infiltrates separated from limbus by a clear zone.[17] This bilateral, often recurrent condition coexists with blepharitis and acne rosacea.

- *Superficial punctuate keratitis:* It occurs due to combination of lens induced mechanical injury, tight lens, lens overwear, dry eye and solution toxicity (Fig. 19.20). Lubricants and topical antibiotics are instituted along with lens discontinuation.

Contributory Factors and Prevention Modalities

The factors which contribute to CLMK are use of extended-wear lenses, sleeping or swimming with lenses, poor lens fit especially steep fit, poor hygiene, poor maintenance of contact lens cases and use of other solutions including tap water for cleaning and storage.[18,22,23]

Overnight lens use has been identified as the single most common risk factor in the developed world.[13] Other contributory factors include bacterial adherence to lens, formation of biofilm on lens/storage case, microbial resistance to disinfection solution, tear stagnation behind the lenses and reduced corneal resistance as a result of hypoxia.[13, 24]

As microbial keratitis almost always results in corneal scarring with some persisting diminution of vision, prevention of infection is aimed at in lens wearers. These precautions

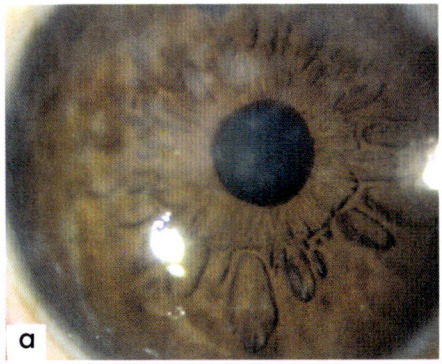
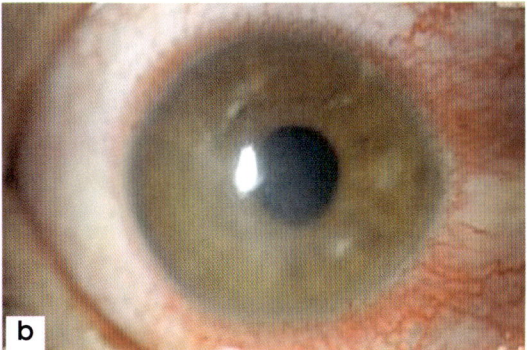

Fig. 19.20: (a) Resolved viral infection causing; (b) Superficial punctate keratitis

include stringent hygiene, lens care measures involving meticulous rubbing and cleaning of lenses with appropriate solution along with case care.[25,26] Patients must be warned not to sleep with CL as this is one of the major risk factors for keratitis.

Cleaning Regimen

Superiority of "rub and rinse" method compared to rinse alone for removing bacteria without consideration to multipurpose solution used or type of contact lens has been repeatedly documented.[27] Tap water has to be avoided at all costs for cleaning of soft lens and if swimming is done without use of protective waterproof goggles, then the lenses must be discarded immediately afterwards.

Lenses have to be stored in a clean case filled with fresh (not "topped off") multipurpose or disinfecting solution. Gram-negative bacteria have been documented to survive at upper inner rim of lens case, due to air–liquid interface biofilms.[28] After removal of lenses in the morning, residual solution in storage case should be discarded, lens case washed in flowing water and left to dry.[5] At weekly intervals, case should be scrubbed with a oil-free detergent using a toothbrush dedicated to this, rinsed and dried for a few hours.

Early treatment in CLMK limits scarring and vision loss with treatment delay by more than 12 hours being detrimental.[10] This underscores the importance of providing patient with a checklist of warning symptoms and instruction to report immediately on occurrence of these signs.[29] Since overnight lens wear/overwear has been identified as common risk factors for CLMK, patients need to be warned never to sleep or nap in their lenses.[13,32] Of the different wearing schedules, daily disposables have been documented as safest with lowest rate of complications.[26]

VII. Others

- *Dimple veiling*: Trapped air bubbles beneath an ill fitting RGP lens cause indentation/desiccation of epithelium manifesting with focal areas of fluorescein pooling. Steep lenses with excessive central pooling and those with edge lift are more prone to cause dimple veiling (Fig. 19.21). Largely asymptomatic, this complication underscores an ill-fitting lens, and flattening of base curve or reducing the overall diameter often resolves the problem.
- *Lens spoilage*: Lenses get spoiled due to ageing, deposits and poor wetting. Scratches on lens are very common and are a result of poor care and handling (Fig. 19.22).

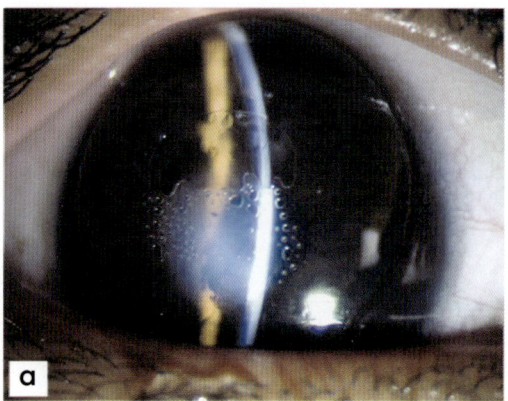 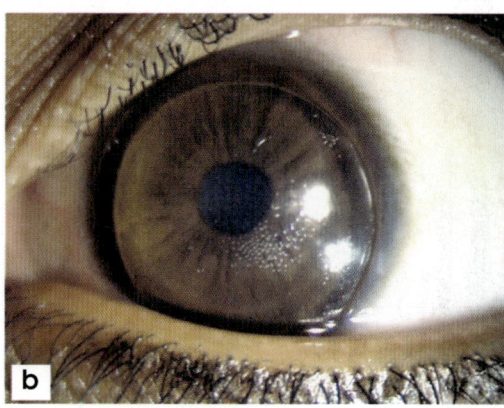

Fig. 19.21: Dimple veiling (a) Central; (b) Paracentral

Spoiled lenses increase inflammatory and allergic lid response leading to lens intolerance. Periodic replacement of lenses at one-year interval for SCL and 2-year intervals for RGP, with periodic edging and polishing of RGP and ultrasonic cleaning of SCL prevent this attrition (Fig. 19.23). Scratches on a RGP lens can be removed by edging and polishing in the laboratory using.

- *Lens Warpage:* This denotes change in base curve from initial parameters which subsequently lead to poor fitting of lens. Cracks or defects are more common in soft lenses and can cause ocular irritation, corneal abrasions and predispose to CLMK.

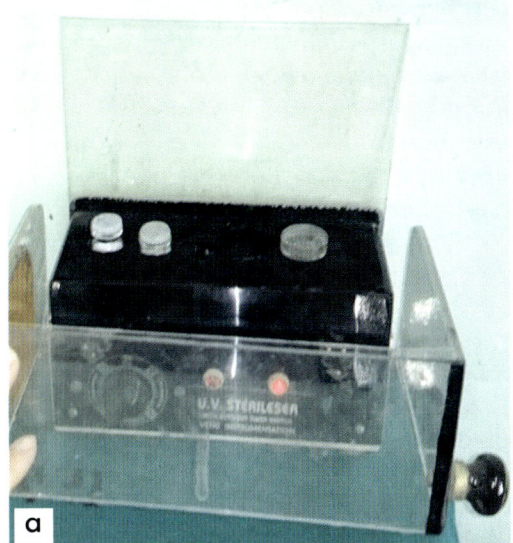

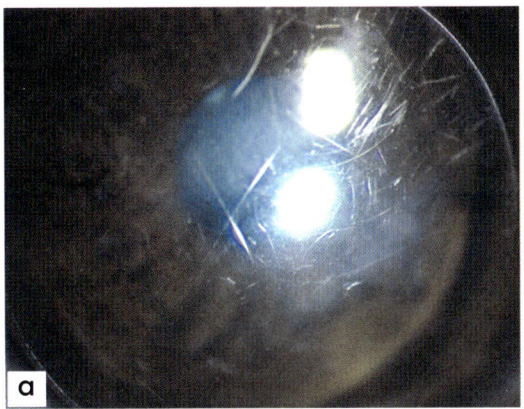

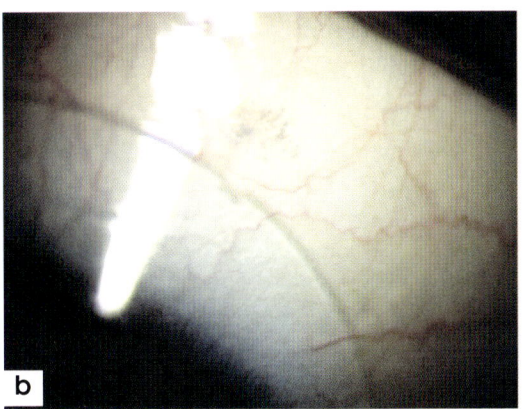

Fig. 19.22: Lens spoilage (a) Scratches on lens; (b) Chipped lens edge, at 2 o'clock position

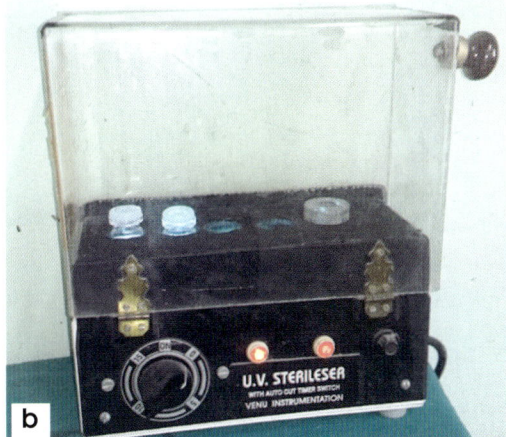

Fig. 19.23: (a) Ultrasonic cleaner with lens in bottle in the designated wells; (b) Ultrasonic cleaning in progress

- *Corneal distortion:* The cornea alters in shape due to mechanical and physiological factors induced by lens wear. The patient presents with blurring of vision which is more marked when the patient switches to his spectacles, the *spectacle blur*. Diagnosis is confirmed by altered keratometry mires and treatment involves switching to higher Dk lenses with better alignment. The condition may be confused with corneal exhaustion and/or wrinkling.

- *Ptosis:* It is occasionally seen in RGP lens wearers especially unilateral wearers. Usually reversible, the condition may become permanent if traumatic lens removal has resulted in lid stretching and damage to levator aponeurosis.
- A strange but not infrequent complication is that seen in Fig. 19.24. It represents a *flipped out* or *inside out* soft lens. Correct lens usage with explanation of lens wearers to the patient, would prevent this complication. As explained before this is done by holding lens on tip of forefinger and squeezing it, to ensure its concavity is actual (Fig 19. 24b). For detail refer to Chapter 21.

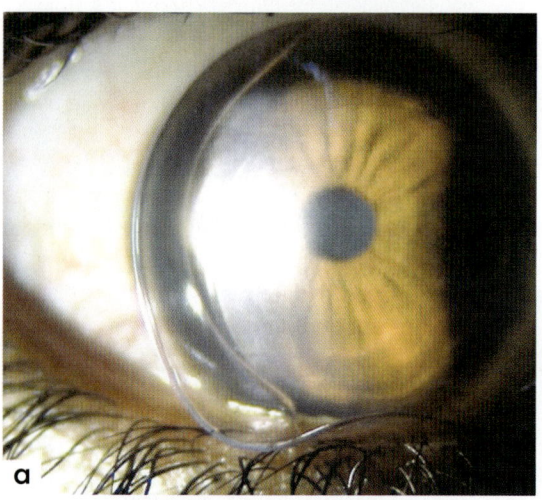
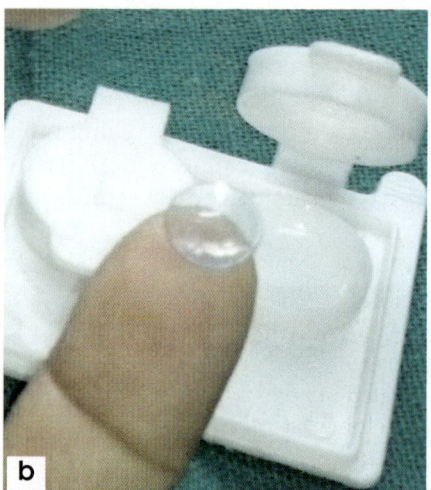

Fig. 19.24: (a) Inside out lens in eye; (b) Ensuring right side up

REFERENCES

1. Key JE. Development of contact lenses and their worldwide use. Eye Contact Lens. 2007 Nov;33 (6, suppl.):343–5.

2. Stapleton F, Keay L, Jalbert I, and Cole N. The epidemiology of contact lens related infiltrates. Optom Vis Sci 2007;84:257–72

3. Jason J. Nichols. Contact Lenses 2012 in *Contact Lens Spectrum*, Volume: 28, Issue: January 2013, 24–29, 52.

4. Sucheki JK, Donshik P, Ehlers WH. Contact lens complications. Ophthalmol Clin North Am. 2003 Sep;16(3):471–84.

5. Forister JF, Forister EF, Yeung KK, Ye P, Chung MY, Tsui A, Weissman BA. Prevalence of contact lens-related complications: UCLA contact lens study. Eye Contact Lens. 2009 Jul;35(4):176–80.

6. Dart JK, Radford CF, Minassian D, Verma S, Stapleton F. Risk factors for microbial keratitis with contemporary contact lenses: a case-control study. Ophthalmology. 2008;115(10): 1647–54.

7. Swanson MW. A cross-sectional analysis of U.S. contact lens user demographics. Optom Vis Sci. 2012 Jun;89(6):839–48.

8. Bruce AS and Brennan NA. A guide to clinical contact lens management. Eds Ciba Vision group of companies. Georgia, USA 1995.

9. Hamano H, Jacob J, Senft C et al. Differences in contact lens induced response in the cornea of Asian and non-Asian subjects. CLAO J 2002, 28: 101–4.

10. Musa F, Tailor R, Gao A, Hutley E, Rauz S, Scott RA. Contact lens-related microbial

keratitis in deployed British military personnel. BR J Ophthalmol. 2010; 94:988–93.

11. Ahn M, Yoon KC, Ryu SK, Cho NC, You IC. Clinical aspects and prognosis of mixed microbial (bacterial and fungal) keratitis. Cornea. 2011; 30:409–13.

12. Stapleton F. Contact lens related microbial keratitis. What can epidemiological studies tell us? Eye Contact lens 2003;29(15): 585–9.

13. Stapleton F, Keay L, Edwards K, et al. The incidence of contact lens-related microbial keratitis in Australia. Ophthalmology. 2008; 115:1655–62.

14. Petroutsos G, Paschides CA, Kitsos G, Drosos AA, Psilas K. Sterile corneal ulcers in dry eye. II. Treatment, complications and course. J Fr Ophtalmol. 1992;15(2):106–11.

15. Fleiszig SM, The Glenn A. Fry award lecture 2005. The pathogenesis of contact lens-related keratitis. Optom Vis Sci. 2006; 83:866–73.

16. Friedman NJ, Kaiser PK, Pineda R. The Massachusetts eye and ear infirmary illustrated manual of ophthalmology. 3rd ed. Philadelphia: Elsevier; 2009. pp. 188–204.

17. Ehlers JP, Shah CP. The Wills eye manual: office and emergency room diagnosis and treatment of eye disease. 5th Ed. Baltimore: Lippincott Williams & Wilkins;2008. pp.62–86.

18. Ibrahim YW, Boase DL, Cree IA. Epidemiological characteristics, predisposing factors and microbiological profiles of infectious corneal ulcers: the Portsmouth corneal ulcer study. Br J Ophthalmol. 2009; 93:1319–24.

19. Hsu HY, Nacke R, Song JC, Yoo SH, Alfonso EC, Israel HA. Community opinions in the management of corneal ulcers and ophthalmic antibiotics: a survey of 4 states. Eye Contact Lens. 2010;36:195–200.

20. Chawla B, Agarwal P, Tandon R, et al. In vitro susceptibility of bacterial keratitis isolates to fourth-generation fluoroquinolones. Eur J Ophthalmol. 2010; 20:300–5.

21. Kanski JJ. Clinical ophthalmology: a synopsis. 2nd ed. Oxford: Butterworth-Heinemann; 2009. pp. 138–50.

22. Al-Yousuf N. Microbial keratitis in kingdom of Bahrain: clinical and microbiology study. Middle East Afr J Ophthalmol. 2009; 16:3–7.

23. Preechawat P, Ratananikom U, Lerdvitayasakul R, Kunavisarut S. Contact lens-related microbial keratitis. J Med Assoc Thai. 2007 Apr;90(4):737–43.

24. Giraldez MJ, Resua CG, Lira M, et al. Contact lens hydrophobicity and roughness effects on bacterial adhesion. Optom Vis Sci. 2010; 87:E426–31.

25. Musa F, Tailor R, Gao A, Hutley E, Rauz S, Scott RA. Contact lens-related microbial keratitis in deployed British military personnel. BR J Ophthalmol. 2010; 94:988–93.

26. Yeung KK, Forister JF, Forister EF, Chung MY, Han S, Weissman BA. Compliance with soft contact lens replacement schedules and associated contact lens-related ocular complications: The UCLA Contact Lens Study. Optometry. 2010; 81:598–607.

27. Zhu H, Bandara MB, Vijay AK, Masoudi S, Wu D, Willcox MD. Importance of rub and rinse in use of multipurpose contact lens solution. Optom Vis Sci. 2011; 88:967–72.

28. Wu YT, Zhu H, Harmis NY, Iskandar SY, Willcox M, Stapleton F. Profile and frequency of microbial contamination of contact lens cases. Optom Vis Sci. 2010; 87:153–8.

29. Chalmers RL, Keay L, Long B, Bergenske P, Giles T, Bullimore MA. Risk factors for contact lens complications in US clinical practices. Optom Vis Sci. 2010; 87:725–35.

30. Ahn M, Yoon KC, Ryu SK, Cho NC, You IC. Clinical aspects and prognosis of mixed microbial (bacterial and fungal) keratitis. Cornea. 2011; 30:409–13.

31. Fleiszig SM, Evans DJ. Pathogenesis of contact lens-associated microbial keratitis. Optom Vis Sci. 2010; 87:225–32.

32. American Academy of Ophthalmology Cornea/ external disease panel. Preferred Practice Patterns Guidelines. Bacterial keratitis. San Francisco, CA: American Academy of Ophthalmology; 2008. Available at: http:// one.aao.org/CE/PracticeGuidelines

Reader's Note

CHAPTER 20

Care Regimens

Success, tolerance and safety of contact lens wear is maximally determined by care taken by its wearer on maintenance and cleaning. The most expert contact lens practitioner faces his Waterloo at hands of the non-compliant lens wearer. To prevent this defeat stringent guidelines in care and maintenance need to be followed. This chapter details the steps of lens care, lens hygiene which would prevent most visually disabling complications associated with lens care.

The three most important steps in lens care are:

- Use of the correct contact lens solution in the correct manner
- Detailed instructions given to patient for lens care
- Periodic monitoring and lens replacement schedules.

By their very nature, contact lenses impede free tear flow and reduce effectivity of eye to cleanse itself of noxious contaminants and bacteria, thereby favoring growth of commensal organisms. Meticulous daily leaning and disinfecting is thus important to prevent visually threatening corneal infections. To a large extent, this action is performed by contact lens solutions. These solutions can be different ones for cleaning and disinfecting but currently multipurpose solutions, which perform all three activities of cleaning, rinsing and disinfection are favored. The acronym given to the sequence of lens care is CRADLE: Clean, Rinse And Disinfect Lenses Everytime.[1]

Aim of Care and Maintenance

- Ensure optimal optics and comfort at all times of wear.
- Prevent/minimise microbial contamination during wear and storage.
- Reduce lens deposits and thereby enhance lens longevity.

Lens Care Protocol

a. Hand hygiene: Handwashing is done with fragrance free soap and hands are subsequently dried with a lint-free towel. This ensures that tap water used for handwashing does not come in contact with the lenses. To reinforce importance of this step, it is advisable to inspect wearer's hands at first visit and then at periodic intervals to ensure cleanliness of hands and nails (Figs 20.1 and 20.2).

The lens is then removed from its case.

b. Cleaning of lens: Lens is then placed on palm of hand and rubbed with forefinger for 15–20 seconds using a to and fro and lateral rolling actions, taking 2–3 drops of cleaning solution. This serves to remove loosely bound cell debris, mucus, lipid, protein, dust, cosmetics and micro-organisms. Rubbing also enhances efficacy of surfactant present in the cleaning solution.

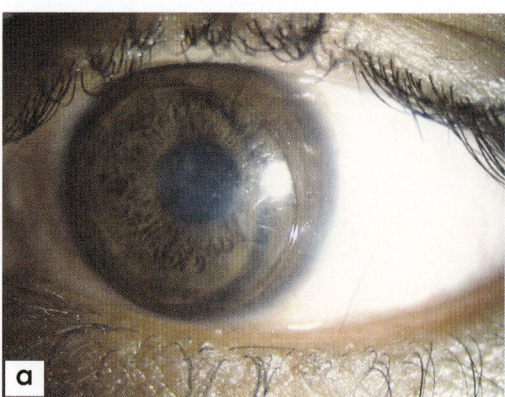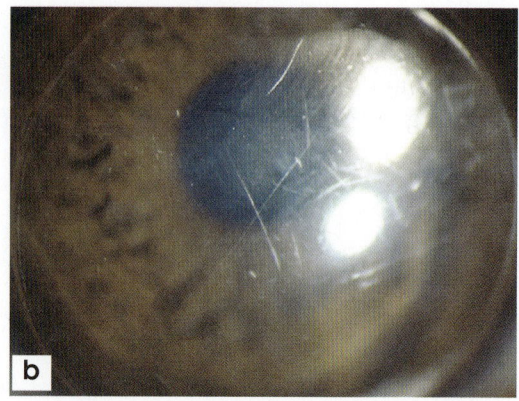

Fig. 20.1: (a and b) Depict scratches on lens due to poor cleaning practices

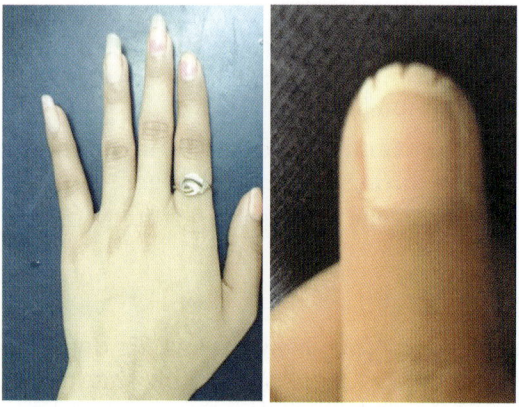

Fig. 20.2: Long-chipped or nails damaged

The components of cleaning solution and their properties are given below:

– *Surface-active agent/surfactant* like isopropyl alcohol, tyloxapol, polyvinyl alcohol, poloxamer-407, amphoteric 10, poloxamine, hexylene glycol, octylphenoxy ethanol, tween 21. These agents emulsify and dissolve loosely bound foreign matter on lens surface like debris, mucus, lipids, proteins, cosmetics, microbes and inorganic deposits by forming a monomolecular layer over the contaminants. The 'coated' contaminants subsequently repel each other mutually or exhibit a lowered surface tension.

– *Hypertonicity* of solution helps to extract soluble contaminants from the soft lens.

– Osmolality adjusting agents and buffer system in solution serve to maintain pH at requisite level, e.g. sodium borate, sodium chloride.

– Preservatives: These are non-ionic or ionic chemicals added to solution.

– Viscosity-enhancing agents like polyvinyl alcohol, methylcellulose facilitate cleaning. Products with lower viscosity, for example, Bausch & Lomb sensitive eyes daily cleaner, are easier to rinse off the lens than those with higher viscosity.

– Mild abrasives or polymeric beads help in removing deposits (present in Opti-Clean II, Opti-Free Daily Cleaner). However a word of caution, excessive rubbing with cleaning solutions incorporating such abrasive cleaners can cause scratches on lens, induce minus power and is to be strictly avoided.

– Certain specific solutions are used for their specific properties, e.g. isopropyl alcohol cleaners like MiraFlow for wearers with propensity to lipid deposits.

c. *Rinsing of lens:* This step is followed by thorough rinsing of cleaner solution with sterile isotonic buffered solution of preserved, unpreserved saline (pH of 7.2, similar to tears). *Homemade saline or tap water should never be used for this step.* Rinsing removes excess of cleaning solution, loosened deposits and microbes. Buffered isotonic saline is preferred to un-buffered since absorption of atmospheric carbon dioxide lowers pH in the latter.

d. **Disinfecting the lens**: Special disinfecting solutions or systems serve to deactivate potentially pathogenic organisms (bacteria, fungi, viruses, amoeba) and maintain lens hydration. These disinfectants reduce microbial level to a safer level but do not eliminate them. For effective disinfection, lenses need to be soaked in disinfecting solution for a minimum of four hours. Since effectivity of disinfectant wanes with time, lenses stored in solution *for more than 3 days* need to be removed, cleaned and re-disinfected using fresh solution for at least 4 hours prior to insertion.

e. **Lens case care:** After inserting the lenses on the eye, all remaining solution in lens case is thrown away. The empty lens case is dried with a clean lint-free towel and allowed to air dry, before being needed again for holding the lenses in it. *An extra dry clean case must be at all times be present with the wearer.*

Types of Lens Disinfection

I. *Thermal Disinfection*

Heat in the range of 70–120°C deactivates all living lens contaminants. Heat disinfection for a period of 20–30 minutes is highly effective against all microbes including spores and Acanthamoeba cysts. In addition, it does not give rise to any allergic side effects.

The technique involves placing of each cleaned lens into a compartment of a storage case filled with preservative-free saline, which is then placed into a heating unit and temperature is increased to a specific level for a prescribed time. The disadvantages of procedure, however, outweigh benefits and currently thermal disinfection is relegated to history pages of lens care. The reasons of this technique being discarded are: Daily heating *alters optical properties* and fit of high water content soft lenses by altering fluid components. Lens spoilage, ageing and discoloration occur as a consequence of protein denaturation, in addition, RGP lenses can warp on heating. Requirement of specialized thermal units, which need to be regularly inspected for damage, cracks or leaks is a further deterrent.

II. *Cold Disinfection Systems*

This is the most commonly performed method and involves use of chemical disinfections or hydrogen peroxide.

A. Chemical Disinfectants

The method entails soaking and storing lens in disinfecting solution for a prescribed period of time. The methods of disinfection utilize oxidation, molecular mechanism and targeting microbial proteins. Use of **Oxidizing agents** is a time-tested method to defang microbes and make them non-pathogenic, examples being thimerosal, benzalkonium chloride and chlorhexidine. **Molecular mechanisms** involve cell membrane disruption, enzyme inhibition and disruption of cell metabolism with examples being benzalkonium chloride, thimerosal. Another method is targeting of **microbial cell proteins** which are then removed from metabolic pathways by coagulation or creation of complexes using chelating agents like EDTA.

It must be remembered that any chemical inimical to microbes is by nature also inimical to cornea or ocular surface. Inadequacy in washing off or neutralizing such solutions from contact lens surface has a potential danger of causing ocular toxicity. In addition, chemicals often lead to burning, stinging, diminished wearing time, conjunctival hyperaemia, intolerance to lens wear depending on extent of solution induced irritation. Sensitivity to a key ingredient is another inherent risk while using chemical disinfection. To avoid these sensitivity reactions, solutions now marketed have less sensitizing disinfecting preservatives like sorbic acid, Polyquad, TrisChem and Dymed. However, flip side of use of safer preservatives is their reduced efficacy against fungi and protozoa.

Some common chemical disinfectants used in contact lens solutions:

- *Thimerosal* (0.001–0.004%): This is a mercurial antibacterial whose mercury ions form covalent bonds with sulphydryl groups of bacterial cell enzymes (proteins) and incapacitate them. The agent also has intrinsic antifungal properties in addition to antibacterial ones. Due to small molecular size of 1.3 nm, it readily penetrates lens matrices of 3–5 nm pore size. It is negatively charged ionic form binds to positively charged lysozyme protein deposits on lens resulting in prolonged exposure to thimerosal with a dirty lens *in situ*. This is one of the reasons for contact lens induced GPC being more common with dirty lenses as the disinfectant gets bound to deposits. Thimerosal's cytotoxicity to corneal epithelium and its activity are both diluted on combination with EDTA/chlorhexidine. The disinfectant is incompatible with BAK and as it is decomposed by light exposure, the solution is marketed and stored in light-proof containers.

- **Chlorhexidine gluconate (CHG 0.001– 0.006%):** A biguanide antimicrobial it gets adsorbed on the siloxane acrylate material of lens in the form of monolayer and can cause corneal toxicity.[2,3] A formidable combination of Thimerosal with chlorhexidine combines superior antifungal action of former with superior antibacterial properties of latter, with effectivity against both trophozoite and cyst forms of Acanthamoeba. These chemicals, however,

have a propensity to bind with protein deposits on lenses and increase ocular irritation.[4]

- **Benzalkonium chloride (BAK** 0.002– 0.01%): A surface active cationic surfactant, it acts by disrupting cell membrane of microbes. For this reason corneal exposure should be avoided. A quaternary ammonium compound with positively charged hydrophilic benzene ring, it binds with negatively charged RGP lens and exposes its hydrophobic hydrocarbon end. This explains enhanced hydrophobicity of lens surfaces after being exposed to this preservative over a long period. This chemical is used in conjunction with a wetting and chelating agent to increase its effectivity. Build up of BAK with continuing exposure is again a source of ocular toxicity.[5]

- **Alcohol-based disinfectants:** These very effective antimicrobials are isopropyl alcohol 20% (marketed as Miraflow) and Ethanol 5% (marketed as Barnes Hind Cleaner). Isopropyl alcohol is an extremely effective disinfectant used for all types of rigid and soft lenses. All these chemicals, however, do not act on spores of bacteria like *Clostridium botulinum*, *tetani* and *Bacillus subtilis*.

  – *Benzyl Alcohol:* A bactericidal and viricidal for RGP lens only, it is ineffective against *Pseudomonas aeruginosa* in low concentrations. It behaves like a lipid solvent and has minimal sensitizing activity.

  – *Chlorbutol (trichloroisobutyl alcohol):* A chlorinated alcohol preservative with broad spectrum of action, it is an unstable, volatile agent with poor bacteriostatic properties and is no longer used.

- **Disodium EDTA:** This chelating agent removes divalent cations such as calcium and magnesium from cell walls of gram-negative organisms and disrupts cell growth. A weak preservative, it serves to potentiate quaternary ammonium compounds against gram-negative organisms but not gram-positive ones. The agent also has a synergistic action with BAK.

Newer Less Sensitizing Chemical Preservatives

- **Sorbic Acid and Potassium Sorbate** (0.1–0.2%): A poor antibacterial with limited antifungal activity, it works best in pH between 4.5 and 6.5 and reacts with lysine in tears to cause yellow/brown discoloration of the lens.

- **DYMED** (0.00005–0.0015% polyaminopropyl biguanide PAPB): A member of biguanide family like chlorhexidine it exhibits 30-fold less binding to RGP lens material.[6] It has traditionally been used as an anti-malarial water treatment and as a swimming pool disinfectant. The agent selectively binds with negatively charged phospholipids of cell wall and causes membrane damage. It is an adjuvant in treatment of Acanthamoeba keratitis and is marketed in B&L's ReNu, Boston's Simplicity Multi-Action Solution, Allergan's Complete and Complete Comfort Plus to mention a few.

- **POLYQUAD** (Polidromium chloride 0.001–0.005%): A high molecular weight (polymeric) quarternary ammonium compound, its large molecular size prevents its entry into lens materials, thereby minimizing ocular irritation. Used with citrate buffer it is marketed as Alcon's Opti-Free, Opti-Free Express, Opti-1, Opti-One and Opti-Soak, Opti-Clean II and Opti-Tears.

- **Chlorine systems:** Poly (dichlorosulphamoyl) benzoic acid. It is supplied as blister packed, anhydrous, effervescent tablets of either stabilized halane (sodium dichloroisocyanurate **Softab**™) or halazone poly (dichlorosulphamoyl benzoic acid **Aerotab**™). A tablet dissolved in 10 mL unpreserved sterile saline makes a disinfecting solution with a pH of 5.5–7.5.

Tablets get hydrolysed in presence of fluid to produce hypochlorus acid which in turn dissociates into hydrogen and hypochlorite ions. It produces chlorine concentrations of 4–8 ppm, and requires lens soaking time of 30 minutes to 4 hours with antimicrobial activity being proportionate to undissociated hypochlorus acid or available chlorine.[2] Lenses must be rinsed thoroughly with sterile saline before disinfection and before insertion to remove residual chemicals. Hypochlorite can also cause bleaching of lenses tinted with reactive dyes, therefore, it should be used to clean cosmetic lenses.

D-Value (Death-Rate Kinetics)

The D-value of a solution defines its antimicrobial ability or time *required to disinfect.* It is time required for test substance/method to decrease number of organisms by one log unit or time required to kill off 90% of originally present organisms. A longer time indicates slower killing rate which may not be same as lower anti-microbial efficacy. Kill rates based on D-value determine soaking time, e.g. low D-value implying slower kill rate, require longer soak time.

B. Hydrogen Peroxide-based/Oxidative System

The antimicrobial property of hydrogen peroxide is due to oxidizing power of generated free oxygen radicals. These free oxygen radicals bind to and destroy cell components very rapidly within 10–20 minutes of soaking time. However, this disinfection process has to be followed by a neutralization step which neutralizes peroxide to non-toxic water and oxygen trace levels. The neutralization process requires use of catalase, sodium pyruvate or sodium thiosulfite solution or is done by catalytic action of a platinum disk. Hydrogen peroxide system has less potential to incite allergic response as it lacks any preservative and is less toxic than chemical disinfectants. The product is marketed in two forms: one-step or two-step.

i. **1-Step Peroxide Systems (AOSEPT/Pure eyes):** In this method a **platinum disc** is used as a catalyst for both disinfection and neutralization. The contact lenses are placed in specially designed vented lens cases over which hydrogen peroxide solution is poured. The process of disinfection and neutralization takes 6 hours and oxygen generated escapes through vents in the lens case. Suboptimal disinfection can occur due to rapid neutralization of peroxide surrounding the disc without allowing sufficient time for disinfection. Platinum disc efficacy gradually decreases over time due to surface contamination and paradoxically gives rise to enhanced disinfection since poor catalyst performance leads to slower neutralization. This *disc failure* may then cause a peroxide *burn* on cornea as a result of poor action/non-replacement of disc, preventing complete neutralization of the peroxide. Thus the manufacturers recommend disc replacement after 100 uses or 3 months, whichever occurs earlier.[7,8]

After neutralization by catalyst, only non-preserved solution remains in case, so lenses remaining in this case for several days are susceptible to bacterial contamination. Therefore, any lenses stored in neutralized AOSEPT for greater than 24 hours require a repeat disinfection cycle.

ii. **2-step systems (Ultracare/Oxysept):** In this method neutralization is performed as a separate step. The first step involves overnight lens soaking in *peroxide solution.* This solution contains a bicarbonate buffer which alters pH, to ensure slow decomposition into water and oxygen. The second step done next morning uses *catalase delayed release tablets* or *sodium thiosulfate* solution for neutralization.

The Ultracare system incorporates additional use of delayed-release neutralizing tablet containing cyanocobalamin, to the peroxide solution, at beginning of disinfection cycle. This cyanocobalamin moiety turns solution pink and serves to remind patient of presence of the tablet. Over a period of two hours, disinfection and neutralization occur. Two hours is deemed as adequate time necessary for optimal activity against Acanthamoeba. It has to be emphasized to patient that before use, tablet must be thoroughly inspected for any cracks on its surface. Cracked tablet must be discarded; otherwise it will start neutralization process much before adequate disinfection has occurred. Newer models come with 30 tablets (one month use).

Disadvantages of peroxide system include multiple solutions use, multiple steps and risk of inadequate neutralization. Forgetfulness on part of patient to perform neutralization step results in insertion of lens with residual peroxide solution causing **peroxide burn**. Such a patient presents with acute pain, photophobia, redness, and possibly corneal epithelial damage. The lens wearer employing this method of disinfection is pre-warned about this complication and cautioned to remove lens and wash eye copiously with sterile saline solution if and when it occurs.

Table 20.1 lists some common solutions available.

C. Multipurpose Solutions

The earlier era of using separate solutions for surface active cleaning, protein removal, and disinfection has been gradually replaced by more convenient trend of using a single multipurpose solution performing these functions. Examples include ReNu multi-plus multi-purpose solution, ReNu multi-purpose disinfecting solution, Opti-Free Express,

Table 20.1: Common lens solution and preservatives used

Chemical disinfection (manufacturer)	Functions	Preservative
Opti-Free express/Opti one multipurpose solution (Alcon)	Cleaning, disinfection, storage	Polyquad
Opti-Free (Alcon)	Disinfection, storage	Polyquad
Allergan hydrocare (Allergan)	Cleaning, disinfection, storage	Thimerosal, bis (2-hydroxy-ethyl). Ammonium chloride
Complete multipurpose (Allergan)	Cleaning, disinfection, storage	Polyhexamethylene biguanide
ReNu/ReNu multiplus multi-purpose solution (Bausch & Lomb)	Cleaning, disinfection, storage. Protein cleaning added in multi-plus	Dymed
Solocare (Ciba vision)	Cleaning, disinfection, storage	Polyhexamide
Silklens (MPS)	Cleaning, disinfection, storage	Polyquad

Silklens MPS, SOLO-care, complete and concsept (Fig. 20.3). All of these solutions are indicated for surface active cleaning of lens, for disinfection with some solutions also performing action of protein removal.

The major problem with a multipurpose solution is that ingredients required in its formulation perform different and somewhat incompatible functions. In addition, it is difficult to include requisite concentrations of ingredients such as surfactant cleaners to be truly effective since required concentrations result in ocular irritation. Also lenses stored overnight in a solution containing a surfactant cleaner, cause build up of the detergent on lens surface leading to irritation. Current multipurpose solutions are thus at best a compromise of adequate function with activity being inferior to use of separate solutions, but the convenience of use makes it the most attractive option.

The ingredients and properties of a multi-purpose solution are:

- *Surfactant/non-ionic or ionic chemical compounds*: These are amphoteric compounds with a positive or negative charge.
- *Antimicrobial agent which* acts as preser-

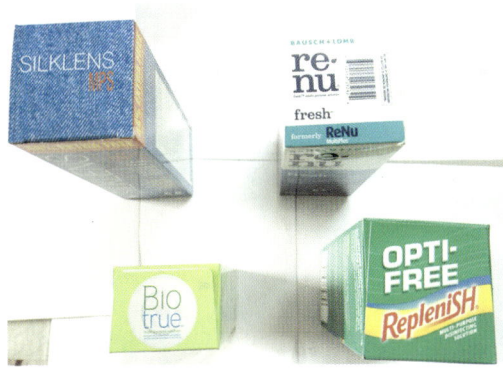

Fig. 20.3: Some multipurpose solutions

vatives to prevent contamination after being opened.

- *Buffer system* (acetates/borates/bicarbonates/citrates/phosphates) which serve to stabilize and maintain solution pH under varying conditions. They adjust both pH, tonicity and for ocular comfort maintain a pH between 6.6 and 7.8. A decrease in pH, decreases water content of hydrogel lenses and causes tight lens fit. Extremely acid/basic solutions cause brittleness, discoloration and even spoilage of lens. In addition, performance of preservatives is pH dependent, i.e. chlorhexidine and thimerosal are stable at neutral pHs, whereas chlorobutanol is more effective in acidic conditions.

- *Chelating agent* acts to remove calcium contaminants in the lens, e.g. EDTA
- *Viscosity-enhancing agent* increases contact time of solution with the lens during use.
- *Mildly abrasive particles* (polyamide polymeric beads) perform friction-enhancing mechanical cleaning.
- *Alcohols* serve to dissolve lipids and enzymes
- *Osmolality:* Normally tears are hypertonic relative to blood plasma at 0.94–0.97% and most soft lens solutions are isotonic.

Solutions must not be used after expiry date or after discard time (after initial opening). For semi-tropical/tropical countries every 10°C increase in temperature, doubles rate of chemical reactions and expiry time for solutions stored in warmer climates should be brought forward.

D. Saline Solutions

Isotonic saline is the basic solution used for rinsing, thermally disinfecting, and storing soft contact lenses after disinfection. Since thimerosal and chlorhexidine can cause sensitivity reactions or irritation in many patients, sorbic acid, Polyquad and Dymed preserved products are preferred for such sensitive eyes. Prepared saline is available as preserved or preservative-free. Preservative-free buffered saline is available in unit-of-use containers (single use), in multi-use bottles (to be discarded after 14 days of use) and as aerosol sprays. *Intravenous normal saline should be avoided as it is acidic for use with soft contact lenses.* In the past, some wearers prepared their own preservative-free homemade saline using salt tablets which caused Acanthamoeba keratitis and this practice needs to be strictly discouraged.

III. *Additional Regimens: Protein/Enzymatic Cleaners*

Protein cleaning is often required for soft and RGP lenses to loosen tightly bound protein deposits. Commonly marketed in tablet form, these preparations dissolve protein deposits by hydrolyzing polypeptide bonds. Chemical based preparations are marketed as ready-to-use liquids. For efficient enzyme cleaning initial cleaning with surface active cleaner is mandatory since presence of lipid or non-proteinaceous deposit would render enzymatic cleaners ineffective. Enzymes include papain, subtilisin, pronase and pancreatin, lipase, amylase to dissolve lysozyme, albumins and immunoglobulins deposits. Papain preparations have a slightly unpleasant odor due to cysteine included as an enzyme stabilizer, e.g. Icon Optizyme, Polyzym, Opti-Free Enzymatic Cleaner. Proteolytic pronase and polysaccharide specific amylase target mucin protein. Subtilisin A and B are formulated for use in peroxide and chemical systems respectively, e.g. B and L sensitive eyes thermal protein removal tablets (Subtilisin B), Allergan Ultrazyme (Subtilisin A). Typically, they contain a low concentration of a non-ionic surfactant to promote cleaning, a polymer to lubricate the lens, a buffering agent and a preservative.

The technique is as follows. An enzyme tablet (papain, pancreatin, subtilisin, pronase, amylase, lipase, and hydroxyalkyl phosphonate) is placed in a solution recommended by manufacturer and lens is placed in this freshly prepared solution for 15 minutes (for high-water content lenses) to overnight (for low-water lenses). The enzymatic cleaner is then thoroughly rinsed off the lens, to remove loosened deposits and prevent sensitization and/or irritation. It is to be noted that Papain is not compatible with hydrogen peroxide lens care.

Weekly enzymatic cleaning is usually sufficient to supplement daily cleaning with surface active products. Heavy protein depositors, especially ionic high water material lens wearers, may require an increased frequency (Fig. 20.4). Heat disinfected lenses require frequent use of protein removers. Since enzyme action loosens protein, it is imperative to instruct the patient to clean lenses by rub and rinse technique upon completion of deproteinizing process. It also needs to be emphasized that enzymatic treatment is *not a substitute* but **only an add-on to the disinfection protocol** and must be followed by regular disinfection procedure before using the lens.

Some enzymatic regimens can be employed simultaneously with thermal or chemical disinfection. A combination like *Thermal Enzymatic Cleaner* (Bausch & Lomb) uses enzyme added into lens case containing saline and soft lens during process of thermal disinfection. *ReNu 1-Step enzymatic tablets* (Bausch & Lomb) can also be placed directly in ReNu multipurpose solution along with soft lenses to simultaneously enzymatically clean and disinfect the lens. Unizyme and Ultrazyme tablets may be added to hydrogen peroxide disinfecting solutions, e.g. Ultra-Care and Oxysept. Supra-Clens liquid containing pancreatin, can be added directly to Opti-Free or Opti-Free Express disinfecting solution. Hydranate (hydroxyalkylphosphonate) an active ingredient of ReNu *Multi-Plus* multipurpose solution ensures separation of protein deposits from lens surface by generating repulsive forces between the two.

Storage and Case Care

Lenses must be stored in a clean case using fresh disinfecting solution each time. Each morning the case is rinsed and dried after removing lens. It should be left empty and refilled with fresh solution just prior to re-placing the lens (Fig. 20.5). Soiled lens case is a common cause of microbial contamination, lens discoloration and intolerance.[9] Biofilm or glycocalyx formation on surface of contact lens storage cases can harbour *Pseudomonas aeruginosa* and *Serratia marcesens*.[10] This biofilm produced by the bacteria protects them from chemical or preservative attack and traps nutrient particles and is best removed by use of cleaning with MPS solution, wiping and then air drying.[11]

While cleaning the case, all used solution is discarded and case scrubbed with a dedicated toothbrush with oil-free soaps or detergents. Subsequently case is rinsed with hot/clean water and rubbed dry a clean tissue/lint free cloth dedicated for this purpose. Scrubbing disrupts the biofilm on the

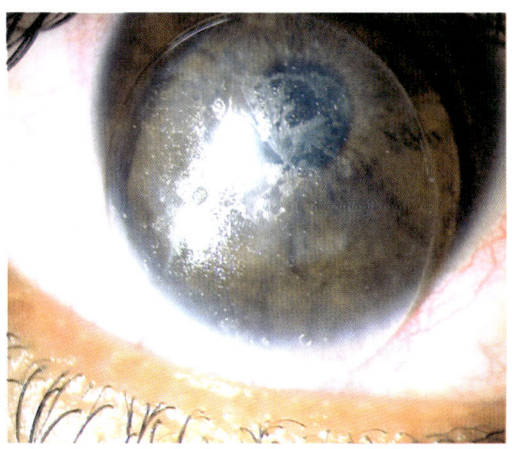

Fig. 20.4: Heavy deposits on lens

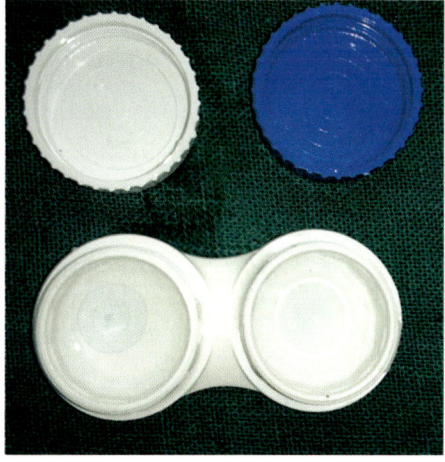

Fig. 20.5: Clean lens case with lens inside

case and hot water of ≥70°C destroys *Acanthamoeba*. Keeping the lens case dry prevents colonization by most micro-organisms, e.g. protozoa that thrive in moist environments. Lens cases that can withstand boiling, e.g. polycarbonate of Bausch & Lomb can be boiled in a water for 10 minutes once a week. Cases should be replaced at frequent intervals (monthly when a new case is supplied with each bottle of disinfecting solution) to reduce risk of contamination/biofilm build-up. Vented storage cases are not recommended and cracked cases must be discarded.

Lens discoloration: Cosmetics, nicotine (cigarette smokers), iron (rust), mercurial deposits (Thimerosal), phenylephrine cause black, grey or brown discoloration of the lens and require removal with an oxidizing agent (sodium perborate, hydrogen peroxide with or without heat). Use of tetracycline or thermal disinfection causes yellow discoloration and use of henna dye (a hair/hand coloring agent) an orange one.

Soft Contact Lens Incompatibilities

• Mixing of a disinfection solution with chlorhexidine and thimerosal with a solution containing quaternary ammonium compound (Allergan Hydrocare), causes toxic keratopathy, known as *mixed solution syndrome.*

• Chemical disinfection with chlorhexidine if additionally subjected to hydrogen peroxide causes small, black precipitates on lenses due to residual chlorhexidine in lens matrix.

• Barnes Hind Daily Cleaner if mixed with cleaner containing poloxamer 407 (Mira Flow/Pliagel) forms cloudy precipitates on lens.

Drugs and Soft Lenses

A. Topical
– Sodium sulfacetamide, pilocarpine: These drops cause dehydration and or/disfigurement of a soft lens.

– Acidic pH cause dehydration with subsequent lens (tighter fit), alkaline pH promotes hydration and subsequent flattening (looser fit).
– Gel and oil formulations: Can alter surface relationship of lens with cornea.

B. Systemic
– *Dryness, altered optics of SCL*: Is caused by oral contraceptives, antihistamines, antimuscarinics, phenothiazines, some beta blockers, diuretics, tricyclic antidepressants
– *Discoloration*: Is seen with use of rifampicin, sulfasalazine, tetracycline
– *Corneal oedema*: Can occur with oral contraceptive, digoxin, primidone
– *Lens deposits:* Oral contraceptives, chlorpromazine, disopyramide, alcohol, sprays
– Reduced eye movement/blinking: These are a result of anxiolytics, hypnotics, antihistamines, muscle relaxants and cause altered lens fit/dynamics.
– Increased lacrimation: Occurs with use of ephedrine, hydralazine.

RGP LENS CARE

The care for the more robust rigid gas permeable lens is less stringent. Infections occur infrequently with RGP lens wear, since micobial lodgement is limited due to their impermeable hydrophic surface. This hydrophobic nature imparted by siloxane, however, prevents easy wettability by tears and gives rise to deposits. The problem is exacerbated by drying due to poor blinking and/or poor fitting of the lens. Microorganisms which normally cannot readily attach to RGP lens surfaces can now be easily attached to these *deposit laden* lenses. This aspect of RGP lens dictates different care regimens for these lenses versus soft hydrogels.

a. Solutions used for RGP disinfection need to combine elements of enhancing lens wettability to negate hydrophobicity of the siloxane material. Disinfecting/soaking solutions for RGP lenses can be classified as multipurpose since they soak, wet and disinfect.

b. Only chemical systems should be used to disinfect RGP lenses since thermal disinfection can cause lens warpage. Peroxide is not preferred as it lacks significant wetting function.

c. Deposits are a major issue with RGP lens wear. They need to be mechanically removed by rubbing with a surfactant cleaner using a rub *rinse technique* (Fig. 20.6a to e). This should include a 10 seconds minimum rub followed by a saline rinse. The wearer is instructed to use a rolling movement of fingers, while rubbing backwards and forwards, left to right to ensure cleaning of lens periphery. Alcohol-based surfactant cleaners are preferred for extensive deposits and surface polishing/edging or resurfacing for recalcitrant deposits.

d. Lens case care is similar to that of soft lenses.

• Cleaning with alcohol-based cleaner immediately after use.

• Placing lens *concave-up* in a flat clean container to prevent lens attachment to case floor ('sucking' on) (Fig. 20.7).

Trial Inventories

• **Storage for** can be dry or wet type. The solutions used comprise of antimicrobial agents, wetting agent, viscosity-enhancing agent, buffer system, e.g. Allergan Total, Boston Simplicity, CIBA SOLO-care-Hard.

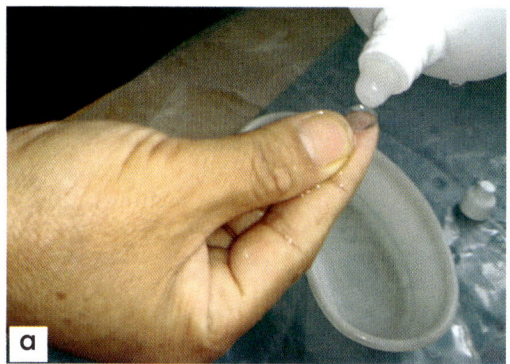
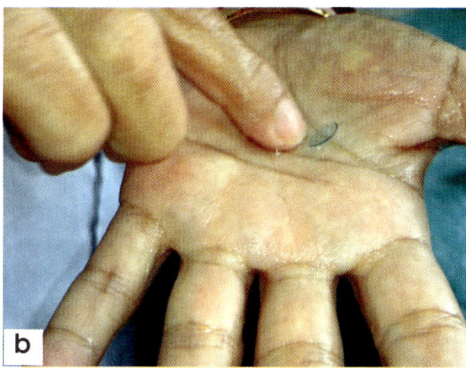
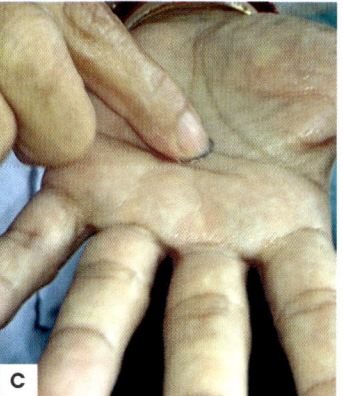
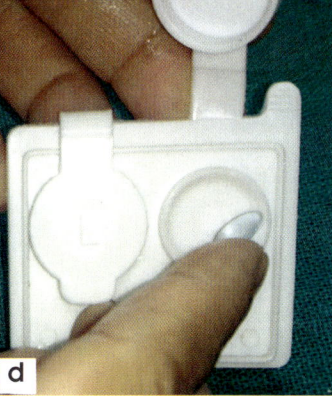
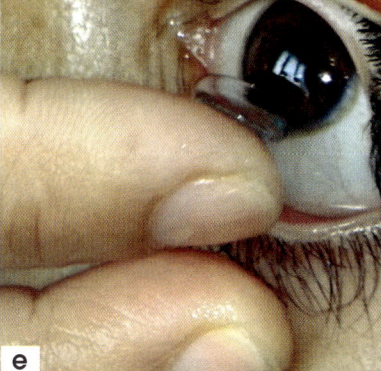

Fig. 20.6: (a to e) Steps of RGP lens care: Wet, rinse, rub, rinse, store, followed by remove, clean, insert.

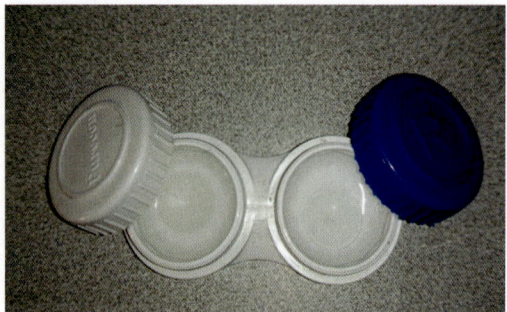

Fig. 20.7: Lens placed *concave-up* in lens case

Solution toxicity is uncommon as preservatives are not normally absorbed by lenses. Viscous agents may adhere to lens surface and cause blurry vision.

- *Wet storage*: Trial inventories used very frequently can be stored wet with solutions being changed every month. Keeping one fixed day of month for cleaning cases and changing solution allows compliance in regular cleaning. Lenses stored by wet storage, are easier to fit.

- *Dry storage*: This is more convenient and removes all potential media for microbial growth. Lenses stored 'dry' may not wet as well during the trial fitting. In addition, drying can cause some alterations like flattening of BOZR.

Disinfection procedures for trial lens inventory:

- *Heater/stirrer units with/without oxidizing agents:* Precaution is required while using hydrogen peroxide, especially hot, as it causes instant skin burns on inadvertent splashes.

- *Standing waves:* Vertically oriented high energy standing waves are generated by a vibrating plate and cause low-frequency agitation of a lens vial containing the lens in a cleaning solution. The resultant turbulence cleans by dislodging contaminants.

- *Ultrasound*: High frequency 15–20 kHz waves create intense agitation of small bubbles at lens surface called cavitation effect. It destroys cell walls of microbial contaminants and is more effective for low water content hydrogels. Ultrasonic cleaning is not as useful for high water content SCL or RGP due to reduced effectiveness of acoustic interface between saline and high water content lens. An example is Sonasept ultrasonic cleaner.

- *Ultraviolet system:* Ozone produced by ultraviolet emitting discharge tube kills microbes by breaking bonds and cross links between nucleic acids. It is effective in disinfecting both SCLs and RGPs (Fig. 20.8).[13]

- *Microwaves:* A type of heat disinfection it kills microbes but also reduces longevity of lenses. A 2.5 GHz unit at 500 watts requires 5 minutes exposure and can handle a large number of lenses simultaneously. Vented lens containers need to be used to allow escape of steam generated by boiling saline and lenses need to be re-hydrated in saline after irradiation.[14]

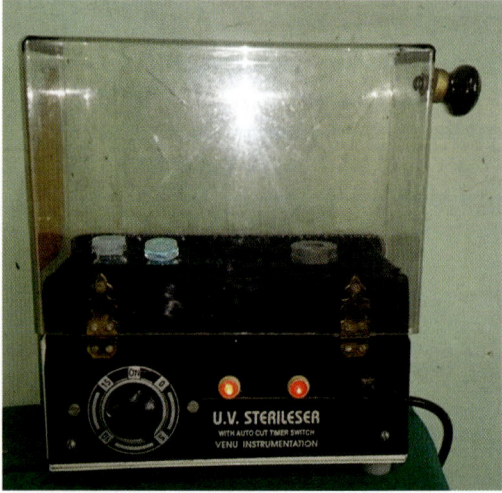

Fig. 20.8: Ultraviolet disinfection unit

REFERENCES

1. Sylvie Sulaiman CRADLE – Clean, Rinse And Disinfect Lenses Everytime. IACLE Contact Lens Course, 1998.Module 5: Units 5.1, 9.

2. Rosenthal P, Chou MH, Salamone JC. *Preservative interaction with GP lenses*. Optician. 1986; (5076): 33–8.

3. Tripathi BJ, Tripathi RC, Kolli SP *Cytotoxicity of ophthalmic preservatives on human corneal epithelium*. Lens Eye Toxic Res. 1993, 9(3&4): 361–75.

4. Davies DJG, Anthony Y, Meakin BJ. *Evaluations of the anti-Acanthamoebal activity of five contact lens disinfectants*. ICLC.1990,17(1):14–20.

5. Chapman JM, Cheeks L, Green K. *Interactions of benzalkonium chloride with soft and hard contact lenses*. Arch Ophthalmol-Chic.1990;108:244–6.

6. McLaughlin WR, Hallberg KB, Tuovinen OH. *Chemical inactivation of microorganisms on rigid gas permeable contact lenses*. Optometry Vision Sci. 1991; 68(9): 721–7.

7. Chalmers RL. Hydrogen peroxide in anterior segment physiology: a literature review. Optom Vis Sci. 1989 Nov;66(11):796–803.

8. Chalmers RL, McNally JJ. *Ocular detection threshold for hydrogen peroxide: Drops vs. lenses*. ICLC. 1988, 15(11): 351–7.

9. Larkin DFP, Kilvington S, Easty DL. *Contamination of contact lens storage cases by* Acanthamoeba *and bacteria*. Brit J Ophthalmol.1990; 74: 133–5.

10. Driebe WT. *Contact Lens Cleaning and Disinfection*. In: Kastl PR (Ed.). *Contact Lenses, The CLAO Guide to Basic Science and Clinical Practice*. 1995. Kendall/Hunt Publishing Company, Dubuque.

11. Vijay AK, Willcox M, Zhu H, Stapleton F. Contact lens storage case hygiene practice and storage case contamination. Eye Contact Lens. 2015 Mar;41(2):91–7.

12. Boltz RL, Leach NE, Piccolo MG, Peltzer B (1993). *The effect of repeated disinfection of rigid gas permeable lens materials using 3% hydrogen peroxide*, ICLC. 20(11&12): 215–21.

13. Harris MG, Fluss L, Lem A, Leong H. *Ultraviolet disinfection of contact lens*. Optometry Vision Sci. 70 (10): 839–42. Optom Vis Sci. 1993 Oct;70(10):839–42.

14. Harris MG, Harris MG, Rechberger J, Grant T, Holden BA. *In-office microwave disinfection of soft contact lenses*. Optometry Vision Sci. 1990; 67(2): 129–32.

Reader's Note

CHAPTER 21

Instructions to Patient

- Wash hands thoroughly with mild soap (oil and fragrance free), rinse and dry using lint-free towel before handling lenses.
- Avoid use of moisturizers, lotion, or oily cosmetics before handling lenses.
- Avoid touching lenses with fingernails. Keep fingernails trimmed to prevent lens damage and ensure hygiene.

A. Lens Removal from Case

i. Blister packing:
- Peel covering foil after supporting package on a flat surface (table), to avoid sudden splashing of lens solution and popping out of the lens.
- After opening foil, first inspect storage case. If solution/inside of blister is dirty do not insert the lens. Open spare set of lenses or use spectacle correction.
- By default mode open/insert lens for right eye first. This habit ensures correct lens placement on correct eye. However, in cases of anisometropia handle lens for eye with poorer vision or higher refractive error first. Most manufactures color right and left case tops differently for easy identification (Fig. 21.1).

ii. Storage case packing:
- Remove lens from storage case. Ensure it is moist, clean, clear, and free of visible tears/scratches/deposits/

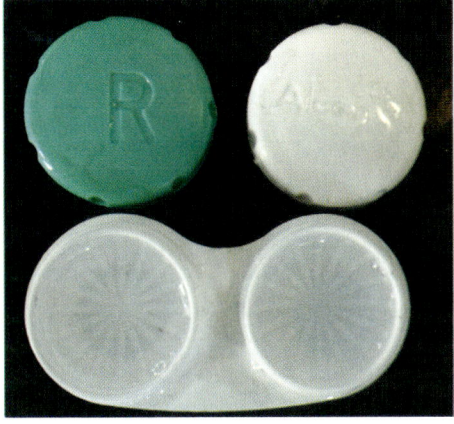

Fig. 21.1: Lens case with right case colored teal green and left white, for easy identification

discolorations. If the lens appears damaged or dirty do not insert. Open spare set of lenses if present or use spectacle correction.

- For soft lenses: Verify lens is not turned inside out by placing on index finger and checking its shape. Normal lens assumes a natural, curved, bowl-like shape. If lens edges tend to point outward, lens is inside out. Another way of ensuring is to squeeze the lens gently between thumb and forefinger. Edges of a normal lens turn inward and for an inside out the edges will turn slightly outward. This is called *Taco test* (Fig. 21.2).

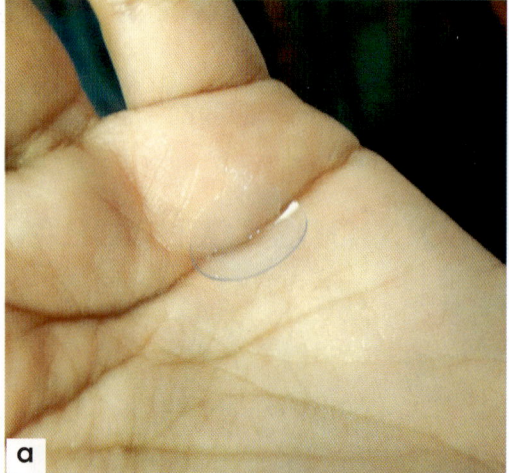

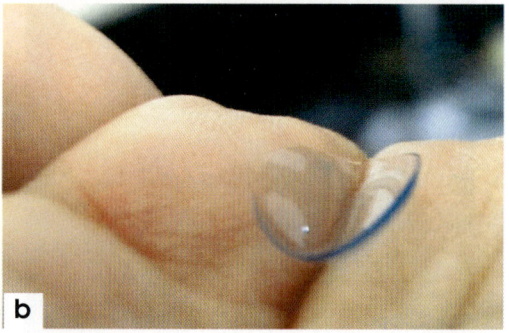

Fig. 21.2: Taco test; (a) Right side up lens; (b) In-turning of lens

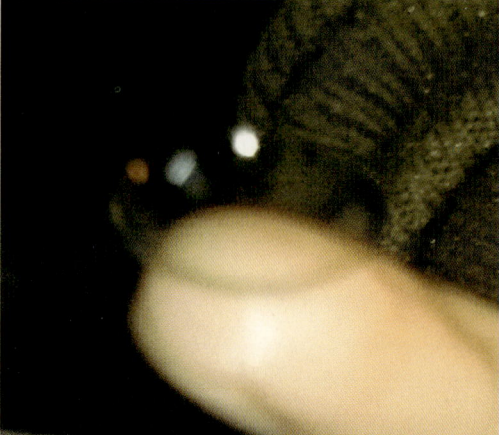

- For RGP lenses: Some manufacturers color right lens differently from left lens for instant identification. Others mark it R and L. Before cleaning check lens edge with the sensitive pad of fingertip to ensure no cracks or uneven edges.
- Clean lens with fresh drop of lens solution.

B. Lens Placement on Eye

Again start with right eye by default to avoid confusion. Use right hand for right lens placement and left hand for left eye lens placement (Figs 21.3 and 21.4).

• Place lens on tip of right forefinger
• With middle finger of right hand, pull down lower lid of right eye.

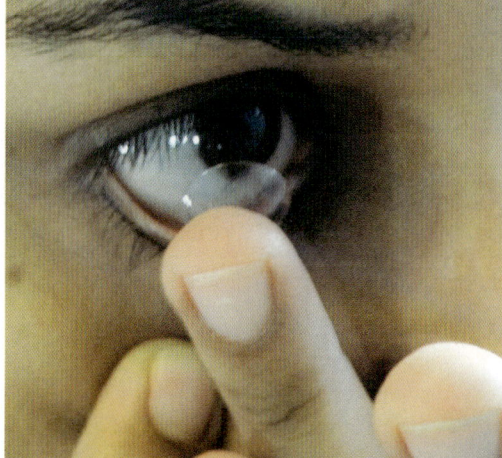

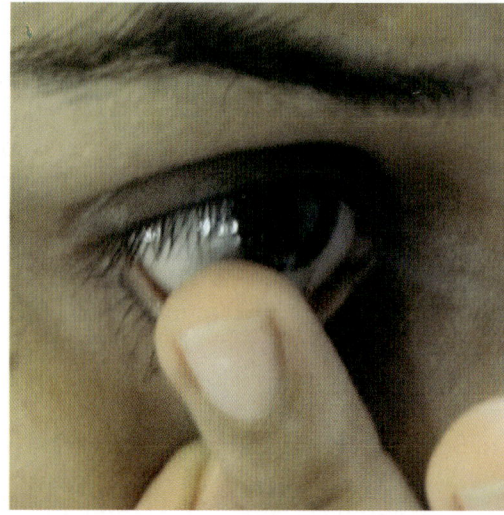

Fig. 21.3: Sequential insertion of soft lens

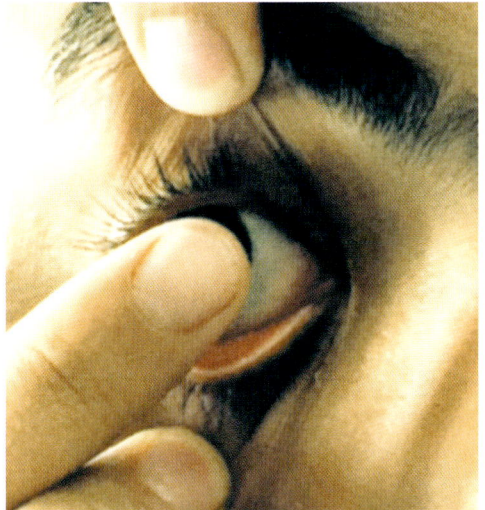

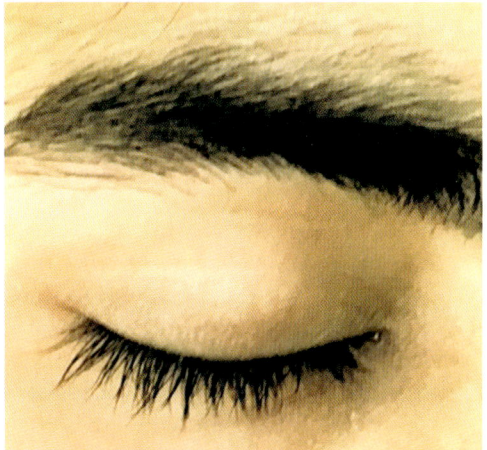

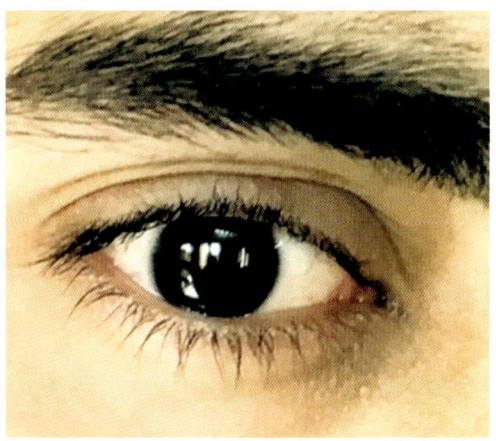

Fig. 21.4: Sequential insertion of rigid gas permeable lens

- Lift upper lid of right eye with index finger of left hand.
- Insert lens in eye like while looking/staring at it. This ensures centration on cornea and prevents reflex lid closure.
- Gently release lids, blink and feel the lens settling down.
- Keep eye gently closed to allow lens to equilibrate and watering of eye to stop. *Do not squeeze eyes shut.*
- Repeat for left eye using left hand.

  For rinsing lenses before insertion, use fresh **sterile saline solution, never boiled water or tap water.**

Checklist After Lens Placement

Check vision of individual eye separately after inserting both lenses.

It is important to understand the common causes of blurred vision, which are decentered lens, wrong lens in wrong eye or inside out lens.

- Decentered lens: This occurs during initial learning period of lens insertion due to defective technique. In case of decentration of lens blink gently 2–3 times (never forcefully as that may further destabilize it). If this does not work, close eyelids and gently massage lens into place through the closed lids. If this also does not work open eye wide, look into a mirror and move off-centered lens onto cornea, using gentle finger pressure through upper/lower lid.

- Inside out lens occurs only with soft lenses and such a lens if inserted would be very uncomfortable in addition to causing blurred vision. In this scenario remove lens, confirm side and then perform *Taco test* to confirm correct shape and then reinsert. If blur persists, remove lens and consult lens practitioner/ophthalmologist.

Do not wear a lens causing blurred vision as it may compromise eye safety in addition to causing problems in daily activities. Surrender your pride and wear your customary spectacles.

C. Lens Care During Wear

– Remember to **blink frequently** to lubricate your lenses with wet mopping action of lids. This keeps lens clean, moist and provides crisp, stable vision. It also ensures prevention of dry spots and reduces lens induced discomfort. During initial weeks of lens wear, wearers often forget to increase their blinking frequency from pre-lens wear states. This causes red eye, burning and discomfort due to dry spots appearing onto the lens and cornea within a few hours. The mantra is *Think blink* and do *Complete blink* (Fig. 21.5). Watch your blinking in the mirror to ensure the completeness of blinking in this initial weeks of lens wear.

– Computer/video terminal users and those working in air-conditioned rooms vitiated with re-circulating air often contaminated with cigarette smoke suffer from *sick building syndrome (SBS)*. These situations commonly cause dry eye syndrome. Wearers in these environs need to blink more frequently and preferably take short break after an hour and look at a distance object, through the

window. This relaxes accommodation, reduces eye fatigue and restores normal blinking.

D. Lens Removal

– Wash, rinse and dry hands thoroughly as for lens insertion
– Always remove right lens first by habit.
– Ensure lens is on cornea before attempting removal. This is done by checking vision of each eye separately. Blurred vision indicates decentration of lens. To locate the vagrant lens, pull up upper lid and lower lid in sequence while looking into a mirror.

Remove soft lens by pinch method or forefinger thumb method.

  i. **Pinch method:** Sit on a chair with a table or flat top in front. Place lens case and multipurpose solution bottle on table. Ensure that case is both clean and dry. Dry it out with a tissue if still wet. For the initial few days, a self-supporting mirror placed on table/surface is helpful. Refill lens case with a few drops of lens solution. To remove lens look upwards, slide lens down to lower part of eye using forefinger and gently pinch lens between thumb and forefinger and remove it off the eye (Fig. 21.6a).

  ii. **Forefinger and thumb method:** Place hand or clean handkerchief under the eye. Bow head down over your hand. Place index finger of same side hand on center of upper lid and thumb of same hand on center of lower lid. Press in and *force* a blink. The lens will drop down on the hand (Fig. 21.6b). Again sitting down posture is helpful. Never attempt this if you have long fingernails.

Never remove or insert lenses on a sink with running water. Many lenses get lost or contaminated this way.

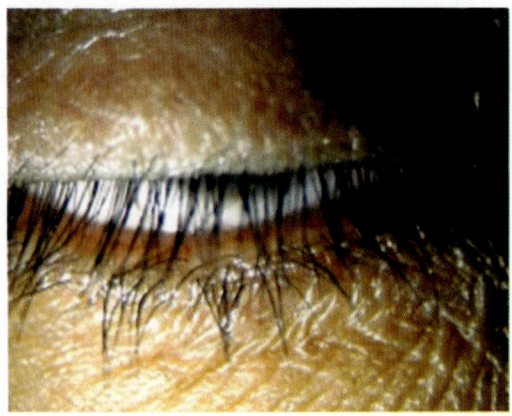

Fig. 21.5: Incomplete and complete blink

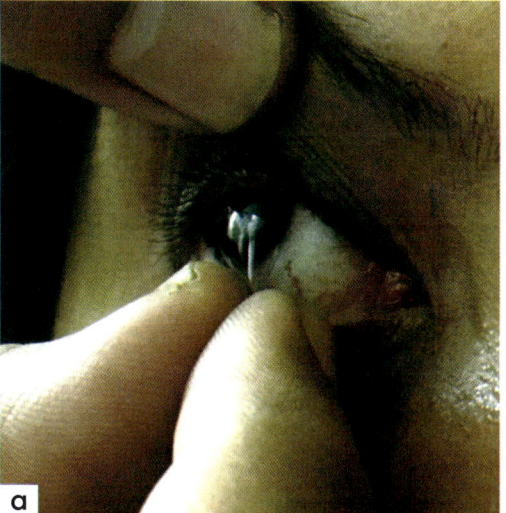 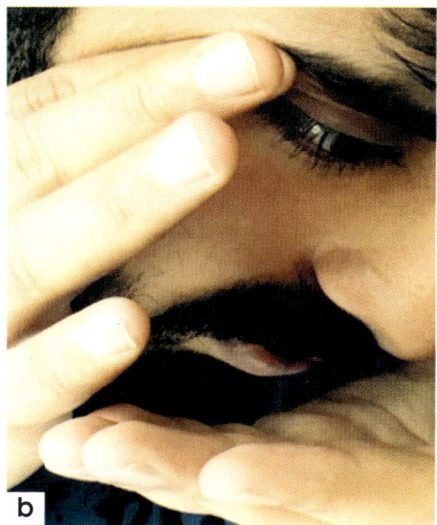

Fig. 21.6: (a) Soft lens removal by pinch method; (b) RGP lens removal

E. Lens Care

This can be easily remembered with the mnemonic.

CRADLES sequence (**C**lean → **R**inse → **D**isinfect → **L**enses **E**very time → *then* **S**tore till next use).

i. **Cleaning of lens:** This is to be done immediately on removal and not deferred later for insertion time. A dirty lens stored invites bacterial growth and deposits. Lenses require to be cleaned individually on the palm of hand instead of between fingers. Place a few drops of solution on lens surface, rub with forefinger for 15 seconds each side using 'to and fro' and lateral left to right motion (Fig. 21.7). *Rub, clean and rinse* is the refrain for lens cleaning regimen. Rigid lenses are cleaned by rubbing center to edge and in a circular motion to remove tear debris like mucus, secretions, films or deposits. For soft lens circular pill rolling motions are sufficient. Both surfaces of lenses need to be cleaned for a minute.

ii. **Rinsing:** After cleaning, lens is thoroughly rinsed with recommended saline or disinfecting solution.

• Subsequently lens is placed into correct cell of the storage case, i.e. right eye lens in right cell and left eye lens in left cell.

• Procedure is repeated for second lens.

• Fresh solution is poured over the lens to completely submerge it. Only specified solution as recommended by lens manufacturer must be used, for lens compatibility issues.

iii. **Disinfecting**: After cleaning, disinfect lenses using system recommended by practitioner. Multipurpose solutions do the job of cleaning, storing and disinfecting simultaneously.

Chemically disinfected lenses may absorb ingredients from the disinfecting solution which may be irritant to the eye. Therefore, rinsing a lens disinfected by chemicals with fresh sterile saline solution is a must prior to placement in the eye. If hydrogen peroxide lens care systems are used, lenses **must be neutralized before wearing.**

F. Case Care

• After lens application, lens storage case is emptied of all solutions, rinsed with

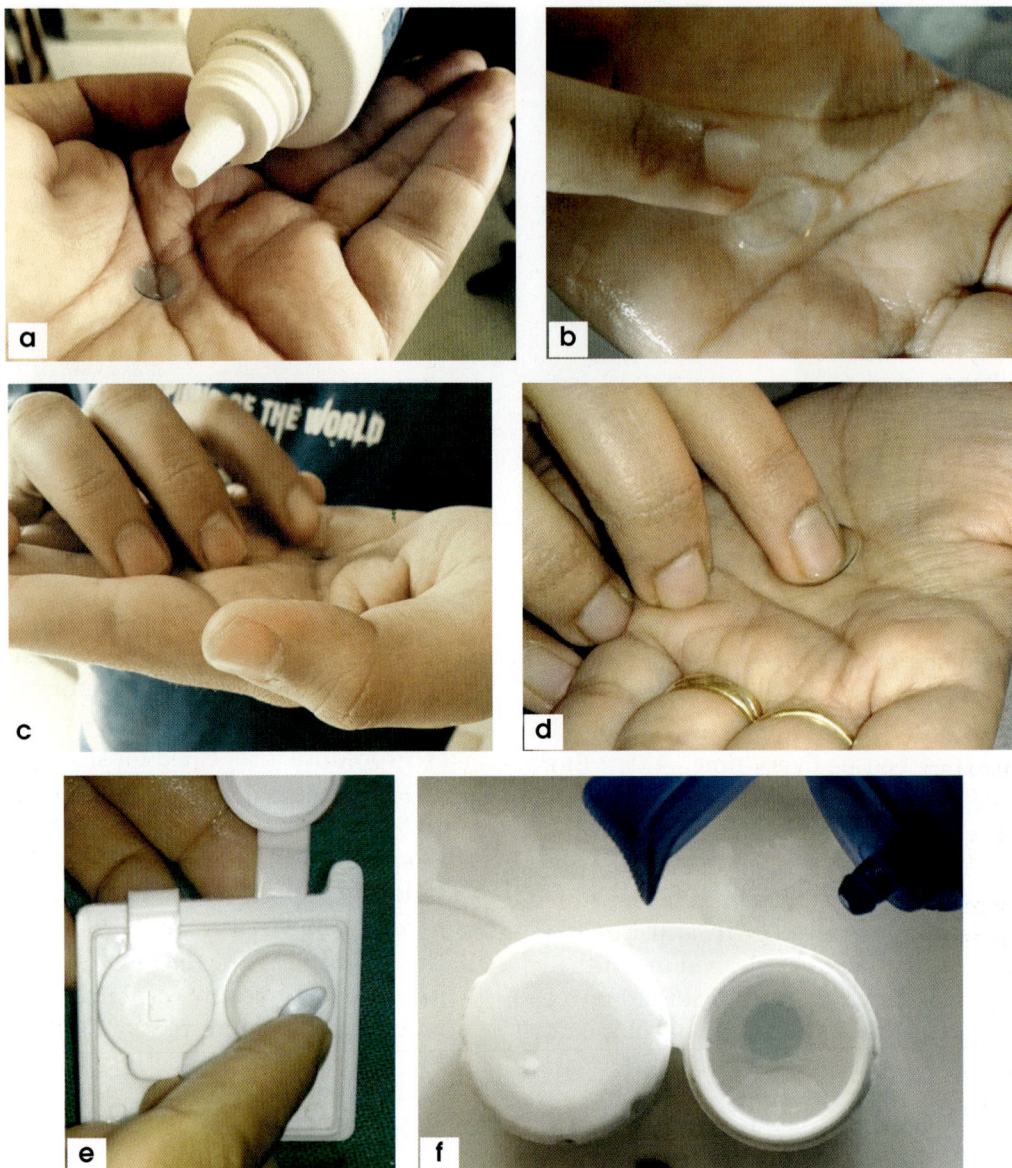

Fig. 21.7: CRADLE sequence of lens disinfection: Remove lens; (a) Place a few drops of cleaning solution; (b and c) Clean with forefinger, using to and fro motion; (d) Reinsert lens in case; (e) Top up with multipurpose solution and store till next use

fresh solution and dried with tissue or clean cloth designated for this purpose. Air drying of case is preferred but requires time. To get benefit of both types of drying it is advisable to keep 2–3 empty clean cases with each set of lenses. Allow used one to dry at home environment and carry spare one in handbag for emergency use in case lens removal is required.

• Replace lens case at regular intervals.

• Keep lenses completely immersed in a recommended disinfecting solution when lenses are not being worn.

On each Sunday or weekly holiday lens case including well and screw cap is scrubbed with a soft toothbrush dedicated for this purpose, rinsed and then allowed to air dry for 24 hours in clean dust free environs. The lenses may be stored in a separate case for that day.

G. After Care

- **Lubricating/rewetting** solutions which are preservative free can be used to enhance comfort during lens wear.

- For a stuck on/non-motile lens, a few drops of lubricating drops in eye recommence lens movement.

- Never rinse/store lenses in tap water as it is not sterile and alters optical properties of soft lenses. Even boiled water should not be used since it is not pH compatible with lens material and can alter lens optics and shape.

- **Cosmetics care:** Lenses need to be inserted before application of eye cosmetics and removed before cleaning off cosmetics. *Lens is first thing in and first thing out* (Fig. 21.8). Water-based cosmetics are preferred to oil based. Iridescent/metallic eye shadows flake off onto lenses and are best avoided. Hair dye, henna should not be applied in presence on lenses *in situ*. Kajal inside the eye is a strict **No No** as it discolors lenses and encourages lens deposits. Hand creams/moisturizing lotions should be applied after lenses are inserted keeping eyes gently closed. Hair spray is used after ensuring eyes are firmly shut or preferably before lenses are inserted if visibility permits.

H. Follow up/After Care Visit

Wearing regimen: Initially lenses are worn for 2–3 hours and wear time is gradually increased by 1–2 hours daily until 8 hours of wear.

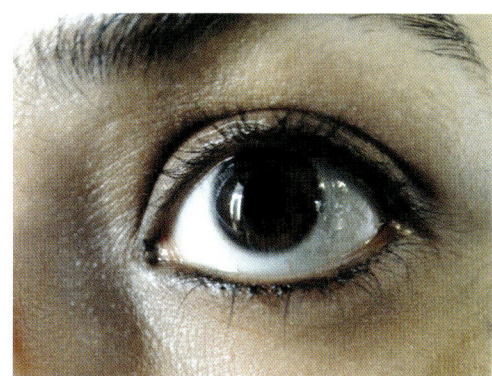

Fig. 21.8: Eyeliner and mascara have been applied after insertion of lens

Lenses should be worn 3–4 hours prior to after-care visit, if no apparent contra-indication (e.g. pain, redness, stinging). Practitioner should **evaluate lenses** *in situ* on slit lamp bio-microscope. Visual acuity, dynamic and static lens fit should be evaluated and upper lid must be everted to rule out papillary congestion.

A minimum of 2–3 follow-up visits is required in first few months for trouble shooting any teething problems and learning modalities of safe lens wear. Contact lenses are viable for one year. Gift yourself one lens pair each birthday. Rigid lenses can be used safely for 2 years with proper handling and frequent edging and polishing. Before replacing lenses annually a check for any change in power or fit is the preferred practice.

I. Emergencies

Splashing of eyes while wearing lenses with any chemicals (household products, gardening solutions, laboratory chemicals, etc.) is to be followed by immediate copious washing of eye with any available clean water including tap water. Subsequently lenses are removed, placed in the case and discarded if damaged. Eyes should be washed again. In case of persisting pain or redness contact lens practitioner is to be consulted.

In case of **redness, secretion, visual blurring, or pain** (RSVP), **remove** contact lenses **at once**. If symptom subsides, lenses are cleaned and reinserted. If symptoms persist or reappear upon lens reinsertion, remove lenses immediately and check with lens practitioner.

DO's and DON'Ts

DO

- DO keep soft lenses moist to prevent tearing.
- DO add a rewetting drop before removing contact lenses.
- DO wet lenses with saline before picking them up from a dry surface or cleaning them to prevent tearing or warpage.
- DO discard eye makeup three months after opening. The exception is pencil eyeliner that is sharpened to a fresh supply.
- DO insert lenses BEFORE applying cosmetics (to see better).
- DO remove lenses BEFORE removing cosmetics (to prevent lens spoilage).
- DO keep your contact lens case clean. Scrub lens case weekly with toothbrush and daily cleaner.
- DO carry a case with you with fresh bottle of lens solution at all times.

DO NOT

- DO NOT touch solution bottle tip of your bottles with fingertip.
- DO NOT hold a rigid gas permeable lens by edges. Hold it front to back.
- DO NOT slide a rigid gas permeable lens across a flat surface.

- DO NOT use hair spray when your lenses are in. Spray your hair BEFORE inserting your lenses.
- DO NOT sleep in your lenses.
- DO NOT use cosmetics or contact lenses if your eyes are irritated or red.
- DO NOT share cosmetics.
- DO NOT apply eyeliner or kajal to inner margin of your eyelid. Chronic use of this cosmetic with lenses on can cause deposition in palpebral conjunctiva and cause lens intolerance (Fig. 21.9).
- DO NOT use waterproof mascara. It is very difficult to clean off lenses.

RGP lenses

- As infection and GPC are much less in RGP wearers versus SCL wearer, a less stringent care regimen can be used for RGP lenses. These lenses have no water content and do not support microbial growth within their polymer matrix.
- Cleaning is easier as surface debris do not invade the lens substance.

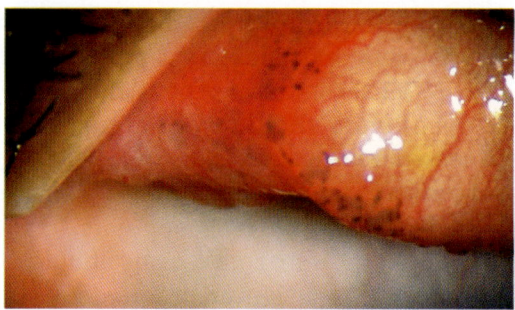

Fig. 21.9: Kajal deposits in the conjunctival papillae

Reader's Note

Reader's Note

Annexures

Radius Conversion Table

(for converting keratometry values to base curve of a contact lens)

Lens Power (Steeper Add Minus: Flatter Add Plus) Sam : Fap
Conversion Formula [337.5/mm or D = or mm]

Dioptres	Millimetres	Dioptres	Millimetres	Dioptres	Millimetres
37.25	9.06	48.75	6.92	60.25	5.60
37.50	9.00	49.00	6.89	60.50	5.58
37.75	8.94	49.25	6.85	60.75	5.56
38.00	8.88	49.50	6.82	61.00	5.53
38.25	8.82	49.75	6.78	61.25	5.51
38.50	8.77	50.00	6.75	61.50	5.49
38.75	8.71	50.25	6.72	61.75	5.47
39.00	8.65	50.50	6.68	62.00	5.44
39.25	8.60	50.75	6.65	62.25	5.42
39.50	8.54	51.00	6.62	62.50	5.50
39.75	8.49	51.25	6.59	62.75	5.38
40.00	8.44	51.50	6.55	63.00	5.36
40.25	8.39	51.75	6.52	63.25	5.34
40.50	8.33	52.00	6.49	63.50	5.31
40.75	8.28	52.25	6.46	63.75	5.29
41.00	8.23	52.50	6.43	64.00	5.27
41.25	8.18	52.75	6.40	64.25	5.25
41.50	8.13	53.00	6.37	64.50	5.23
41.75	8.08	53.25	6.34	64.75	5.21
42.00	8.04	53.50	6.31	65.00	5.19
42.25	7.99	53.75	6.28	65.25	5.17
42.50	7.94	54.00	6.25	65.50	5.15
42.75	7.89	54.25	6.22	65.75	5.13
43.00	7.85	54.50	6.19	66.00	5.11
43.25	7.80	54.75	6.16	66.25	5.09
43.50	7.76	55.00	6.14	66.50	5.08
43.75	7.71	55.25	6.11	66.75	5.06
44.00	7.67	55.50	6.08	67.00	5.04
44.25	7.63	55.75	6.05	67.25	5.02
44.50	7.58	56.00	6.03	67.50	5.00
44.75	7.54	56.25	6.00	67.75	4.98
45.00	7.50	56.50	5.97	68.00	4.96
45.25	7.46	56.75	5.95	68.25	4.95
45.50	7.42	57.00	5.92	68.50	4.93
45.75	7.38	57.25	5.90	68.75	4.91
46.00	7.34	57.50	5.87	69.00	4.89
46.25	7.30	57.75	5.84	69.25	4.87
46.50	7.26	58.00	5.82	69.50	4.86
46.75	7.22	58.25	5.79	69.75	4.84
47.00	7.18	58.50	5.77	70.00	4.82
47.25	7.14	58.75	5.74	70.25	4.80
47.50	7.11	59.00	5.72	70.50	4.79
47.75	7.07	59.25	5.70	70.75	4.77
48.00	7.03	59.50	5.67	80.00	4.75
48.25	6.99	59.75	5.65		
48.50	6.96	60.00	5.63		

Annexure II

VERTEX CONVERSION TABLE (Average 12 mm Distance)

For Minus Powers Read left to right & for Plus Powers Read right to left

–	+	–	+	–	+
3.25	3.00	8.50	7.75	18.00	14.50
3.50	3.25	8.75	8.00	18.12	14.75
3.75	3.37	9.00	8.25	18.50	15.00
4.00	3.75	9.25	8.37	18.75	15.25
4.25	3.87	9.50	8.62	19.00	15.50
4.50	4.12	9.75	8.75	19.50	15.75
4.75	4.50	10.00	9.00	20.00	16.00
5.00	4.75	10.25	9.12	20.50	16.50
5.12	4.87	10.50	9.25	21.00	16.75
5.37	5.00	10.75	9.37	21.50	17.00
5.50	5.12	11.00	9.62	22.00	17.37
5.62	5.25	11.25	9.75	22.50	17.75
5.75	5.37	11.50	10.00	23.00	18.00
5.87	5.50	11.75	10.25	23.50	18.25
6.00	5.62	12.00	10.37	24.00	18.50
6.12	5.75	12.50	10.75	24.50	18.75
6.37	5.87	12.75	11.00	25.00	19.00
6.50	6.00	13.00	11.25	25.50	19.50
6.62	6.12	13.50	11.50	26.00	20.00
6.75	6.25	13.75	11.75	27.00	20.50
6.87	6.37	14.00	12.00	27.50	21.00
7.00	6.50	14.25	12.25	28.00	21.50
7.12	6.62	14.75	12.50	29.00	22.25
7.37	6.75	15.00	12.75	30.00	23.00
7.50	6.87	15.50	13.00	31.00	24.00
7.62	7.00	15.75	13.25	33.00	25.00
7.75	7.12	16.25	13.50	35.00	26.00
7.87	7.25	16.75	13.75	38.00	27.00
8.00	7.37	17.00	14.00	41.00	28.00
8.12	7.50	17.25	14.25	43.00	29.00
8.25	7.62	17.62	14.37	45.00	30.00

Annexure III

CL proforma created and used by author

M.P. C.L. J. 834—1000 15-9-2010—www.medonine gov.in

गुरू नानक नेत्र केन्द्र, नई दिल्ली
GURU NANAK EYE CENTRE, NEW DELHI
कान्टैक्ट लैंस इकाई
CONTACT LENS & LOW VISION AID UNIT

नाम NAME _____	क्लि॰ सं॰ CI. No. _____
उम्र एवं लिंग वर्ष पुरुष/स्त्री Age & Sex : Year _____ Male/Female _____	
पता Address _____	ओ॰पी॰डी॰ सं॰ O.P.D. No. _____
दूरभाष सं॰ Telephone No. _____	
उद्यम (वृत्ति) Occupation _____	(रोग निदान) Diagnosis _____
शिक्षा का स्तर Education level _____	

ए.   का॰ लैं॰ की जरूरत
A. **Indication for CL use Cosmetic:**

[सही निशान (√) जो उपयुक्त हो]
[Tick (√) wherever applicable]

चश्मे की जरूरत Refractive	एनिसोमेट्रोपिया ए/1 Anisometropia A/1	एस्टिगमेटिज्म ए/2 Astigmatism A/2	उच्च नं॰ का चश्मा ए/3 High refractiverror A/3
एफेकिया ए/4 Aphakia A/4	सुडोफेकिया ए/5 Pseudophakia A/5	कोर्निया पर निशान ए/6 Corneal opacity A/6	स्कार्स ए/7 Scars A/7
विशेष मामले : कैरेटोकोन्स ए/8 Special cases : Keratoconus A/8	एनिरिडिया ए/9 Aniridia A/9	पुतली बदलने के बाद ए/10 Post PK A/10	ऑपरेशन के बाद का चश्मा ए/11 Post refractive surgery A/11

बी.   का॰ लैं॰ के प्रयोग हेतु इतिहास .
B. **History of prior use of CL:**

[निशान (√) जो उपयुक्त हो]
[Tick (√) wherever applicable]

का॰ लैं॰ के प्रयोग संबंधी इतिहास
Relevant history of CL use:

एलर्जीज—पलक की सूजन बी/1 Allergies—Blepharitis B/1	नजले की बीमारी बी/2 Sinusuitis B/2	अन्य बी/3 Others B/3
शल्य चिकित्सा—मोतिया बी/4 Surgery—Cataract B/4	काला मोतिया बी/5 Glaucoma B/5	भैंगापन बी/6 Squint B/6
आँखों का ऊपरी हिस्सा Ocular Surface Disorder	सूखापन बी/7 Dry Eye B/7	पलक का जुड़ना बी/8 Symblepharon B/8
	नखूना बी/9 Pterygium B/9	अन्य बी/10 Others B/10

(1)

(2)

कोर्निल सेन्सेशन
Corneal Sensation:

न्यूरोपैरालिटिक बी/11
Neuroparalytic B/11

जल जाने के पश्चात् बी/12
Post Burns B/12

पोस्ट हर्पीस बी/13
Post Herpes B/13

दवाई
Medication:

आँख की बी/14
Topical B/14

शारीरिक बी/15
Systemic B/15

गठिया या अन्य कोई शारीरिक विकलांगता में सही कान्टैक्ट बी/16
Arthritis or other handicap in fitting CL B/16

शरीरिक बीमारियाँ
Systemic Diseases:

मुधमेह बी/17
DM B/17

गिल्लड़ बी/18
Thyroid B/18

दमा बी/19
Br. Asthma B/19

दिल की बीमारी बी/20
CAD B/20

अन्य
Others

सी. परीक्षण
C. Examination:

चेहरे का आकार
Facial Anatomy:

एसिमेटी सी/1
Asymmetry C/1

पलक का झपकना/आँख की चौड़ाई सी/2
Lid Blinking, Palpebral aperture C/2

पलक गिरना सी/3
Ptosis C/3

नीली पलक सी/4
Lax lids C/4

आँख के मांसपेशियों की गति सी/5
EMO Movements C/5

भैंगापन सी/6
Stabismus C/6

कोर्मियल आकार सी/7
Corneal Size C/7

छूना, महसूस करना सी/8
Sensation C/8

निशान सी/9
Opacity C/9

खून की नस्लियां सी/10
Vascularization C/10

पुतली का आकार (कम लाईट में जांच) सी/11
Pupil Size (measured in dim light) C/11

एक्सेंट्रिसीटी सी/12
Eccentricity C/12

लिम्बल एनामोली—डेलेन, फलिकटेन ब्लेब, पिंगेकुला इत्यादि सी/13
Any limbal anamoly—Dellen, filtering bleb, pingecula etc. C/13

सक्रिय कंबंकटिवल बीमारियां—फैपिलरी या फालिकुलर सी/14
Active conjunctival disease—Fapillary or follicular C/14

(3)

आँसु स्थिति-बी यू टी सी/15
Tear film **staus**—BUT C/15

स्लिट लैम्प परीक्षण सी/16
Slit lamp **exam.** C/16

नजर की जांच
Visual Acuity:

दांयी आंख
Right Eye

बांयी आंख
Left Eye

नग्न आंख
Unaided

चश्मे के साथ
Aided (pt spectacles)

नये चश्मे के साथ
With new refraction

नजदीकी
Near

चश्मे का नं॰
Refraction:

दांयी
RE

बांयी
LE

केरैटोमेटरी
Keratometry:

दांयी
RE

बांयी
LE

लैंस का नाप
Trial lens:

निशानें
Remarks

(4)

ट्रायल सं॰
Trial No.:

दांयी आँख	बांयी आंख	फिट
Right Eye	Left Eye	Fit

प्रथम
First:

द्वितीय
Second:

तृतीय
Third:

चतुर्थ
Forth:

कोर्नियल टोपोग्राफी
Corneal Topography:

दांया नेत्र	बांया नेत्र
Right Eye	Left Eye

ओवर रेफरेक्शन
Over Refraction:

का॰ लैं॰ की गति
Movements of the CL:

फ्लोरेसन   आकार/मुलायम लैंस फिट
Fluorescein   Pattern/Soft Lens fit:

दांयी आंख	बांयी आंख
Right Eye	Left Eye

लिखा गया लैंस
Lens Prescribed:

एक	दो	तीन	चार	पांच
1	2	3	4	5

(5)

लैंस के प्रकार
Type of lens:

आर जी पी-डी के 20, 30, 60   मुलायम-आम/लगातार, पहना हुआ   टोरिक/स्फेरिक इत्यादि
RGP—DK 20, 30, 60, specify   Soft—Regular, extended wear   Toric/Aspheric/Piggy Back etc.

वर्गीकरण
Specification:

दांयी आंख   बांयी आंख
Right Eye   Left Eye

बेस कर्व
Base Curve _____

ऑप्टिकल डायमीटर
Optic Diameter

अंक शक्ति
Dioptric Power

पूर्ण डायमीटर
Overall Diameter

ऑप्टिक जोन
Optic Zone

पेरीफेरल मोड़
Peripheral Curves

एज डिजाइन
Edge Design

पहली बार पहनना
First Wear:

दृष्टि
Vision:

दा॰ ने॰   बा॰ ने॰
RE _____   LE _____

सहना
Tolerance:

एक   दो   तीन
1   2   3

मनोवैज्ञानिक एडजस्टमेंट
Psychological Adjustment _____

(6)

उन्नति रिपोर्ट
Progress Report:

एफ यू वी FUV	तिथि I Date	तिथि II Date	तिथि III Date	तिथि IV Date	तिथि V Date
पहनने का समय (घंटे) Wearing Time (Hrs.)					
सबसे अधिक पहनने का समय Max. Wear Time					
लैंस की जगह Lens Pstn.					
का॰ लैं॰ गतिविधि CL Movement					
जी.पी.सी. GPC					
कोर्नियल स्टेनिंग Corneal Staining					
चुभन Irritation					
पानी बहना Watering					
कंकड़ महसूस करना FB Sensation					
लैंस गिरना Lens fall out					
लैंस हिलना Decentration					
फ्लेयर Flare					
घोस्टिंग/दो दिखाना Ghosting/Diplopia					
एज फ्लेयर Edge Flare					
खुजली Itching					
लीड रिएक्शन Lid Reaction					
कोर्नियल सूजन Corneal Edema					
मनोवैज्ञानिक एडजस्ट Psychological Adjustment					
अन्य Others					

GMGIPMRND—893GEC(S3)—16.09.2011.

Reader's Note

Reader's Note

Glossary

AEL/AEC: Axial edge lift/clearance

BOZD: Back optic zone diameter

BOZR: Back optic zone radius

HVID: Horizontal visible iris diameter

BVP: Back vertex power

CG: Centre of gravity

CL: Contact lens

ODTD: Overall total diameter

OD: *Oculus dexter*, Latin for right eye

OS: *Oculus sinister*, Latin for left eye

OU: *Oculus uterque*, Latin for both eyes

OZ: Optic zone

PCR: Peripheral curve radius

RGP: Rigid gas permeable lens

SCL/Hydrogels: Soft contact lens

TC: Central lens thickness

TLT: Tear lens thickness

Reader's Note

Index